Future Aspects in Contraception
Part 1   Male Contraception

Future Aspects in Contraception

Part 1   Male Contraception
Part 2   Female Contraception

Future Aspects in Contraception

Proceedings of an International Symposium held in Heidelberg, 5–8 September 1984

Part 1   Male Contraception

Edited by B. Runnebaum, T. Rabe and L. Kiesel

WKAP ARCHIEF

1985   **MTP PRESS LIMITED**
a member of the KLUWER ACADEMIC PUBLISHERS GROUP
BOSTON / THE HAGUE / DORDRECHT / LANCASTER

Published in the UK and Europe by
MTP Press Limited
Falcon House
Lancaster, England

British Library Cataloguing in Publication Data

Future aspects in contraception: proceedings
of an international symposium held in
Heidelberg, September 5–8, 1984.
1. Contraception
I. Runnebaum, B.   II. Rabe, T.   III. Kiesel, L.
613.9′4   RG136

Published in the USA by
MTP Press
A division of Kluwer Boston Inc.
190 Old Derby Street
Higham, MA 02043, USA

Library of Congress Cataloging in Publication Data

Main entry under title:

Future aspects in contraception.

  Includes bibliographies and index.
  Contents: pt. 1. Male contraception—pt. 2. Female
contraception.
  1. Contraception—Addresses, essays, lectures.
I. Runnebaum, B. (Benno), 1933–   .   II. Rabe, T.
III. Kiesel, L. [DNLM: 1. Contraception—trends.
WP 630 F996]
RG136.F87 1985   613.9′432   85–11622

ISBN-13: 978-94-010-8675-2   e-ISBN-13: 978-94-009-4910-2
DOI: 10.1007/978-94-009-4910-2

Contents of Part 1

Principal contributors to Parts 1 and 2

Principal contributors to Parts 1 and 2

Nancy J. Alexander
Reproductive Biology and Behavior
Oregon Regional Primate Research Center
505 North West 185th Ave
Beaverton, Oregon 97006
USA

Hugh Allen
Department of Obstetrics and Gynecology
University of Western Ontario
and
Suite 201
111 Waterloo Street
London, Ontario
Canada

Deborah J. Anderson
Division of Immunogenetics
Dana-Farber Cancer Institute and Department of Pathology
Harvard Medical School
44 Binney Street
Boston, Massachusetts 02115
USA

Etiènne E. Baulieu
Hormones Laboratory
INSERM U33
94270 Bicêtre
France

Alain Belanger
Departments of Medicine and Molecular Endocrinology
Le Centre Hospitalier de l'Université Laval
Quebec G1V 4G2
Canada

Professor Dr B. Berić
Department for Obstetrics and Gynecology
Faculty of Medicine
University of Novi Sad
S.V. Markóvica 15
YU-21000 Novi Sad
Yugoslavia

Marc Bygdeman
Department of Obstetrics and Gynecology
Karolinska Hospital
S-104 01 Stockholm
Sweden

André Demoulin
Department of Obstetrics and Gynecology
University of Liège
81, Bd de la Constitution
B-4020 Liège
Belgium

Egon Diczfalusy
Reproductive Endocrinology Research Unit
Karolinska Institute and Hospital
Box 60500
S-104 01 Stockholm
Sweden

H. Donat
Department of Obstetrics and Gynecology
Medical Academy of Magdeburg
Gerhart-Hauptmann-Strasse 35
3060 Magdeburg
German Democratic Republic

Klaus-Wolf von Eickstedt
Department of Pharmacology and Toxicology
Bundesgesundheitsamt Berlin
Gebweiler Strasse 15
Berlin 33
West Germany

Norman R. Farnsworth
College of Pharmacy and PCRPS
The University of Illinois at Chicago
Room 310
833 South Wood Street
Box 6998
Chicago, Illinois 60680
USA

David L. Gardner
Polymer Science and Technology Section
Battelle
Columbus Laboratories
505 King Avenue
Columbus, Ohio 43201-2693
USA

A. A. Haspels
Academische Kliniek
Department of Gynecology
Catharijnesingel 101
Utrecht 3585 CP
The Netherlands

Walter L. Herrmann
Hôpital Cantonal Universitaire de Genève
Départment de Gynécologie et d'Obstétrique
32 bis, Bd de la Cluse
CH-1211 Geneva 4
Switzerland

Ilpo Huhtaniemi
Department of Clinical Chemistry
University of Helsinki
Meilahti Hospital
SF-00290 Helsinki
Finland

Natwar R. Kalla
Department of Biophysics
Basic Medical Sciences Building
Panjab University
Chandigarh 160014
India

Louis G. Keith
Department of Obstetrics and Gynecology
The Medical School
Northwestern University
and
Prentice Women's Hospital and Maternity
  Center
333 East Superior Street
Chicago, Illinois 60611
USA

Ludwig Kiesel
Division of Gynaecological Endocrinology
Department of Obstetrics and Gynaecology
University of Heidelberg
D-6900 Heidelberg 1
West Germany

Hans Kopera
Department of Experimental and Clinical
  Pharmacology
University of Graz
Universitätsplatz 4
A-8010 Graz
Austria

F. Krassnig
Department of Dermatology
University of Munich
Frauenlobstrasse 9-11
D-8000 Munich 2
West Germany

H. Kuhl
Universitäts-Frauenklinik
Abteilung für Gynäkologische
  Endokrinologie
Theodor-Stern-Kai 7
D-6000 Frankfurt am Main
West Germany

F. Labrie
Endocrinology of Reproduction
St François D'Assise Hospital
Department of Molecular Endocrinology
Laval Medical Center
10 Rue de l'Espinay
Quebec G1L 3L5
Canada

André Lemay
Department of Gynecology/Obstetrics
Laval University
Hôpital St-François d'Assise
10 Rue de l'Espinay
Quebec G1L 3L5
Canada

Guo-Zhen Liu
Department of Urology
Capital Hospital
Peking
China

Thomas J. Lobl
Biopolymers Research
The Upjohn Company
Kalamazoo
Michigan 49001
USA

K. Loewit
Institute for Medical Biology and Genetics
University of Innsbruck
Schöpfstrasse 41
A-6020 Innsbruck
Austria

Marianne Mall-Haefeli
Social-Medical Department
University Clinic of Obstetrics and Gyne-
  cology
Schanzenstrasse 46
CH-4031 Basel
Switzerland

H. G. Massouras
Obstetrician/Gynaecologist
3 Marasli St
Athens 106 76
Greece

Stephen A. Matlin
Department of Chemistry
The City University
Northampton Square
London EC1V 0HB
UK

Wolfgang E. Merz
Department of Biochemistry II
University of Heidelberg
Im Neuenheimer Feld 328
D-6900 Heidelberg 1
West Germany

Marcella Motta
Department of Endocrinology
University of Milan
Via Andrea del Sarto 21
I-20129 Milan
Italy

Zvi Naor
Department of Hormone Research
The Weizmann Institute of Science
P.O. Box 26
Rehovot 76 100
Israel

Mary V. Nekola
Department of Medicine
Tulane Medical School
1430 Tulane Avenue
New Orleans, Louisiana 70112
USA

F. Neumann
Hauptdepartment Endokrinpharmakologie
Schering AG
Müllerstrasse 170–178
Postfach 65 03 11
1000 Berlin 65
West Germany

S. J. Nillius
Section for Reproductive Endocrinology
Department of Obstetrics and Gynaecology
Academic Hospital
S-751 85 Uppsala
Sweden

Willem A. A. van Os
St Elisabeth's Grote Gasthuis
Boerhaavelaan 22, Postbus 417
2000 AK Haarlem
The Netherlands

Anand O. Prakash
School of Studies in Zoology
Jiwaji University
Vidya Vihar
Gwalior-474011
India

T. Rabe
Division of Gynaecological Endocrinology
Department of Obstetrics and Gynaecology
University of Heidelberg
D-6900 Heidelberg 1
West Germany

Subir Roy
Department of Obstetrics and Gynecology
University of Southern California School of
  Medicine
1240 North Mission Road
Los Angeles
California 90033
USA

B. Runnebaum
Division of Gynaecological Endocrinology
Department of Obstetrics and Gynaecology
University of Heidelberg
D-6900 Heidelberg 1
West Germany

J. Sandow
Hoechst AG
Pharmacology H 821
Postfach 80 03 20
D-6230 Frankfurt am Main 80
West Germany

Joseph G. Schenker
Department of Obstetrics and Gynecology
Hadassah University Medical School
P.O. Box 12000
91120 Jerusalem
Israel

Wolf-Bernhard Schill
Dermatologische Klinik und Poliklinik der
  Universität
Frauenlobstrasse 9–11
D-8000 Munich 2
West Germany

P. Senanayake
International Planned Parenthood Federa-
  tion
18–20 Lower Regent Street
London SW1Y 4PW
UK

Vernon C. Stevens
Department of Obstetrics and Gynecology
Ohio State University Hospitals
410 West 10th Street
Columbus, Ohio 43210
USA

H.-D. Taubert
Universitäts-Frauenklinik
Abteilung für Gynäkologische
  Endokrinologie
Theodor-Stern-Kai 7
D-6000 Frankfurt am Main
West Germany

Lourens J. D. Zaneveld
Department of Obstetrics and Gynecology
Rush-Presbyterian–St Luke's Medical
  Center
and
College of Pharmacy
Health Sciences Center
1753 West Congress Parkway
Chicago, Illinois 60612
USA

1
Future aspects in contraception: an overview

T. RABE, L. KIESEL and B. RUNNEBAUM

INTRODUCTION

World population is expanding at an alarming rate of 146 people per minute, 8790 per hour and 210 959 per day. This means a total annual increase of world population of 77 million (Figures 1 and 2). The population of India, amounting to approximately 40% of the world population together with China, increases by 1 million people per month. This rapid expansion continues in spite of war and famine. The problem of overpopulation and the resulting need for birth control are becoming ever more important.

Recent trends indicate that the earliest point of time at which a zero increase in the world population could be expected is the year 2100. At this time approximately 10.5 billion people will live in the world.

The tremendous explosion of world population has caused the political leaders of the nations world wide to look at family planning projects as vital. The problem of overpopulation leads to an increasing deficiency of minerals, which may cause an economic crisis in the industrial sector and famine in the nutritional sector.

The World Health Organization (WHO) encourages the development of contraceptive methods which are safer (Pearl Index), less disturbing and easier to handle. An ideal contraceptive should fulfil the following conditions: (1) high efficiency; (2) easy application; (3) reversibility (=normal fertility after withdrawal of the method); (4) no severe hazards; (5) low costs; (6) easy distributory systems; and (7) acceptability in the light of the religious, ethical and cultural background of the patients.

For the limitation of the exploding population the optimal application of contraceptive methods already available and the development of new ones are necessary. Important modes of action are governmental control of fertility—for example, in China, where parents are given tax concessions after the first child and lose tax and social advantages after the second and third child. The improvement of present and the development of future methods of contraception are mainly based on pharmaceutical research. The pharmaceutical industry is interested in the development of new contraceptive products, because of the large market. Unfortunately, the interest and commitment is much lower, compared with the enormous efforts being

1

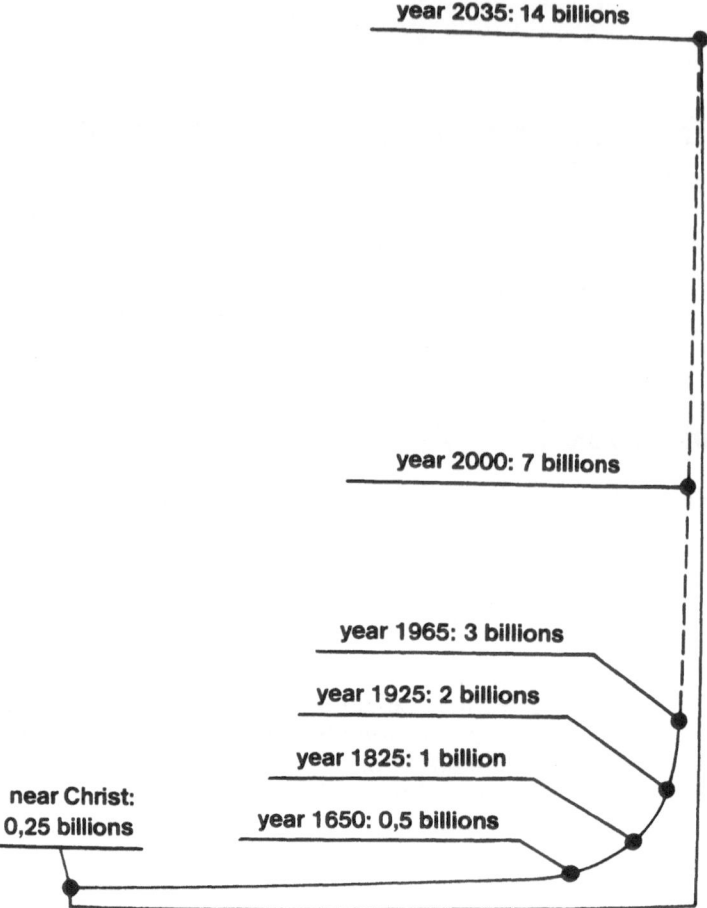

Figure 1   Population development (*Population Reports*, 1983)

made to discover the pathogenesis of and new methods for the treatment of cancer, allergies and asthma.

The importance of research in the field of contraception is clearly demonstrated by the following quotation (Boyarsky and Polaski, 1981): 'The future of mankind does not depend on the victory over cancer, but on the control of human reproduction.'

Di Raddo and Wardell showed in 1981 that, between 1963 and 1976, 956 new substances were developed by pharmaceutical companies in the USA. Of these, only 20 could be applied for contraception and only 17 reached the investigational new drug stage according to the definition of the American Drug Association (Notice of Claimed Investigational Exemption for a New Drug) after animal and clinical research.

The problem of research in the field of contraception arises from the fact that effective control of new substances requires considerable time and expense, as toxicological examinations have to be performed over a long period of time. The drugs should be applied to healthy women and men over a very long period of time without intensive medical observation.

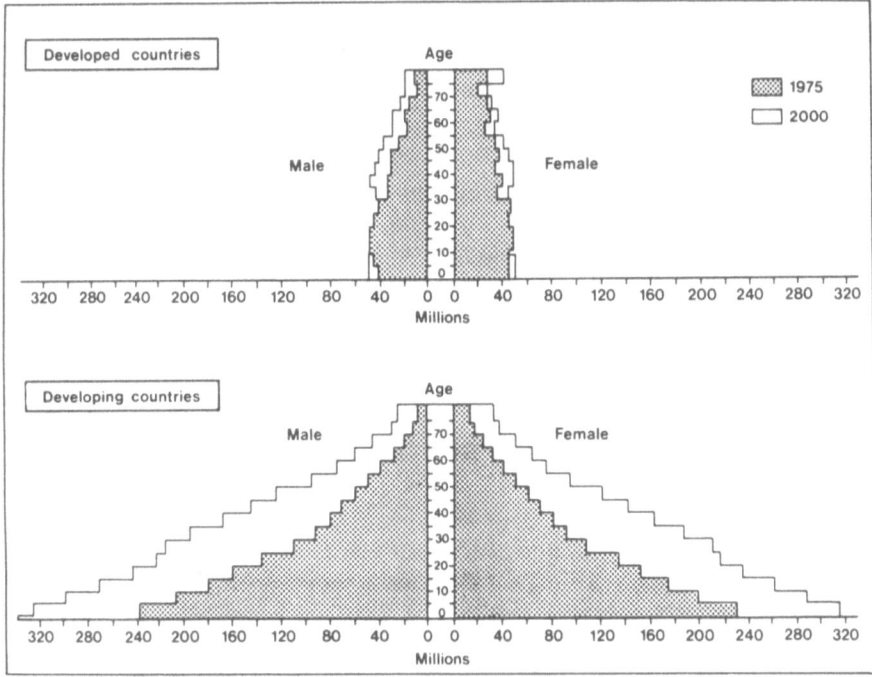

Figure 2   The population pyramid (from Global 2000, 1981)

Therefore, tremendous expenses (40 billion US $) are necessary for research to fulfil the conditions listed above.

In this review the different approaches in female and male contraception are summarized.

The various sites of action of contraception in the female and the male are summarized in Table 1. In the following sections the different approaches in female and male contraception are discussed separately.

Table 1   Sites of action of various contraceptive methods in the female and the male

Sex	Mode of action	Contraceptive action
Female	ovulation	suppression of ovulation
	fertilization	inhibition of a fusion of oocyte and spermatocyte
	implantation	prevention of nidation of the embryo
	pregnancy	interruption of pregnancy after implantation
Male	spermatogenesis	suppression of spermatogenesis
	fertilization	prevention of fusion of oocyte and spermatocyte

One of the most important criteria in the evaluation of contraceptive methods is contraceptive safety. Contraceptive safety can be evaluated either by the Pearl Index or according to the life table analysis. The Pearl Index summarizes the number of undesired pregnancies during application of the method over 1200 woman-years—i.e. the number of pregnancies in 1200 patients applying the method for 1 month or in 100 patients applying the method for 12 months. From this definition it is obvious that the duration of application influences the safety of a method according as the patient becomes acquainted with its performance. Therefore, the life table analysis, in which the frequency of side-effects is analysed in relation to the duration of application, is more reliable. As the data of the life table analysis are only comparable after different time intervals, the contraceptive safety of the available methods is summarized in Table 2 by means of the Pearl Index.

Table 2 Contraceptive safety of various contraceptive methods (Runnebaum and Rabe, 1979)

Method	Pearl Index
No contraception	115–200
Combination pill	0.1–0.9
Sequential pill	0.3–0.9
Progestogen-only pill	0.4–2.5
Morning-after pill	c. 0.5
Three-months injectable	0.2–2.6
Condom	6–28
Cap	c. 7
Diaphragm/cream	3–34
Spermicide vaginal preparations	0.7–7
Basal body temperature	1–3
Time method	14–35
Coitus interruptus	8–38
Intrauterine device	0.5–5
Laparoscopic tubus sterilization	c. 0.3

In Table 3 the approximate frequency of application of various contraceptive methods world wide is analysed.

Table 3 Estimated number (in millions) of couples performing contraception world wide. Arrows indicate increase, exact data not yet available. (From Population Reports, 1978, and Djerassi, 1980)

Method	1970	1977	1980
Oral contraceptives	30	55	60–80
Condom	25	35	↑
Other methods (diaphragms, spermicides, rhythm, coitus interruptus)	60	65	
Voluntary sterilization	20	80	↑
IUD	12	15	60*
Pregnancy termination	40	40	30–40
Total (without abortions)	147	260	

* People's Republic of China: 45 millions

PHYSIOLOGY OF REPRODUCTION

Preconditions for reproduction in the female

Under the influence of pituitary hormones LH (luteinizing hormone) and FSH (follicle stimulating hormone), there is a maturation of primordial to tertiary follicles in the ovary within the first 14 days of the menstrual cycle. The regulation of the gonadotrophin release is controlled by releasing hormones synthesized in the hypothalamus and transported to the pituitary by neurosecretion. The hypothalamus is controlled by cortical centres. In this regulatory process biogenic amines as well as catecholamines may be important.

During the phase of ovomaturation (Figures 3, 4), the pituitary releases both LH and FSH and stores larger amounts of LH in certain granula. The steroid hormone 17β-oestradiol formed by the ripening follicle induces, probably together with low amounts of progesterone, a release of LH out of the pituitary stores and induces an LH peak in the peripheral blood of mid-age. This LH peak triggers ovulation. After ovulation the oocyte is picked up by the fimbria of the fallopian tube. It is unknown whether the fimbria, as suggested earlier, encloses the respective area of the ovary or whether the oocyte is picked up by the fimbria from the Douglas pouch after ovulation. The lifetime of the oocyte is approximately 6–12 h. During oocyte migration through the fallopian tube, fertilization of the oocyte by the spermatocytes occurs; otherwise there will be no implantation. After

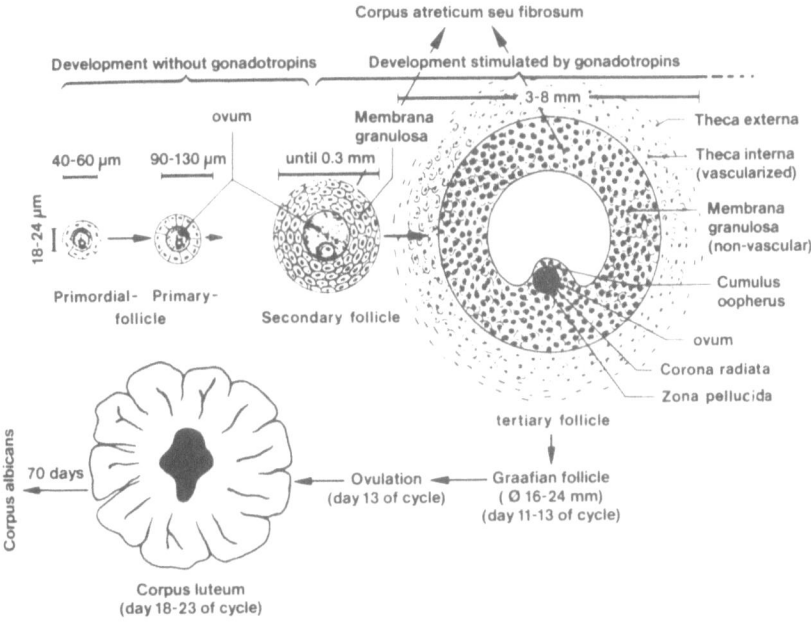

Figure 3 Morphological maturation of oocytes up to the development of the corpus luteum (from Schreiner, 1976)

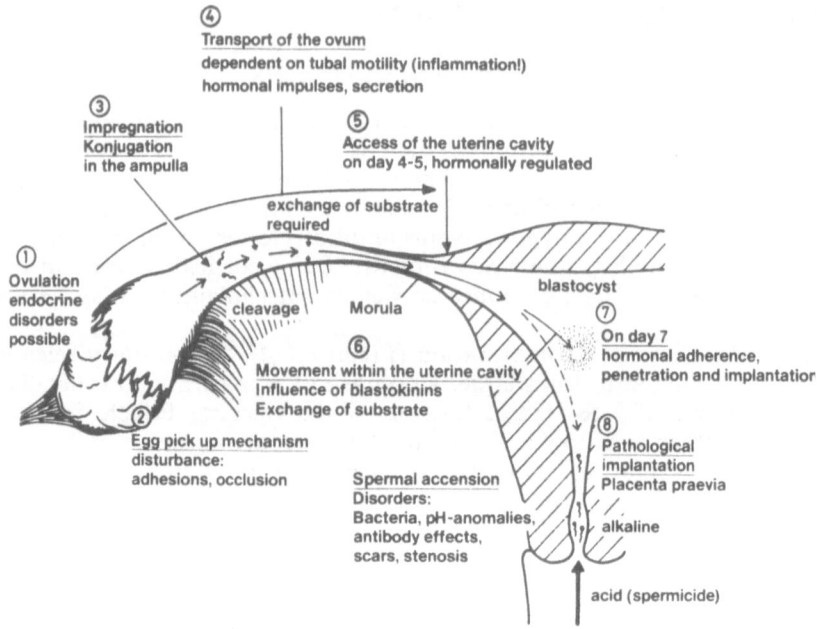

④
Transport of the ovum
dependent on tubal motility (inflammation!)
hormonal impulses, secretion

③
Impregnation
Konjugation
in the ampulla

⑤
Access of the uterine cavity
on day 4-5, hormonally regulated

exchange of substrate
required

①
Ovulation
endocrine
disorders
possible

cleavage   Morula

blastocyst

⑦
On day 7
hormonal adherence,
penetration and implantation

⑥
Movement within the uterine cavity
Influence of blastokinins
Exchange of substrate

②
Egg pick up mechanism
disturbance:
adhesions, occlusion

Spermal accension
Disorders:
Bacteria, pH-anomalies,
antibody effects,
scars, stenosis

⑧
Pathological
implantation
Placenta praevia

alkaline

acid (spermicide)

Figure 4 Migration of the oocyte from ovulation to implantation (from Schmidt-Mathiessen, 1979)

fertilization, the fertilized oocyte during its migration through the fallopian tubes gives some as yet unknown biological signals which induce specific changes in the endometrium. After the implantation hCG synthesized by the trophoblasts prolongs the lifetime of the corpus luteum, which would otherwise be destroyed by luteolytic processes.

Preconditions for reproduction in the male

Male reproductive potency is linked to a normal function of the testes and the epididymis. Morphologically, there is a close neighbourhood between germinal cells and the Leydig cells localized in the interstitial tissue. The Leydig cells are responsible for testosterone biosynthesis (Figure 5). Regarding the formation of spermatocytes, we have to differentiate between spermatogenesis, which includes the total morphological differentiation of the spermatozoa from the spermatogonia, and spermiogenesis, which describes the transformation of the spermatids into spermatozoa. The duration of spermatogenesis is 74 days. The infertile spermatozoa mature during the 12 days' migration through the epididymis passage. It takes, therefore, approximately 90 days for an immature spermatogonium to evolve into a mature, mobile spermatozoon and to reach the ampulla of the vas deferens.

After ejaculation the spermatocytes of the epididymis are transported by the ductus deferens; spermatocytes mix with secretory products of accessory glands (prostate, seminal vesicle). After the liquefaction of the previously

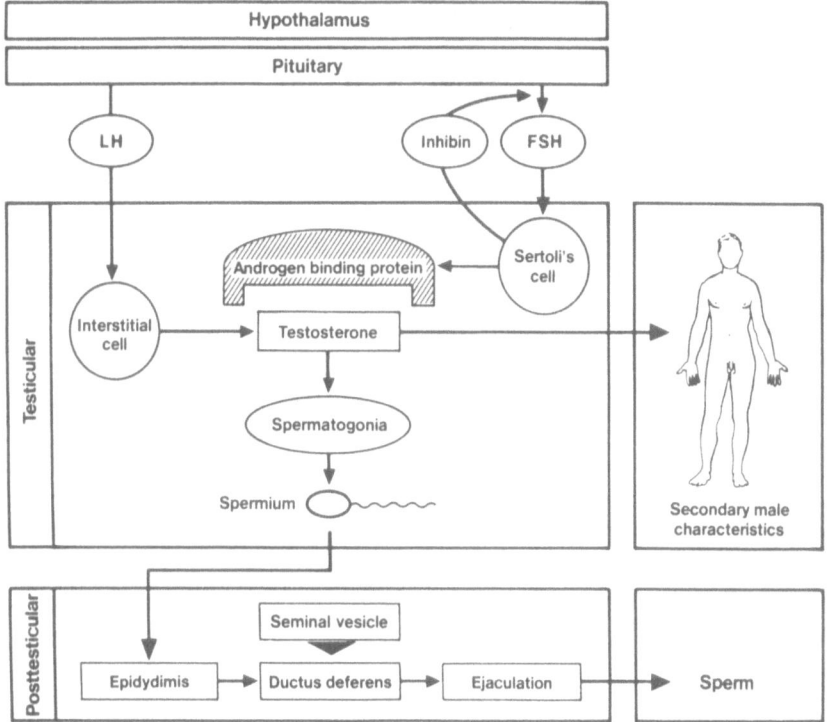

Figure 5 Central and intracellular regulation of testis function. LH, luteinizing hormone. (From Hansson, 1976)

coagulated ejaculate, spermatocytes can penetrate into the cervical mucus. The precondition is an increased peri-ovulatory permeability of the physiological cervix barrier.

In order to obtain the potency for fertilization the spermatozoa follow a potentiation process in the female genital tract. Sperm potentiation includes the liberation of the penetration enzymes from the substances that inactivate them biochemically. The three most important enzymes necessary for penetration are localized in the acrosome of the spermatocyte. These enzymes are necessary for the penetration of the various covers of the oocyte during the fertilization process. After the corona radiata has been digested by a hyaluronidase enzyme the corona radiata is penetrated by a specific corona-penetrating enzyme. The zona pellucida is perforated by means of acrosin, similar to trypsin, which is a key enzyme in this process. For the maintenance of male fertility a complex system of hormones and regulatory mechanisms is required. Under the influence of the hypothalamus releasing hormones are secreted and the anterior pituitary secretes LH and FSH. The Leydig interstitial cells are stimulated to produce testosterone (Figure 6).

FSH targets are the Sertoli cells and the tubuli seminiferi, where FSH activates the transport system for biologically active androgens from interstitial tissue into the tubuli seminiferi by-passing the blood–testis barrier.

Testosterone and its active metabolite, 5α-dihydrotestosterone, are most important stimuli for testicular spermatogenesis. After migration of spermatozoa from the testes into the epididymis the maturation process is under the control of androgens.

Under the influence of FSH the Sertoli cell synthesizes a specific protein (ABP = androgen binding protein). This protein binds androgens and is secreted with the fluid into the tubuli seminiferi. It is suggested that the function of the androgen binding protein is in the transport of active androgens through the blood–testis barrier.

The various site of actions of male contraceptives are summarized in Fig. 7.

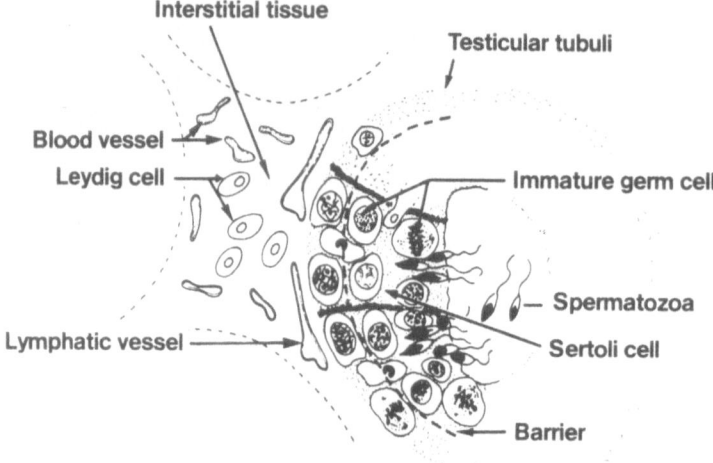

Figure 6 Morphology of the testis (from Hansson, 1976)

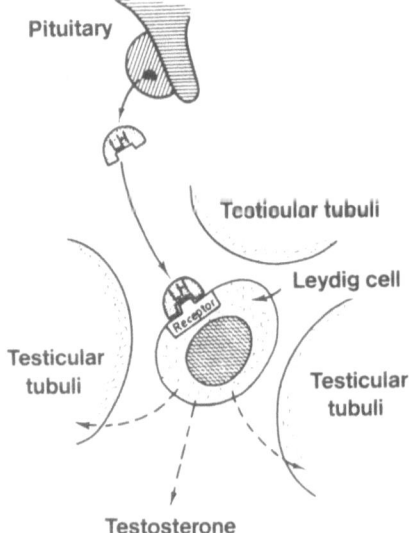

Figure 7 Different approaches for male contraception. Contraceptive methods in the male are divided into those with a testicular and those with a post-testicular mode of action

FEMALE CONTRACEPTION

Ovulation inhibition

Various approaches in female contraception by inhibition of ovulation are summarized in Tables 4 and 5.

Table 4   Oral contraceptives: assessment of substances used for ovulation inhibition

Site of action	Mechanism of action	Route	Substance	Assessment
Inhibition of GnRH and gonadotrophin release	steroid hormones inhibit the release of hypothalamic and pituitary gonadotrophins	oral combined pill: sequential pill once-a-month pill	oestrogen– gestogen combination	clinical application for 25 years, at present used by 60 m women
		parenteral: three-months injection	progestogens	clinical application (world-wide)
		implantables	progestogens norgestrel norethisterone	clinical trial
	compounds with antiserotonin activity			trial stage
Inhibition of gonadotrophin release	GnRH agonists	nasal spray implantables	GnRH analogues buserelin	clinical trial
	GnRH antagonists	nasal spray implantables	GnRH antagonists	clinical trial

Oral contraceptives

COMMONLY USED METHODS

Since the development of the Pincus pill its oestrogen and progestin content has been steadily decreasing. Within the past 20 years only two orally active oestrogens, ethinyloestradiol and its 3-methyl ether, mestranol, found clinical application, whereas nine different progestins, derivatives of 17α-hydroxyprogesterone or 19-nortestosterone, could be used in oral contraception. The aim of research in contraception is the development of pure progestins without oestrogenic, androgenic and corticoid residual activity. Such side-effects are responsible for the complications caused by oral contraceptives (e.g. changes in the cardiovascular system as well as metabolic changes in lipid and carbohydrate metabolism). Besides contraception, there are numerous desired side-effects of the oral contraceptives, which could be used therapeutically. For instance, the frequency of benign breast tumours, of cysts of the ovary and of endometrial carcinoma is decreased.

Table 5   Strategies in the development of new oral contraceptives

Aim	Methods	Criteria
Development of specific steroids	progestogens oestrogens: synthetic natural	pure progesterone action central inhibition of ovulation without peripheral side-effects
Reduction of steroid dosage	introduction of new intake schemes triphasic pill mid-cycle pill	contraceptive safety good control of menstrual cycle
Introduction of new application schemes	mid-cycle pill once-a-month pill implantables depot injections contraception plaster	
Improvement of steroid release	releasing systems for oral application: microcapsules microspheres microsponges parenteral application: microcapsules microspheres microsponges liposomes	continuous drug release prevents concentration peaks
Improvement of therapeutic efficacy following omission of pill intake	use of steroids with long half-life use of releasing systems	
Decrease in production costs	paper pill simple large-scale steroid synthesis	simple packing and steroid dosage per day

FUTURE DEVELOPMENTS

In the field of hormonal contraception there will be the following future approaches. As a further decisive decrease in oestrogens and progestins in currently available hormonal contraceptives is not possible, future clinical trials will be concerned with the possibility of combination (e.g. triphasic pill) of the available oestrogens and progestins. Furthermore, the application of natural oestrogens (e.g. oestradiol) will have to be tested for hormonal contraception. In search of pure progestins without oestrogenic and androgenic rest activity, numerous new progestins were synthesized (e.g. norgestrel, desogestrel, norgestimate and gestoden).

Further investigations are necessary to determine whether the continuous application of hormonal contraceptives without a menstrual withdrawal bleeding is accepted by the patient over a longer period of time. In this context a 1-month pill or a 3-month pill would be of interest. The idea of the 1-month pill was suggested in the mid-1950s (Greenblatt, 1967). It was forgotten for some time, but in the People's Republic of China at present a large clinical trial is concerned with a once-a-month pill consisting of a long-acting oestrogen (cyclopentyl ether of ethinyloestradiol) in combination with a short-acting progestin (e.g. levonorgestrel). This clinical trial is being carried out mainly in the province of Tianjin, where more than 340 000 cycles have been observed (Fan, 1980). Furthermore, long-acting pills free of oestrogen were tested in Shanghai (Yang, 1979). The problem, however, is that frequent disturbances of the menstrual cycle (bleeding pattern and menstrual disturbances) occur.

The application of an oestrogen–progestin combination on cellulose acetate or ester foils (e.g. paper pill) for developing countries remains to be checked clinically.

A new galenic form of oral contraceptive combinations, the so-called paper pill (Figure 8), has been tested clinically since 1977 (Damm, 1979). The paper pill consists of a number of cellulose stamps (rice-flavoured) soaked with a carefully titred mixture of progestins and oestrogens. In the

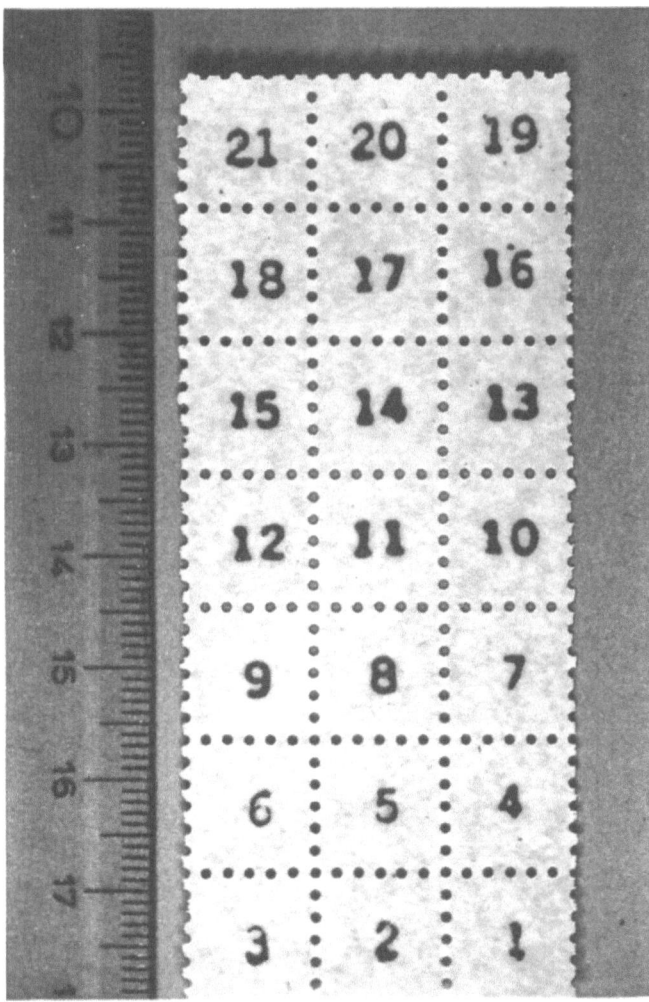

Figure 8 The paper pill (Schering AG, Berlin)

state of Durango, Mexico, approximately 138 patients without prior experience in hormonal contraception were treated with a long-acting steroid in the form of a conventional tablet for 3 months, alternating with the new paper pill. Before changing the mode of application and at the end of the clinical trial, objective and subjective parameters were analysed. Seventy-eight per cent of all patients persisted to the end of the study. The first questionnaire after 3 months showed a side-effect rate of 5.5% in the paper pill group and of 5.7% in the tablet group. More than 90% of the patients in both groups would like to maintain the same mode of application. Safety and ease of application were judged to be better in the conventional tablet form (Damm, 1979). The further development of the new galenic form would, according to the authors' view, only be possible provided that there is a cost reducing production (Damm, 1979).

By microencapsulation of oestrogens and progestins in oral contraceptives a continuous release and the occurrence of a peak concentration of steroid hormones in the peripheral blood can be avoided.

A further possibility for the suppression of ovulation consists of an application of progestins at the time of the expected ovulation to block

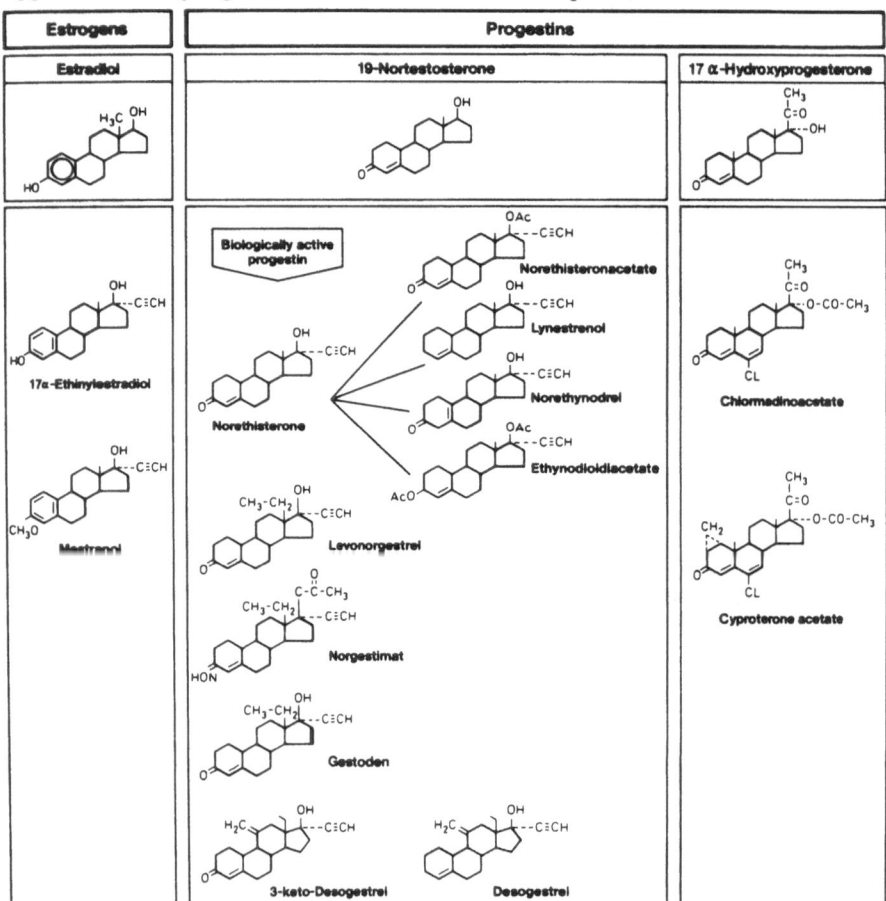

Figure 9 Contraception with synthetic oestrogens and progestins

ovulation (Raynaud *et al.*, 1975). The so-called mid-cycle pill with the gestogen R-2323 has been clinically tested in France (Sakiz and Azadian-Boulanger, 1971).

Steroid hormones used for oral contraceptives depend on a mixture of synthetic oestrogens and progestins. The synthetic oestrogens are derivatives of oestradiol, whereas the synthetic progestins are derivatives either of 19-nortestosterone or of 17α-hydroxyprogesterone (Figure 9).

The aim of the development of progestins is to obtain pure progestins, i.e. substances without androgenic, oestrogenic or corticoid residual activity. The progestins developed most recently are desogestrel, which becomes active after 3-reduction, and a levonorgestrel derivative, 3-ketozim-levonorgestrel (norgestimate: $\text{D-}13\beta$-ethyl-17α-ethinyl-17β-acetoxy-gon-4-en-3-on-ozim). Norgestimate is based on levonorgestrel after chemical modification of the keto group in position 3 into an ozim derivative and of the hydroxyl group in position 17β into the acetyl derivative. Tests with the derivative of levonorgestrel, desogestrel, showed a slightly lower moderation of the lipoprotein metabolism (De Visser *et al.*, 1977). This gestogen is approximately twice as potent as levonorgestrel. Another new gestogen is a derivative of levonorgestrel after introduction of a double bond at C-15 which leads to gestoden.

It can be assumed that natural oestrogens (e.g. oestrone, oestradiol) are less potent than synthetic oestrogens in causing cardiovascular and metabolic hazards. Owing to nausea and disturbances of the menstrual cycle, these natural oestrogens have not fulfilled expectations (Ratnam and Prasad, 1980).

The problem in developing synthetic oestrogens is to find substances

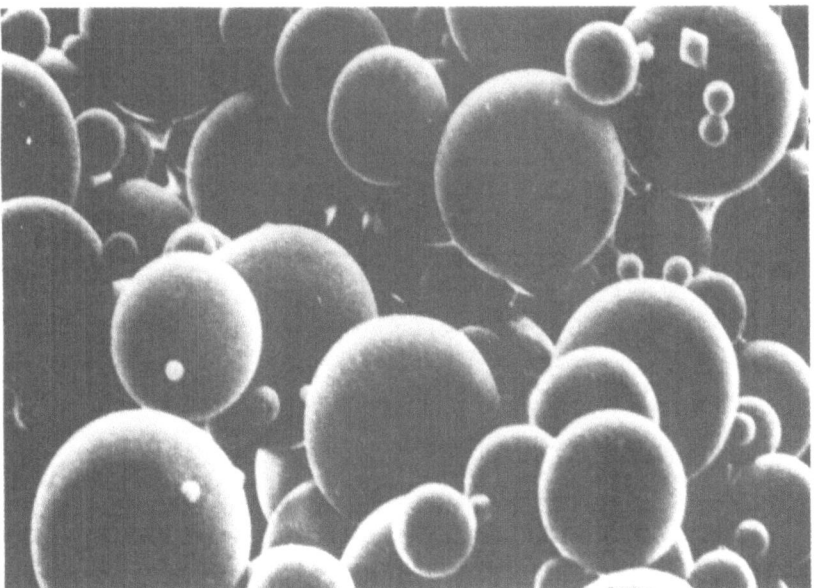

Figure 10 Grid electron microscopy of poly(DL-lactate acid) microcapsules containing 22% progesterone (from Beck *et al.*, 1983)

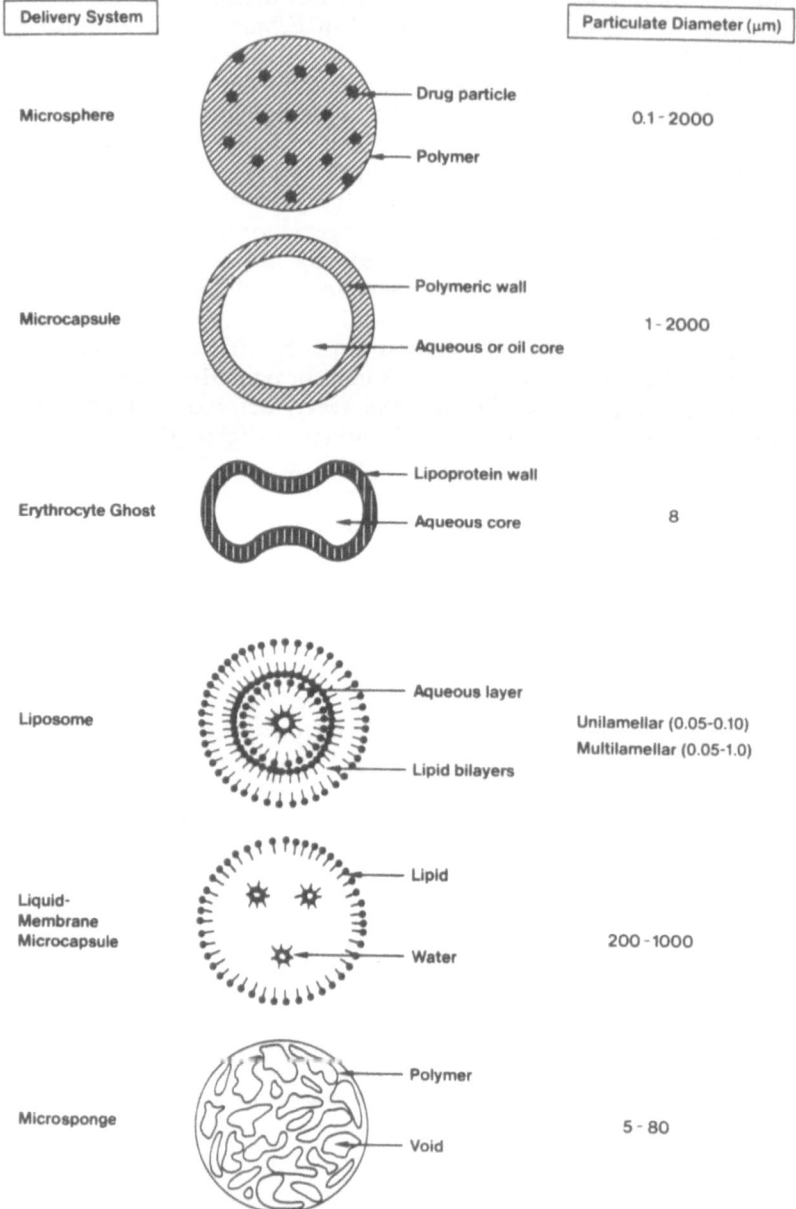

Figure 11 Bio-delivery systems for contraceptives (from Gardner, 1980)

which inhibit ovulation in a small dose without peripheral oestrogen-dependent side-effects. At present the only synthetic oestrogens are ethinyloestradiol and its 3-methyl ether, mestranol. Mestranol metabolizes into ethinyloestradiol by demethylation. So far, no synthetic oestrogens which can be applied for hormonal contraception have reached the stage of clinical trials.

Implantables

GENERAL REMARKS

Implantables use bio-delivery systems containing microencapsulated steroid hormones which are released continuously after subcutaneous implantation over a longer period of time. Various bio-delivery systems are summarized in Figures 10 and 11 and Table 6.

Table 6 Bio-delivery systems for contraceptives (from Gardner, 1980)

Delivery system	Description	Probable mode of administration	Particulate diameter (μm)
Microcapsule	a solid polymeric membrane surrounding an aqueous or oil core which contains the solubilized or suspended contraceptive agent	oral, parenteral, vaginal	1–2000
Microsphere	a solid polymeric particle which contains the contraceptive agent dispersed throughout the particle or attached to the particle	oral, parenteral, vaginal	0.1–2000
Erythrocyte ghost	a natural erythrocyte (devoid of its haemoglobin) which has been resealed with the contraceptive agent enclosed within an aqueous core	parenteral	8
Microsponge	a solid polymeric particle which contains voids filled with a solution or suspension of the contraceptive agent	oral, parenteral	5–80
Liposome	a collection of concentric lipid bilayers in which the contraceptive agent could be located in either the aqueous or lipid bilayers	parenteral	unilamellar (0.05–0.10) multilamellar (0.05–1.0)
Liquid-membrane microcapsule	a stable double emulsion (oil-in-water-in-oil or water-in-oil-in-water) in which the contraceptive agent is dissolved in the internal phase	oral, vaginal	200–1000

During the past 13 years various implantables containing different compounds were tested for contraceptive efficiency. Most investigations and clinical trials were performed with Silastic implants in Brazil, Chile and India. The respective progestogens were microencapsulated and implanted subdermally in the form of silastomere capsules. The hormone is released by diffusion and maintains a constant blood level for a longer period of time. Where contraception is no longer desired, the subdermal capsule can be removed (Norplant) (Figure 12).

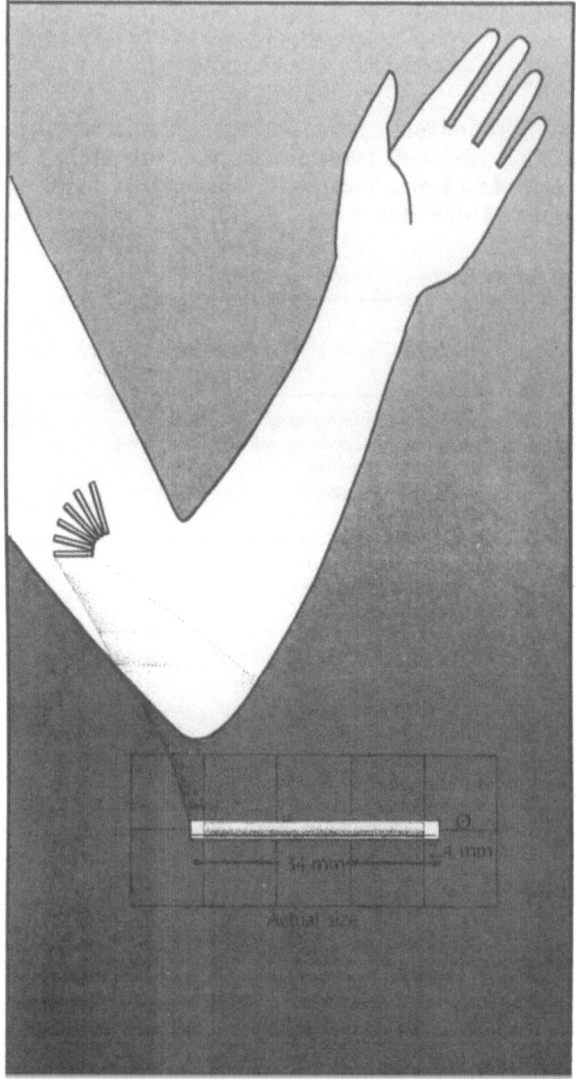

Figure 12   Norplant: levonorgestrel-containing implants (6 × 36 mg) for contraception up to 5 years (Leiras, Product Information)

GESTOGENS

Long-acting steroid contraceptive systems can be divided in those releasing the drug systemically and those releasing it locally. A controlled release of drugs from biologically degradable polymers can depend on two different modes of action (Heller *et al.*, 1983). First, a drug can be released by diffusion through a polymer membrane. An erosion which occurs later leads to the decomposition of the capsule. The other mechanism depends on a release of a drug by erosion of the polymer and, under ideal conditions, release of the drug and the polymer erosion occur simultaneously, so that

Table 7 Progestins which can be applied as implantables used for contraception (Coutinho, 1978)

Compound	Release rate ($\mu g/cm^{-1}$ day^{-1})	No. of capsules	Expected lifetime (cycles)	Efficacy in clinical trials
Norgestrienone (R-2010)	13	6	920–1470	18 months
Gestrigon (R-2323)	20	6	400–640	12 months
Megestrol acetate	14	4	600–960	15 months
Norgestrel	4	6	3000–4800	5 years
ST-1435	40	1	300–480	6 months
Lynoestrenol	60	5	200–320	8 months
R-1364	20	4	600–960	15 months

no polymer will remain in the tissue after the drug has been used up. Poly (ortho ester) is a polymer used for capsule membranes.

Different modes of action are possible for the development of long-acting steroidal contraceptive systems. The pharmacological approach includes investigation of long-acting steroid compounds: specific biological actions of drugs, including the solubility of the injection in various body fluids, affinity to receptors in body fluids and tissues, metabolization rate and excretion from the body, determine the effective life. New technologies are concerned with the application of biologically inert carrier systems controlling the rate and the duration of drug release.

Megestrol acetate   Megestrol acetate is a derivative of 17α-hydroxyprogesterone (Figure 13). It was the first compound to be used as an implantable, owing to its excellent release rate *in vivo* and the low tissue reaction near the site of the implantation. Studies with megestrol acetate had to be abandoned, however, because of the occurrence of mammary tumours in beagles after long-term application (Coutinho, 1978).

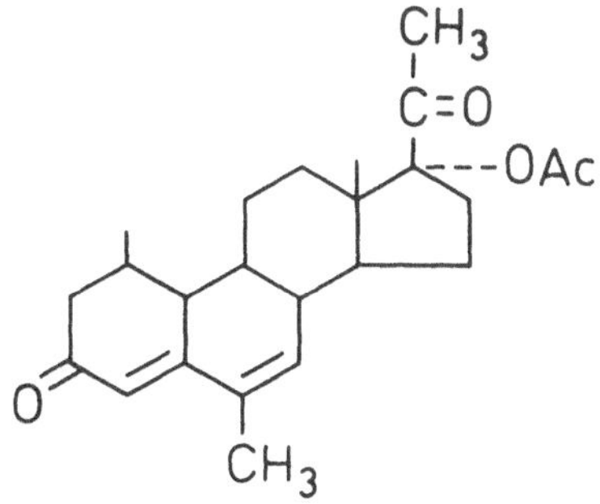

Figure 13   Megestrol acetate

Norgestrienone (R-2010)   Norgestrienone is a 17β-hydroxy-17α-ethinyl-4,9,11-oestrien-3-one (Figure 14). Coutinho (1978) performed a clinical trial with implants releasing norgestrienone (R-2010) in a group of 1448 patients. These were observed over a period of 21 783 cycles. The patients were treated with 1–6 capsules containing 30–47 mg of this compound implanted subcutaneously. The Pearl Index was approximately 0.6 within the first year

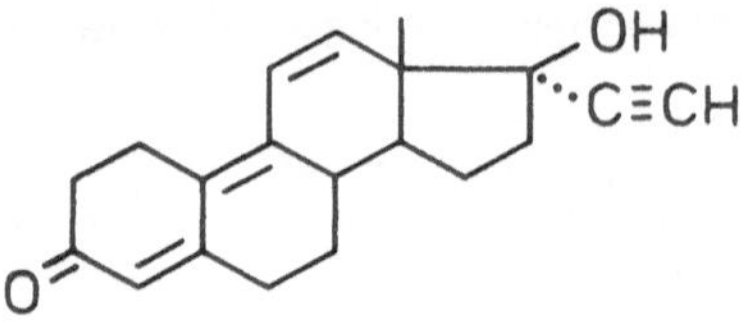

Figure 14   Norgestrienone

and about 1.2 after an application period of 18 months, and increased after a longer period of application (2 years). In all patients disturbances of the menstrual cycle occurred within the first 6 months. The probability of amenorrhoea increased with the number of implanted capsules. Most of the patients had regular menstrual bleedings (bleeding-free interval 29.5 days; bleeding period 2–6 days).

Gestrigon (R-2323)   The compound gestrigon, which is identical with ethinyl norgestrienone, or R-2323, is an anti-oestrogen and antiprogestogen. The anti-oestrogenic effect of R-2323 is not yet fully understood, as this compound acts as an anti-oestrogen at the uterus without occupation of the oestrogen receptors. On the other hand, gestrigon occupies the androgen receptors without any antiandrogenic effect. This is the reason why gestrigon can be used successfully for suppression of spermatogenesis. In clinical trials of Coutinho *et al.* (1975) it had been expected that the contraceptive action of 3–5 capsules would persist for 9–12 months. The clinical investigations could show clearly that the contraceptive action of 3, 4 and 5 implants persists for 9 months or longer. The Pearl Index depends on the number of capsules implanted and was, for 3, 4 and 5 capsules, 1.7, 2.3 and 4.9, respectively. The most important side-effect, amenorrhoea, occurred in patients within the first 5 months. In 44% and 50% of all patients who had 3 or 5 capsules implanted, onset of amenorrhoea could also be observed in the third month. This amenorrhoea persisted in one group of the patients until 8 months after removal of the implantable. Endometrial biopsies in these women showed different degrees of endometrial atrophy. Other side-effects, such as a decrease in breast circumference and improvement of acne and hirsutism, occurred in only 5% of the patients observed.

Levonorgestrel   D-norgestrel, or levonorgestrel, is a derivative of 19 nortestosterone (Figure 15). Coutinho (1978) investigated the contraceptive action of norgestrel in males and females after implantation of a delivery system

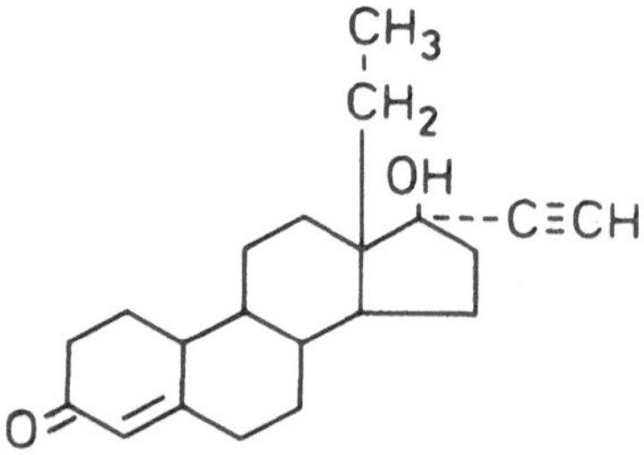

Figure 15   Norgestrel

containing levonorgestrel. This implantable released the contraceptive progestin in a constant dose over 1–3 years and was completely resorbed after exhaustion of the hormone depot. The implantable consisted of 85% levonorgestrel and 15% cholesterol in a 1 cm large sphere which had to be implanted subcutaneously. The new levonorgestrel implant had 15% cholesterol as an additive to prolong its dissolving at room temperature. In animal tests levonorgestrel implantables with 20 mg of steroid released 35 µg/day within the first 10 days; from the 10th day after implantation on, the release rate decreased continuously to 15 µg/day; and after 75 days it dropped to 10 µg/day.

The other clinically investigated subcutaneous implantables consisted of 15–20 mm long silicon capsules which cannot be resorbed after exhaustion of the steroid depot and have to be removed.

The calculated costs for continuous contraception by progestin implantables are only 10% of the costs for oral contraceptives. This new mode of preparation has been expected to provide an improved compliance and a continuous effect. Especially in developing countries, this could provide contraception with high drug safety and long-lived action.

Lynoestrenol and R-1364 Lynoestrenol is, like levonorgestrel, a derivative of 19-nortestosterone (Figure 16). Lynoestrenol and R-1364 were tested in a clinical trial in Bahia (Coutinho, 1978). Both compounds meet the preconditions for application over a short period of time. Capsules with lynoestrenol and a drug release rate of 60 µg per cm per day have a lifetime of only 200–300 days. Four or five capsules are sufficient for safe contraception for approximately 6–8 months.

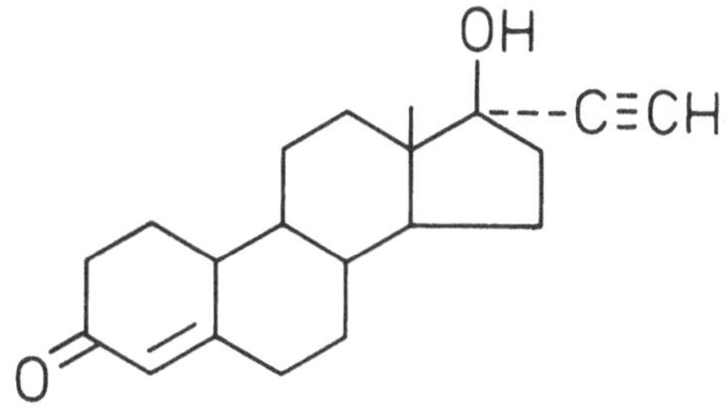

Figure 16 Lynoestrenol

In a pilot study with 60 patients over 556 cycles in which five capsules with lynoestrenol were implanted, no pregnancies occurred (Coutinho, 1978). In tests with R-1364, 13 out of 220 patients became pregnant (Coutinho, 1978). Clinical trials with both compounds had to be stopped because compounds such as R-2010, R-2323, norgestrel and ST-1435 showed better release rates. Despite the release rates, both compounds could be used as implantables for short-term contraception.

ST-1435 The compound ST-1435 (16-methylene-17α-acetoxy-19 norpregn-4-en-3,20-dione) is a derivative of 19-nortestosterone with androgenic and antiandrogenic actions. ST-1435 has a high release rate. The lifetime of this implantable is limited to 300 days. The contraceptive action of ST-1435 is higher than that of norethindrone and norgestrienone, which results in the reduction of the number of capsules to one or two per patient.

The first clinical trials were performed in Bahia with a group of 285 patients. Each patient was given 3–5 capsules, which were implanted subcutaneously. Altogether, 3174 cycles were observed (Coutinho, 1978). In 52 women with three capsules (530 cycles) and in 48 patients with four capsules (502 cycles) no pregnancy occurred. In the largest group of 185 patients, who received 5 capsules each and were observed over 2142 cycles, two pregnancies occurred. In a more recent study one capsule containing ST-1435 was implanted in 205 women. In these patients only a short-time observation over 6 months could be carried out. During these 1014 cycles no patient became pregnant.

After implantation of a single implantable ST-1435 capsule the most important side-effect was amenorrhoea. In 50% of the patients this amenorrhoea persisted for the whole of the 6-month application period of the implantable. Hormone analysis could prove suppression of LH and an absence of the progesterone increase in the second phase of the cycle. This suggests that low steroid liberation suppresses ovulation. Amenorrhoea can be regarded as a consequence of the inhibition of ovulation.

THERAPEUTICAL APPLICATION

In contrast to the treatment with contraceptives or hormone injections, the advantage of bio-delivery systems applied in the vagina or in the cervix for hormone release is that these systems cause low and continuous concentrations of the drug and its metabolites in the peripheral blood and in the respective target organ. One progestogen which can be released by silicon rubber implants in the female reproductive system is 6–125 times more effective than an injection and 13–26 times more effective than in oral application (Chang and Kincl, 1979).

In various clinical studies the individual steroids were tested regarding their contraceptive efficiency. The following steroids were tested clinically: norgestrienone (R-2010), gestrigon (R-2323), megestrol acetate, levonorgestrel, ST-1435, lynoestrenol and R-1364. In the various clinical trials different numbers of implants were tested. The possible period of action, which depends on the dose and the release rate of the capsules, varies between 6 months and 6 years. The results of these studies (Coutinho, 1978), in which 5000 patients were tested over 8 years, showed a high degree of efficacy and acceptability. One major disadvantage is based on disturbances of the menstrual cycle.

To avoid possible androgenic side-effects resulting from the prolonged application of oestrogen-free implants, a combination of oestrogens and progestogens in the form of capsules was investigated.

Emperaire and Greenblatt (1969) reported an excellent contraceptive efficiency after the implantation of four capsules containing oestradiol (25 mg per capsule), which were implanted at intervals of 6 months. Asch et al. (1978) performed tests with subcutaneously implanted oestradiol capsules, and these authors found that this method is easy to handle, effective and acceptable to the patients and has only minimal side-effects. Additionally, an orally potent progestin was used each month to trigger a withdrawal bleeding. The schemes of the treatment started with the implantation of four capsules and were followed by a dose reduction down to one capsule every 6 months. Altogether, 236 patients were observed over 6360 cycles (489.2 woman-years). During this treatment two pregnancies occurred. The Pearl Index was calculated to be 0.37. No side-effects were observed (Asch *et al.*, 1978).

Beck (1983a) analysed the pharmacokinetics of a long-acting microcapsule delivery system in ten patients. The microcapsules consisted of a biocompatible and biodegradable polymer poly(DL-lactide-co-glycolide) (Figure 10) with a diameter of 60 or 90 μm and a steroid content of 22% norethisterone. This steroid blocked the ovarian function and ovulation in all patients for 3 months. The norethisterone levels could be detected even 20 weeks after the start of the treatment. After the injection an increase in norethisterone and a slow decrease over 8-10 weeks occurred. After 10-20 weeks from the beginning of the treatment a second increase and fall in norethisterone occurred. This treatment led to suppression of the endometrium for 3 months and, apart from breakthrough bleedings and irregular cycles, no side-effects occurred.

Combined pills Table 8 summarizes the results of investigations of Coutinho *et al.* (1970, 1972).

Table 8 Comparison of implantables with different progestins in progestin–oestrogen combinations (Coutinho, 1978)

Compound	No. of patients	No. of cycles	Pregnancies	Pearl Index
Norgestrienone	453	7830	28	4.2
Norgestrienone oestradiol	183	3485	16	5.5
Megestrol acetate	102	1474	11	8.9
Megestrol acetate oestradiol	55	496	9	21.7
Gestrigon	179	2209	4	2.1
Gestrigon oestradiol	82	995	6	7.2

Injectables

GENERAL REMARKS

The injectables at present most commonly used contain either medroxyprogesterone acetate (DMPA) or norethisterone enanthate (NET). These compounds are applied in one single injection with a duration of action of 3 and 2 months, respectively. Alarming reports published recently about side-effects (e.g. endometrium carcinoma in rhesus monkeys) could not be confirmed in large clinical studies.

DMPA induces a significant increase in serum cholesterol level, which might eventually induce coronary thrombosis after long-term application (Kremer *et al.*, 1980). Other problems arising from the application of DMPA are bleedings, amenorrhoea and prolonged recurrence of fertility after withdrawal of DMPA.

The main reason for the development of new steroidal injectables is the fact that the currently available drugs do not release their substances continuously. After an injection, initially high peak values can be observed, which decrease within the following 4 weeks (Weiner and Johannson, 1975). Many of the side-effects of injectables seem to be dependent on their pharmacokinetics.

The aims of contraceptive research in the field of injectables are concentrating on the following subjects: (1) development of new steroids with better releasing profiles; (2) increase in the number of injections with simultaneous application of lower doses of steroids currently available; (3) application of natural oestrogens; and (4) improvement of steroid release by microencapsulation of the steroids.

WHO supports a large number of programmes for the development of new steroids with better releasing profiles. With regard to levonorgestrel, as many as four esters have been synthesized so far. A second approach to increase the number of injections at a low dose has been studied by Prema *et al.* (1981). In this study 20 mg norethisterone enanthate was injected monthly, which showed good contraceptive effects and only a low rate of side-effects.

Combinations of oestrogens and progestins were also tested as injectables. At the present time, a clinical study with Cyclo-Provera (25 mg medroxyprogesterone acetate, 5 mg oestradiol cypionate) and a WHO compound (50 mg norethisterone enanthate, 5 mg oestradiol valerate) is being carried out, in which the latter injectable seems to have the better prospects from the point of view of pharmacokinetics.

Another approach for the stabilization of the drug release rate is the encapsulation of steroids in polymer microspheres. By this mode of application it is possible to prolong the active period of norethisterone from 60 days to 2 years (Beck *et al.*, 1981). The drug release rates are better than those of conventional injectables. Norethisterone doses of 0.267 mg/kg do not affect ovarian function and menstruation after 6 months' use. In contrast, norethisterone dosages above 2.3 mg/kg suppress ovulation and cause a prolongation of the bleeding-free intervals of the menstrual cycle.

Oriowo *et al.* (1980) investigated the pharmacokinetic properties of three oestradiol esters: oestradiol cypionate, oestradiol valerate and oestradiol benzoate. The author treated healthy patients with a combination of the oestradiol esters with the progestin norethisterone enanthate as a 1-month injectable. Of these three esters, valerate seems to be most appropriate for contraception, owing to its pharmacokinetic properties. After an injection of 5 mg in 5 ml of an oleous solution the endogenous oestrogens increased in voluntary patients, who had been treated with 150 μg levonorgestrel and 30 μg ethinyloestradiol for 1 month prior to the injection for the suppression of endogenous oestrogens. After the application of oestradiol cypionate the peak values were lower than after the application of the valerate and the benzoate. The peak values of oestradiol and oestrone were reached approximately 4 days after administration of oestradiol cypionate and were observed in a significantly shorter period of time after application of the valerate and the benzoate. The average period of time in which elevated oestrogen levels occurred was shortest in the benzoate group (4–5 days), followed by the valerate group (7–8 days) and the cypionate group (11 days).

Lewis *et al.* (1983) investigated a new long-acting contraceptive which provided a continuous, controlled release of certain steroids including progesterone, norethisterone and norgestimate for 1–6 months. The injectable contraceptives consist of microspheres built of a biologically degradable aliphatic polyester, in which crystals of the steroid, dispersed homogeneously, are incorporated. The microspheres have a diameter of 20–200 μm. The steroid will be released out of these microspheres either by diffusion through the polymer membrane or by erosion of the polymer, and in some cases by a combination of both mechanisms.

Hahn *et al.* (1983) investigated different charges of microcapsules providing a continuous, constant release of norgestimate of from 4 weeks to 8 months. In tests with normally menstruating female baboons the action of norgestimate in the form of microcapsules consisting of a biologically degradable polymer of poly(lactic acid) was investigated; the action on the endometrium was analysed.

THERAPEUTICAL REGIMENS

One-month injectable Various 1-month injectables have been tested clinically. Most of them contained an oestrogen–progestogen combination. Sufficient clinical data are available for only two compounds: 25 mg DMPA plus 10 mg ethinyloestradiol cypionate (Cyclo-Provera) and 150 mg DHPAP in combination with 10 mg oestradiol enanthate (Deladroxat).

Detailed investigations of the compound DHPAP were performed. This compound was injected between days 7 and 9 of the menstrual cycle in monthly intervals. The second combination (Cyclo-Provera) provided nearly 100% contraceptive action in 1167 patients who obtained 11 229 injections.

Three-month injectable Various clinical investigations are concerned with the development and improvement of the 3-month injectables. For all 3-month injectables two compounds can be used for contraceptive purposes: medroxyprogesterone acetate and norethisterone enanthate. The disadvantage of the 3-month injectables lies in the fact that, during the first menstrual cycles, breakthrough bleedings occur and, after repetitive application, amenorrhoea occurs.

Six-month injectable So far, only DMPA as a long-acting steroid has been analysed as a 6-month injectable. Various dosages ranging from 200 to 1000 mg DMPA in 6000 women were tested over 165 000 cycles altogether. The failure rate ranged from 0 to 3.6/100 cycles. It can be assumed that a dose of 300 mg DMPA provides a good and sufficient contraceptive effect.

Releasing hormone analogues

GENERAL REMARKS

Since the discovery of the structure of the gonadotrophin releasing hormone (GnRH) by Schally (Figure 17), attempts have been made to use this substance or its analogues for contraception.

The cyclic pulsatile release of the releasing hormone GnRH occurring

(pyro) Glu - His - Trp - Ser - Tyr - Gly - Leu - Arg - Pro - Gly - NH₂

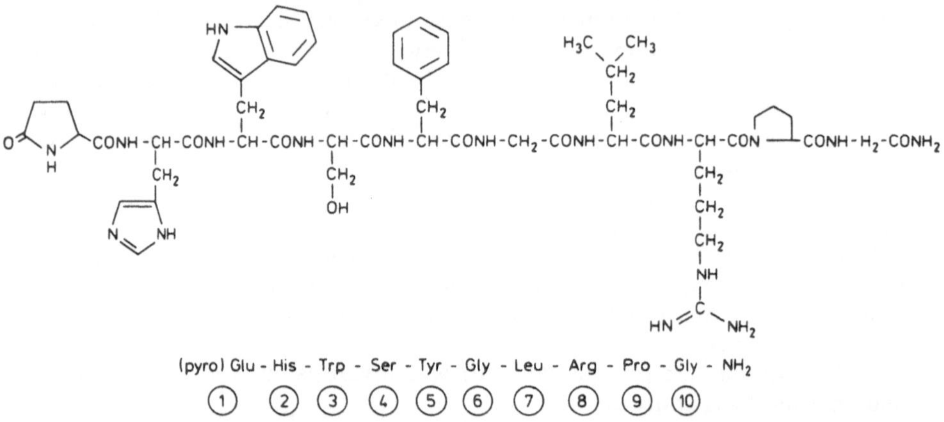

① ② ③ ④ ⑤ ⑥ ⑦ ⑧ ⑨ ⑩

Figure 17 Amino acid sequence of human LHRH

every 90 min in woman is necessary for the normal menstrual cycle. After application of the releasing hormones in a supraphysiological dose (more than 1000-fold the physiological dose) contraception via suppression of the mid-cycle LH can be obtained. Owing to the fact that GnRH analogues are small peptides, this compound can be applied as a nasal spray like oxytocin. The contraceptive effect of the substance is so high that, even with a cold, there is a sufficient resorption of the compound. Besides the naturally occurring releasing hormone, hormone analogues can also be used, which only bind at the receptor binding sites without activating the receptor and which block the GnRH receptor of the pituitary. The most important development in this field is the production of highly active superanalogues, one of which is buserelin, a nonapeptide which is appropriate for fertility control. It could be shown that the ovarian function after repeated application of buserelin cannot be stimulated dose-dependently, but, on the contrary, gonadotrophin secretion of normally ovulating females was reduced within a few days. Berquist *et al.* (1979) found that 400 μg buserelin as a nasal spray is sufficient to suppress ovulation. During continuous application over 6 months Taubert and Kuhl (1981) and Schmidt-Gollwitzer (1981) observed an inhibition of ovulation. Side-effects of this therapy are insufficient control of the menstrual cycle, cycle disturbances, breakthrough bleedings, as well as stimulated endometrium proliferation rate with a tendency to hyperplasia. Sufficient regulation of the menstrual cycle is only possible by additional application of 10 mg norethisterone acetate over 3 days. Fertility control with GnRH at this time provides no acceptable alternative to hormonal contraception, owing to the fact that additional oestrogen–progestogen mixtures are necessary for the stabilization of the menstrual cycle and thus the advantage of the treatment with pure peptide hormones (GnRH analogues) is negated by additional steroid hormone application.

In principle, potent agonists and antagonists of the releasing hormones can be applied for contraception. Whereas agonists inactivate the releasing hormone receptors of the pituitary by means of overstimulation and down-regulation of the receptor sites, antagonists block the receptor competitively without provoking a biological response. A comparison of structure/effect of LHRH and potent analogues is shown in Figure 18.

1. LH-RH: Glu-His-Trp-Ser-Tyr-Gly-Arg-Pro-Gly-NH$_2$

2. Super-Agonist: Glu-His-Trp-Ser-Tyr-D-Trp-Leu-Arg-Pro-NH-C$_2$H$_5$

3. Potent Antagonists: Acetyl-Ala-D-ClF-D-Trp-Ser-Tyr-D-Trp-Leu-Arg-Pro-

Gly-NH$_2$

Figure 18   Structure of LHRH and of potent analogues. D-ClF = D-p-chlorophenylalanine. (Rivier *et al.*, 1981)

The pituitary LH secretion in dependency on LHRH stimulation (physiological and superphysiological LHRH application) is summarized in Figure 19.

The relative receptor binding of GnRH and its analogues has been reviewed by Clayton and Catt (1981) (Table 9).

Table 9   Receptor binding affinity of GnRH and its analogues (Clayton and Catt, 1981)

Peptide	Receptor affinity, K_a (M^{-1})
GnRH superagonists with natural sequence	0.7×10^9
D-Ser(tBu)^{6}des-Gly^{10}-GnRH N-ethylamide	4.8×10^9
D-Trp^{6}des-Gly^{10}-GnRH N-ethylamide	9.0×10^9
D-Leu^{6}des-Gly^{10}-GnRH N-ethylamide	2.5×10^9
TriMe-D-Phe^{6}GnRH	3.4×10^9
Nap$_2$D-Ala^{6}GnRH	4.8×10^9
Nap$_2$D-Ala^{6}des-Gly^{10}-GnRH N-ethylamide	4.8×10^9
Partial agonists	
D-pGlu^{1}GnRH	3.9×10^7
βAla^1,D-Ala^6,Gly^{10}GnRH	3.5×10^7
des pGlu^{1}GnRH	2.1×10^6
Antagonists	
des-His$_2$GnRH	4.0×10^7
D-Phe^{2}GnRH	2.5×10^7
L-αMe-Phe^{2}GnRH	4.6×10^6
D-αMe-Phe^{2}GnRH	4.8×10^6
D-Phe^2,D-Phe^{6}GnRH	1.5×10^8
D-pGlu^1,D-Phe^2,D-Trp^{3,6}GnRH	4.5×10^9
D-pGlu^1,D-Phe^2,D-Trp^{3,6}des-Gly^{10}-GnRH N-ethylamide	8.2×10^9
N-acetylAla^{1}D-p-chloro-Phe^2,D-Trp^{3,6}GnRH	4.3×10^9
N-acetylD-Phe^1,D-p-chloro-Phe^2,D-Trp^{3,6}GnRH	2.0×10^9
Agonist analogues	
des-pGlu^{1}D-Ser-(tBu)^{6}des-Gly^{10}-GnRH N-ethylamide(2-9 octapeptide)	5.8×10^7
des-pGlu^1,desHis^{2}D-Ser(tBu^6)des-Gly^{10}-GnRH N-ethylamide(3-9 heptapeptide)	4.5×10^7
des-pGlu^1,desHis^2,desTrp^{3}D-Ser(tBu)^6 des-Gly^{10}-GnRH N-ethylamide(4-9 hexapeptide)	6.4×10^6

The biological potency *in vitro* as measured by retention times at two different pH values (pH 2.25; physiological pH 7.3) of five GnRH superagonists with the general structure pGlu-His-Trp-Ser-Tyr-X-Leu-Arg-Pro-Gly-NH$_2$ is given in Table 10. The amino acids in positions 2 and 3

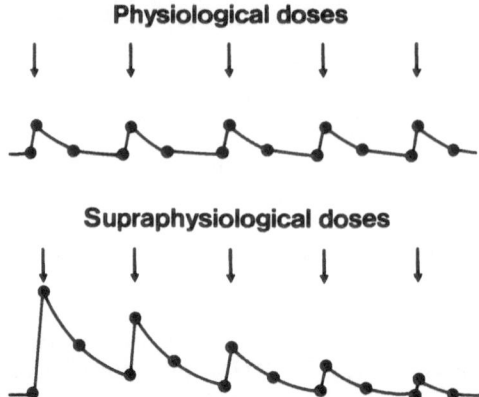

Figure 19   Pituitary LH secretion in dependency on LHRH stimulation. Upper panel: physio-logical LHRH application leads to a pulsatile increase in serum LH. Lower panel: superphysi-ological stimulation leads to an overshooting LH secretion during the first stimulatory doses and a decrease in LH response thereafter. This can be explained by receptor inactivation and down-regulation

are responsible for receptor affinity. The amino acids in positions 6 and 7 are targets for peptidases.

Table 10   Biological potency of five GnRH analogues which were substituted in position 6. The bio-logical potency was estimated by release of LH by rat pituitary cell cultures. (Rivier *et al.*, 1981)

Peptide	Release of LH by rat pituitary cell cultures (n-fold of native GnRH)
X = D-Lys	17
X = D-Leu	15
X = D-Tyr	68
X = D-Trp	144
X = D-His	200

AGONISTS

Under normal conditions the pituitary is stimulated by GnRH pulses to secrete the gonadotrophins LH and FSH. The GnRH is released by the hypothalamus in a pulsatile manner. By use of LHRH agonists a prolonged biological activity can lead to a down-regulation of GnRH receptors of the pituitary and the gonads.

GnRH agonists can be applied orally or as a nasal spray via the nasal mucosa. If the agonist is administered daily at the beginning of the men-strual cycle, an initial stimulatory phase can be observed. Long-term ad-ministration of the agonists decreases the capacity of the pituitary to secrete large amounts of gonadotrophins necessary for follicle maturation and ovu-lation. The administration of the agonists can block the function of both the follicles and the corpus luteum during the normal menstrual cycle (Fraser, 1982).

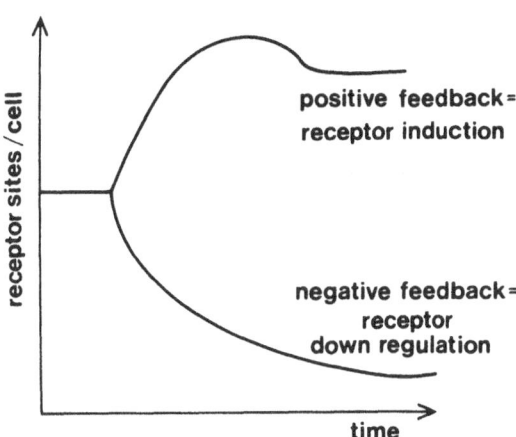

Figure 20 Changes in the receptors according to hormone stimulation. In the presence of a low hormone concentration the number of receptors increases as a result of receptor induction; down-regulation of the receptors can be achieved by prolonged stimulation

The administration of antagonists seemed to be a logical approach to the blockade of gonadotrophin release. Paradoxically, however, the agonists—originally developed for the treatment of infertile patients—show strong inhibitory effects.

GnRH analogues can also be released by injectable polymer microcapsules. This was shown by investigations of Kent *et al.* (1983). As a D-Na(2)[6] analogue GnRH is encapsulated as an injectable, biologically compatible, biologically degradable polymer. This system was effective in rhesus monkeys over a period of more than 1 month.

Sanders *et al.* (1983) investigated the mechanism of release of a D-Nal(2)[6] analogue of GnRH which had been microencapsulated in poly(DL-lactide-co-glycolide). In this study the size of the microcapsules, the molecular weight of the polymer and the composition of the polymer were investigated.

Hoe 766 (Buserelin)   Hoe 766 is an analogue of the natural gonadotrophin releasing hormone GnRH with the formula $C_{60}H_{86}N_{16}O_{13}$ and the following amino acid sequence: L-pyroglutamyl-L-histidyl-L-tryptophyl-L-seryl-L-tyrosyl-*O*-tert. butyl-D-seryl-L-leucyl-L-arginyl-L-proline-ethyl-amide (glu-his-trp-ser-tyr-D-ser(Bu^t)-leu-arg-pro-NH-C$_2$H$_5$) and the terminus (D-ser(Bu^t)[6])GnRH-(1–9)-nonapeptide ethylamide.

In Figure 21 the structures of GnRH and buserelin are compared. The receptor binding is analysed with regard to the various amino acid residues in Figure 22.

The substitution of glycine in position 6 by D-serine (t-Bu) and of glycinamide in position 10 by ethyl amide leads to a nonapeptide with a 20–170-fold higher potency in comparison with native GnRH. By this chemical modification the release of the follicle stimulating hormone (FSH), in particular, can be improved. The therapeutic dose of Hoe 766 could be lowered remarkably when compared with GnRH. Whereas GnRH is mainly

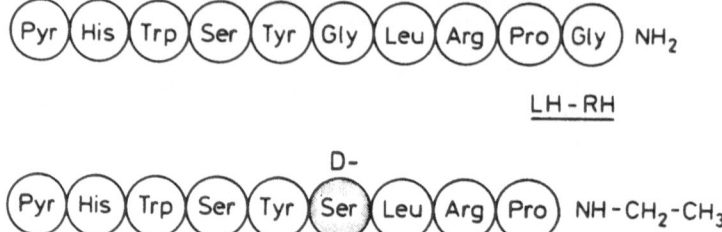

Figure 21   Structure of GnRH and buserelin

applied intravenously, Hoe 766 can be administered subcutaneously and nasally.

Animal tests showed no side-effects on the cardiovascular system, the kidney, the metabolism, the smooth muscles or the central nervous system. In man, no side-effects could be observed.

The distribution of Hoe 766 in the organism correlates with the pharmacological behaviour of native GnRH. After intravenous application of iodine-labelled substance to rats, Hoe 766 was eliminated comparably to GnRH with a half-life of 2–3 min. Sixty minutes after the application of $[^{125}I]$-Hoe 766 a significant increase in radioactivity could be observed in the liver, the kidney and the pituitary, whereas in these organs no labelled native GnRH activity could be detected. This might be caused by a much slower metabolization of Hoe 766. It is known that the cleavage of the

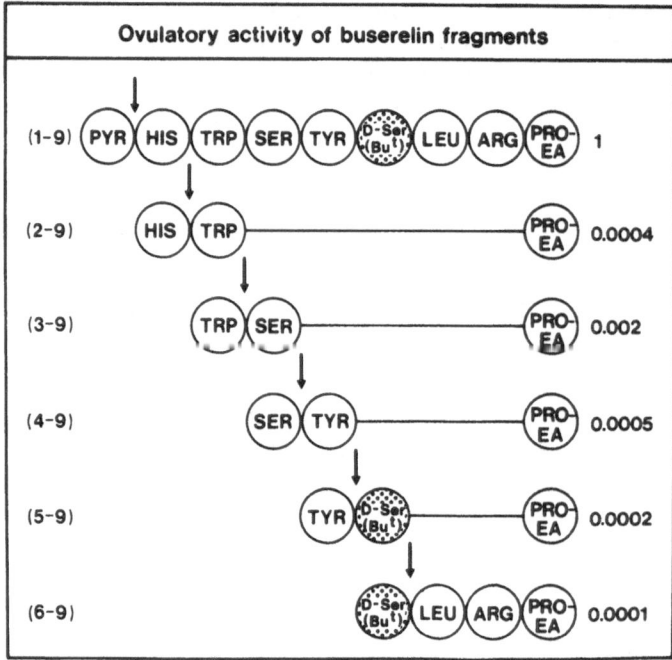

Figure 22   Amino acids of buserelin, the chemical change of which will reduce LHRH inhibition, and also the amino acids which are responsible for receptor binding

Ovulation

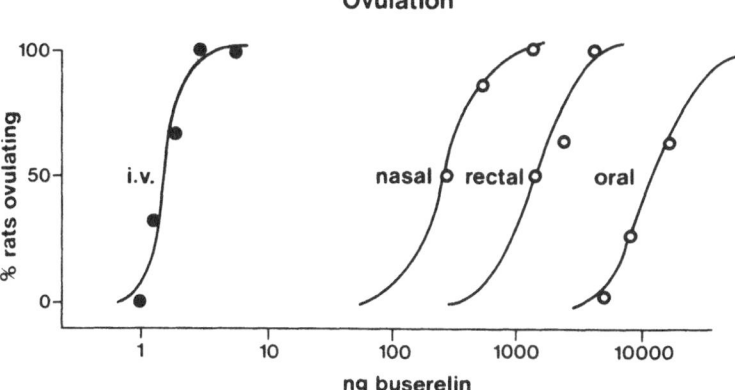

Figure 23 Induction of ovulation in rats by buserelin in relation to the mode of application

peptides 1-6 and 7-9 in Hoe 766 occurs much more slowly because at these positions of the molecule the substitution had been performed.

Toxicological examinations have shown a good acceptability of Hoe 766 in all dosages tested. In a high dosage and with a treatment over several weeks in all animals atrophy and a decrease in function of the genital region (testis and prostate or ovary and uterus) could be observed, which were fully reversible after the withdrawal of the drug. These changes were caused by a feedback mechanism in the regulatory cycle hypothalamus-pituitary-gonads and are manifestations of changing hormonal influence. An embryotoxic effect of Hoe 766 has not been observed.

A prolongation or a prevention of the delivery and a decrease in fertility with a dosage of 0.2-1.8 mg Hoe 766/kg s.c. observed during investigations of the reproductive functions in rats is not to be expected for humans. The rats were treated during the whole time of gestation and their ovarian cycle reacts very sensitively (Figure 23).

The clinical investigations in man have shown that Hoe 766 is approximately 20 times more potent than GnRH. The same dose induces a fourfold increase of LH and FSH in females compared with males. The duration of action measured by LH and FSH excretion in all dosages is comparable and approximately 8 h. Too high dosages and/or too frequent application of Hoe 766 lead to a decrease in the gonadotrophin secretion and, hence, to a decrease in testosterone and oestradiol in the serum.

After application of buserelin in three different dosages Schmidt-Gollwitzer *et al.* (1981a) tested the antifertility effect as well as the frequency of an uncontrolled oestrogen stimulation of the endometrium in man. In all three groups the total number of 70 female volunteers aged between 17 and 42 with ovulatory cycles, who had not taken any oral contraceptives for at least 3 months prior to the test, were treated from the first day of the menstrual cycle by daily nasal application of 400 μg, 200 μg (as one dose or as two sprays of 100 μg each) or 100 μg. Patients in the latter group additionally used mechanical contraception. During the 6 months of the treatment clinical examinations and determinations of FSH, LH, oestradiol and progesterone, as well as a total of 109 endometrial biopsies, were performed. Of the 337 treatment cycles evaluated, contraception by buserelin was effective in that only one pregnancy occurred in a patient who had reduced her own daily dosage from 200 to 100 μg. Anovulation as well as severe corpus luteum deficiency occurred in 97.2%, 84.5% and 69% of the groups treated with 400, 200 and 100 μg buserelin, respectively. The frequency of amenorrhoea was 19 out of 337 treated patients and was independent of the dosage. In one half of the group treated with 400 μg buserelin irregular menstrual cycles occurred. An inhibition of follicle maturation indicated by a low oestradiol secretion could be observed at least at the lowest dosage but not in all patients.

According to Schmidt-Gollwitzer et al. (1981a, b), 200 μg buserelin is effective for contraceptive purposes, but further studies will be necessary to investigate the follicle maturation as well as oestradiol secretion.

Inhibition of fertilization

GENERAL REMARKS

The best methods for a natural inhibition of fertilization (Table 11) depend on the prediction of the point of time of the ovulation and consist mainly in measuring various hormonal parameters and the temperature. Besides these methods, barrier methods by means of mechanical devices as well as in the form of tampon spermicides, vaginal sponges and vaginal rings, are being developed further.

Behavioural methods

CURRENTLY APPLIED TECHNIQUES

Natural family planning is characterized, even under exact performance, by a high failure rate. Nevertheless, it should be mentioned that some women, owing to their religious beliefs, have no other possibilities than the use of these methods. The morning basal temperature method seems to be the most important technique.

By an improvement of the behavioural methods a high contraceptive safety can be achieved. This might be particularly important if several methods are combined, for instance the combination of the basal body temperature measurement with the cervical mucus technique as suggested by Billings.

FUTURE DEVELOPMENTS

The future developments are based on the measurement of the basal body temperature by means of a microprocessor technique and microcomputers measuring and calculating the basal body temperature and giving a signal if the patient is in a fertile or infertile period at the given point of time. These techniques depend on a rise of the basal body temperature by 0.3 to 0.5 °C above the average temperature of the seven days before within 1–2 days due to progesterone secretion by the corpus luteum. During the hyperthermal phase of the menstrual cycle the patient is infertile.

Table 11 Inhibition of fertilization: assessment of clinical methods and drugs which can be applied for inhibition of fertilization

Site of action	Mechanism of action	Route	Substance	Assessment

Behavioural methods	behaviour inhibits the contact of sperm and oocyte	periodic abstention:
		  calendar method
		  basal temperature
		  symptothermal method
		  coitus interruptus
				world-wide use
				world-wide use
				world-wide use
				world-wide use

	amenorrhoea induced by hypoprolactin-aemia	prolonged breastfeeding		

Local applicable methods (non-hormonal)	mechanical aid prevents sperm–oocyte contact	mechanical barrier methods:
		  condom
		  diaphragm
		  cervical cap
		  intracervical device
		chemical methods:
		  ovula, cream
		  vaginal sponges
			spermicide
			spermicide
				world-wide use
				world-wide use
				world-wide use
				world-wide use
				trial stage
				world-wide use
				clinical trial

Tubal passage	tubal occlusion	electrocoagulation surgical interruption clip method chemical sterilization	quinacrine cyanoacryl	world-wide use clinical use clinical use

Hormonal methods	effect on cervical mucus and tubal motility	oral:
		  mini-pill
		local:
		  vaginal ring
			progestogens
			
			progestogens
				world-wide use
				
				clinical trial

Immunological methods	immunization against spermatozoa and oocyte antigen	parenteral immunization:
		  active
		
		  passive
			spermatozoa antigen:
			  LDH-X
			  acrosin
			oocyte antigens:
			  zona pellucida
			monoclonal antibody
				trial stage

Temperature measurements by microcomputers A microcomputer for measurement of the basal body temperature is illustrated in Figure 24. A small thermometer is connected with a small computer which evaluates the change in the basal body temperature. The result is given by a coloured lamp: a green light indicates an infertile, a red light a fertile, period; during the dangerous period interval the light is flashing. WHO supports the development of these devices, especially for developing countries, where many couples had problems with measuring the basal body temperature. A method which allows of the determination of the safe period by measuring the basal body temperature is also accepted by the Roman Catholic Church.

Another microcomputer system for detection of ovulation and non-pharmacological contraception was described by Aref (1983). This microcomputer requires an electronic thermometer which measures the temperature

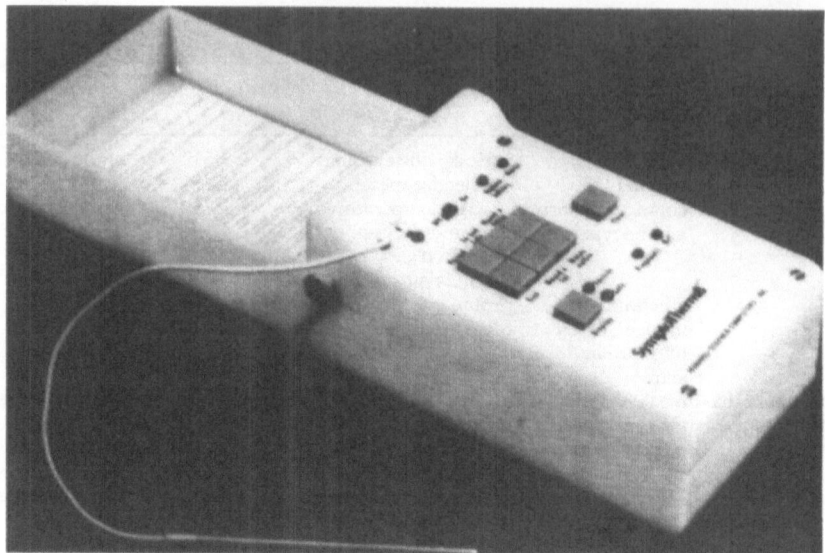

Figure 24   Microcomputer for temperature measurements (Schneider, 1982)

and stores the data. This computer can store up to 12 cycles. The basal body temperature curve is indicated by a liquid crystal screen.

Schneider (1982) described a microcomputer system for the measurement of the basal body temperature with the advantage that the duration of the sleeping period is considered for calculation. The microcomputer system measures the temperature orally and allows of the input of additional information concerning, e.g., menstruation, sickness and vaginal discharge; later it signals whether the patient is fertile. If the basal body temperature does not return to its initial value within 20 days, possible pregnancy is indicated by a light signal.

The Bioself 101 system (Figure 25) is also based on the measurement of the temperature according to the method of Vollmann and Knaus-Ogino.

Ovulometer   The ovulometer, for measuring the viscosity of the cervical mucus, is only mentioned in passing here, as clinical trials failed to show any useful advantage in contraception.

Determination of urine LH peak   Diagnostic methods for the detection of forthcoming ovulation have been analysed. One is the rapid determination of the LH peak in the urine by means of an OvuStick (Kasper *et al.*, 1984). After the LH peak, ovulation occurs between 24 and 36 h later. The disadvantage of the determination of the LH peak in the urine is that non-detection of the LH peak could lead to a misinterpretation of the ovulation point and, thus, to an unwanted pregnancy. Furthermore, the time interval between the LH peak and the ovulation is very short for safe contraception, which can only be performed 3 days after detection of the LH surge. The combination of this technique and basal body temperature measurement, however, seems to be promising.

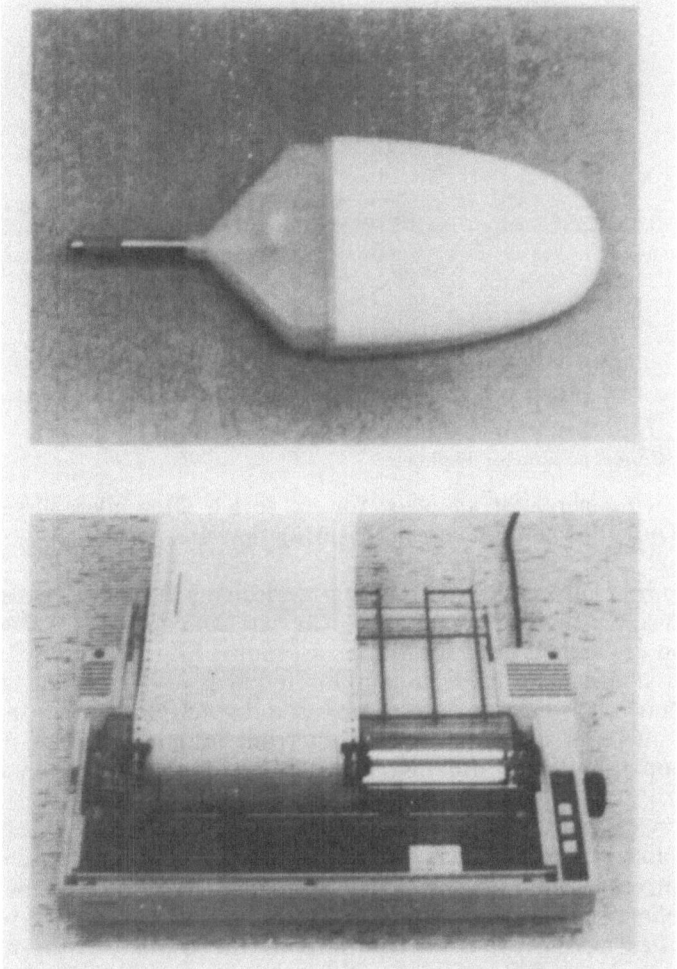

Figure 25   Bioself 101 microcomputer for measurement of basal body temperature

BARRIER METHODS

Barrier methods have several disadvantages. One is their low efficacy and disturbance during sexual intercourse by the necessary manipulations.

Diaphragm   The diaphragm is a rubber cap with a metal ring which is placed tilted in the vagina and covers the cervix (Figure 26). It is a mechanical barrier and prevents the sperm from entering the uterus. Its efficacy can be supported by a spermicidal jelly. The diaphragm must be placed in the vagina before intercourse. If it is properly adapted, it seems to be reliable. The diaphragm is available in various sizes. The advantage of this method lies in the fact that it is, unlike oral contraceptives and intrauterine devices, only used when necessary and not over a period. Also, the diaphragm is cheap and can be used for a long time. A disadvantage is the

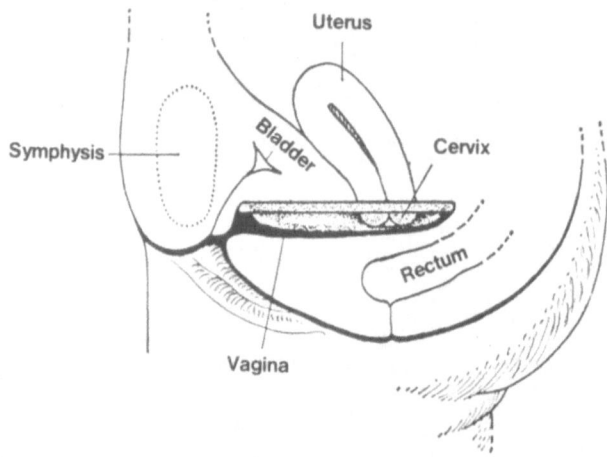

Figure 26   Correct position for diaphragm

fact that it must remain in place for up to 8 h after intercourse and the patient is not allowed to have a bath during that time.

Cervical cap   The cervical cap also is a mechanical barrier, which covers the cervix like a thimble (Figure 27). The cervical cap remains fixed on the cervix and prevents the spermatocytes ascending into the uterus. It is made of rubber and can be used in combination with a spermicidal gel. After some practice it is easy to insert. Like the diaphragm, the cap is inserted prior to intercourse. Patients suffering from inflammation of the cervix should not apply this form of contraception until the inflammation has healed.

The cervical cap must be left on the cervix for at least 8 h after intercourse. Later it must be washed out with warm water and stored dry. This contraceptive method, too, is cheap and can be used for a long time.

Freese and Goepp (1983) manufactured cervical caps for the individual patient after having evaluated the size of the cervix. In this way they achieved a higher efficiency. It is still unknown whether the individually fitted cap is of great importance.

Future developments   Future developments in the field of fertilization inhibition are based on the investigation of new spermatocides and new

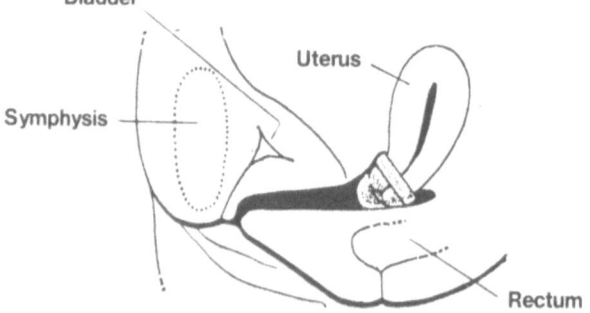

Figure 27   Exact position of cervical cap

administration schemes (e.g. tampon spermatocides, vaginal sponges) or the local application of progestins by means of vaginal rings.

The most important *spermatocides* are nonoxynol-9 and TS 88. These drugs are safe, but they cause vaginal irritation. Improvements are not expected in the near future. However, they have already been used in vaginal rings and collagen sponges. This new generation of vaginal contraceptives consists of sponges and tampons produced from different materials such as collagen, polyurethane, polyester or cotton.

Recent studies have shown that the beta-blocking propranolol can also be used as a locally effective spermatocide. Propranolol has been investigated in its steric as well as in its D-isomeric form and has been proved to be an effective inhibitor of sperm motility. Propranolol is resorbed by the vagina and, in addition, is, in small amounts, secreted by the sperms. It is suggested that a vaginal application of propranolol will lead to a rate of undesired pregnancy of 3–4% per 100 woman-years in a fertile population group (Pearson *et al.*, 1983).

The role of benzalkonium chloride as a spermatocide cannot be evaluated at present. Recent studies of benzalkonium chloride (Pharmatex Cones) have been published by Barwin (1983) and by Erny *et al.* (1983).

Medicated tampons which are placed into the vagina were described by the ancient Egyptians. In the last 50 years, however, this form of contraception has hardly been used, owing to the development of other contraceptives. Owing to the side-effects of oral contraceptives and intrauterine devices, this contraceptive method has, however, gained some importance lately.

Page (1981) performed clinical trials with a tampon containing a spermatocidal solution (Figure 28). In tests with 26 volunteers who used this tampon during intercourse the method proved to be acceptable and practicable, although 4 patients had difficulty in removing the tampon. Postcoital examination of the cervical mucus at the time of ovulation failed to reveal motile spermatozoa (Page, 1981).

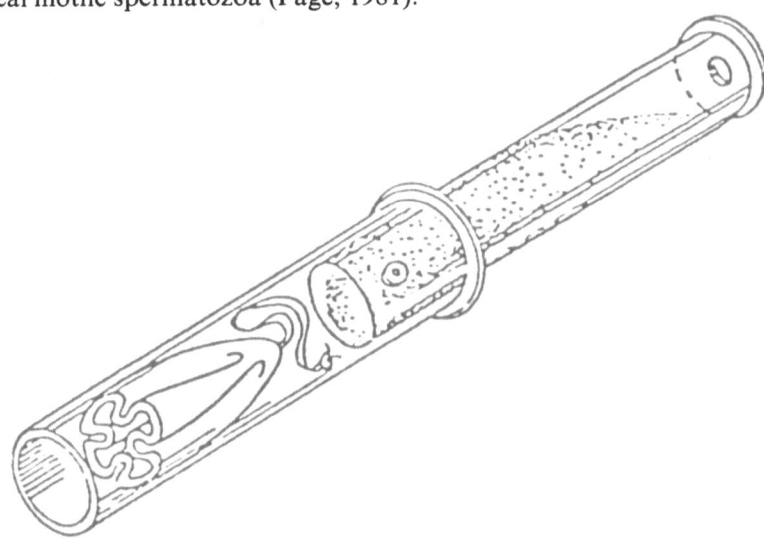

Figure 28 Tampon applicator (Page, 1981)

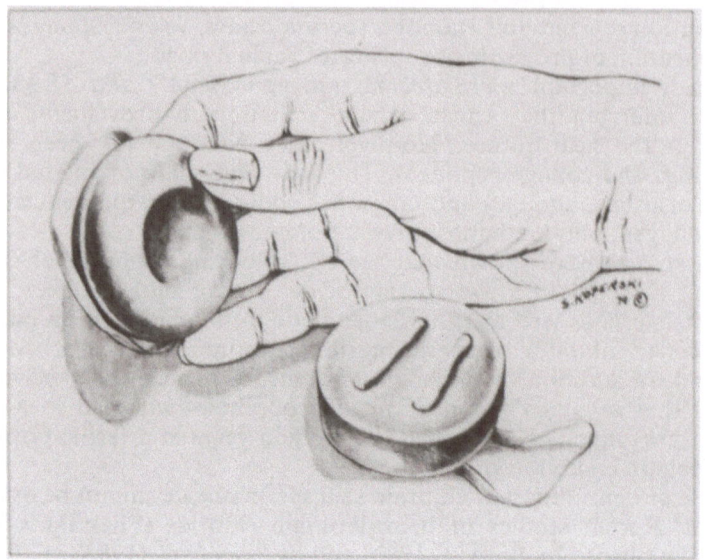

Figure 29   Vaginal sponge (Jackson, 1982)

Vaginal sponges consist of a soft polymer which is loaded with a spermatocide during fabrication (Figure 29). The 'two-day vaginal contraceptive sponge' (VLI Corporation) developed by Vorhauer (1980) is a vaginal sponge loaded with nonoxynol-9. Its action depends on the following mechanisms: (1) the spermatocide kills the sperms when in contact with the sponge; (2) sperms remaining alive are blocked in their ascent into the uterine cavity by absorption into the sponge. After application, the contraceptive potency of the vaginal sponge is stated to last for up to 48 h.

Recent studies on the efficiency of vaginal sponges are available only for polyurethane nonoxynol-9 sponges (Vorhauer, 1980). This author confirms an efficiency of 96-98% in 1000 women in different countries.

At present a local application of progestins near the cervix is only possible by means of *vaginal rings* (Figures 30, 31). It is not yet possible to

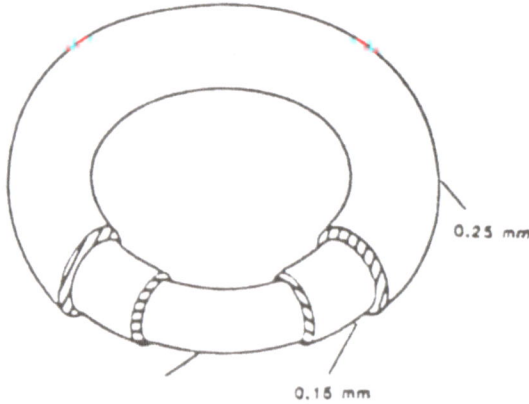

Figure 30   Vaginal ring (Mishell, 1982)

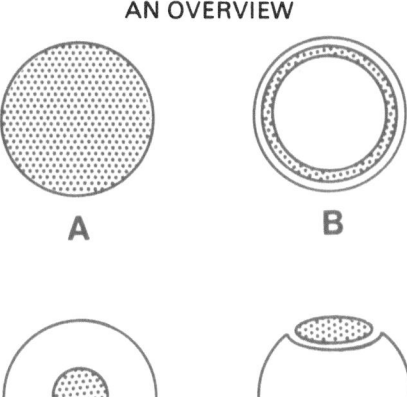

Figure 31 Cross-sections of different types of ring. The dark ground represents the crystalline steroids. A, homogeneous ring; B, hollow ring; C, ring with central hormone loading; D, ring with enclosure. (From Mishell, 1982)

evaluate whether sponges loaded with progestins will play an important role in future contraception.

Vaginal rings are slowly releasing progestins (levonorgestrel, chlormadinone acetate, R-2323 or progesterone) or progestogen–oestrogen mixtures near the cervical os, whereby the viscosity and the structures of the cervical mucus are changed, similar to the action of the progestin-only pill. The mucus becomes thicker and stickier, and the penetration of the sperms is blocked. The contraceptive effect is based on the suppression of ovulation.

Since the development of the first vaginal rings in 1968, which contained medroxyprogesterone, various steroids, carrier substances and ring forms have been investigated. Vaginal rings are expected to have a long-term contraceptive effect with good control of the bleeding pattern, without additional application of other drugs or dangerous side-effects.

The vaginal ring has a diameter of 56 mm and a thickness of 9.5 mm. It is made out of an elastic material and should fulfil two conditions: on the one hand, a local contraceptive effect with a fixed, constant daily release rate of progestins should be achieved; on the other hand, the present duration of action during continuous use should be increased from 90 days to 1 year or more. The release rate of vaginal rings depends on the size of the ring's surface, the solubility of the steroids, the diffusion constant and the distance the steroid has to cover from the crystal reservoir to its release from the ring.

At the moment four types of vaginal ring are being investigated in clinical trials all over the world (Figure 31). The four different types of vaginal ring are compared in Table 12.

In an internal comparison study vaginal rings with levonorgestrel and oestradiol (Nordette) have been compared with oral contraceptives. Both methods reduced the menstrual blood flow and the duration of bleeding (Sivin *et al.*, 1981).

The main advantage of progestin-loaded vaginal rings is a weak meta-

Table 12 Comparison of different vaginal rings

Ring model	Advantages	Disadvantages
Homogeneous ring	simple structure; easy application	exhaustion of the reservoir causes changes of the release rate
Hollow ring	minimal diffusion changes of the initial to the exhaustion phase by hormone loading in the same distance to the external ring circle	see above
Ring with central hormone loading	central grouping, see hollow ring; advantageous when slow release is desired	see above
Ring with steroid setting	setting in the interior and the exterior of the ring; loading with two different steroids possible; possibility of reloading without exchange of the entire ring	see above

bolic side-effect. In studies by Robertson *et al.* (1981) and Ahren *et al.* (1981) the effect of levonorgestrel/oestradiol vaginal rings on lipoproteins and apolipoproteins was investigated. Ten healthy female volunteers with regular menstruation were admitted to this trial. After 21 days of application and 7 days of non-application of the ring over 6 months, the concentrations of cholesterol, HDL cholesterol, triglycerides and LDL cholesterol were significantly higher than the control values: cholesterol by 25%, HDL cholesterol by 28%, triglycerides by 435% and LDL cholesterol by 24%.

In a prospective study performed by Ahren *et al.* (1981) the metabolic effect of a contraceptive vaginal ring releasing levonorgestrel (290 µg/day) and oestradiol (180 µg/day) was compared with that of an oral contraceptive containing 30 µg ethinyloestradiol and 150 µg levonorgestrel. The glucose-tolerance test showed no change. The early insulin response to glucose tolerance increased by 50% in the group of patients with contraceptive rings after 1 year, whereas in the group of patients taking oral contraceptives no change could be observed. All other insulin tests showed no change. The liver enzymes showed normal values, apart from alkaline phosphatase, which slightly increased in both groups.

The action of vaginal rings on the vaginal flora was investigated by Roy *et al.* (1981). Comparing the effect of vaginal rings and oral contraceptives, they found that vaginal rings cause a rapid increase in or an occurrence of pathogens.

The advantage of vaginal rings is that this contraceptive method can be applied easily, does not lead to permanent expense and has only minor systemic side-effects. The disadvantage is that vaginal rings in the form of the models tested in clinical trials have to be replaced monthly, and they are not generally available, since they are still in the phase of clinical trial. Furthermore, wrong positioning and an insufficient release of steroid may lead to undesired pregnancy.

The cervical os is a natural barrrier for the migration of the sperms from the vagina to the uterine cavity. Therefore, the cervical canal is another

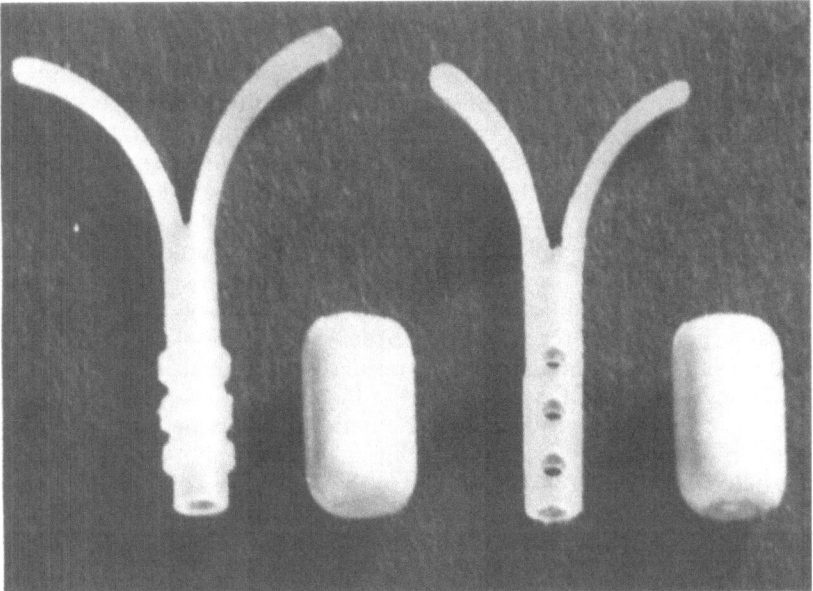

Figure 32 Intracervical pessary

possibility for contraception in the form of an intracervical pessary (Figure 32). A precondition is the fact that the pessary does not impede menstrual bleeding and can be inserted more easily than the commonly used IUDs. A problem seems to be the individual fitting, since the cervical canal of multiparas differs in size from that of a nullipara. One of the intracervical pessaries which are now undergoing clinical trial consists of a polypropylene tube containing a reservoir which can release drugs such as quinine and emetine and steroids such as norgestrel and norethindrone. Reservoirs with a drug release rate of 25 μg/day can have a lifetime of many years.

Gould and Ansari (1983) showed that the penetrability of the cervical mucus is increased by anions and lowered by cations. This effect depends directly on the valency of the ions. Sodium, calcium and chloride ions do not induce changes of the cervical mucus, if the mucus shows a good penetrability. Bivalent ions are much more effective, as shown in investigations with Fe^{2+}, Sn^{2+} and sulphate ions. Change in the cervical mucus achieved by means of *electrolytes* seems to be an interesting aspect of research into non-hormonal, reversible methods for fertility control.

Immunization

GENERAL REMARKS

The development of a pregnancy-specific immunization has been the subject of much scientific discussion. Immunization for contraceptive purposes is possible by raising antibodies against spermatozoa, seminal plasma antigens, antigens against the oocyte, against hormones of the trophoblast as well as trophoblast antigens. By an immunization against antigens of the oocyte a fertilization, by an immunization against trophoblast antigens an implantation of the fertilized oocyte can be prevented. The spermatocyte antibodies cause an inactivation of the ascending spermatozoa and prevent fertilization. Immunization against specific oocyte antigens causes irreversible damage of the oocyte. It cannot be predicted whether an autoimmune reaction in the ovary can occur. Several investigations are concerned with the experimental immunization of female animals against antigens of the male reproductive organs which cause reduction of fertility.

Until 1920–1934, 12 clinical publications were concerned with immunological contraception. Rosenfield (1926) tried to immunize three patients by multiple subcutaneous injections of human spermatocytes. In two of the patients a light local reaction was observed. Serological investigations proved an immunization against the spermatozoa, but the titres and specificity of the antibodies have not been sufficient for contraception. Baskin (1932) reported a clinical trial with 20 patients receiving 5–20 ml of fresh human semen in weekly injections for 3 weeks. In all cases a humoral sperm cytotoxicity was induced with a duration of 12 months. No pregnancy occurred, while the serological reactions were positive.

Another possibility for immunological suppression of female fertility consists of immunization against enzymes of spermatozoa, of which in the case of mammalia only 20% could be demonstrated in the acrosome. Tests with the spermatozoa-specific enzyme LDH-X are of great promise (Goldberg, 1974). This enzyme is localized in the middle-piece of the spermatozoa and has also auto- and isoantigenic properties. Antibodies against the LDH-X are blocking sperm penetration and are reducing the fertility rate in female animals.

The most important problems in the production of pregnancy-specific vaccines are the exact identification and isolation of spermatospecific antigens and the characterization of the specific immune reaction causing sterility. The number of sperm antigens is relatively high, and most of them occur ubiquitously in other tissues. To avoid undesired effects, especially reaction with other cells, a high specificity of these vaccines is necessary.

Besides active immunization for the regulation of fertilization there is the possibility of passive immunization by the use of monoclonal antibodies. The availability of human monoclonal antibodies with a high antigen-specificity leads to a revolution in the role of passive immunization for the prevention and for the treatment of human diseases.

Human monoclonal antibodies play the following role in the future regulation of fertility:

(1) Termination of early pregnancy by a systemic and intrauterine application of antibodies with a specific activity against embryonal or placental antigens or of other factors necessary for the maintenance of pregnancy.

(2) Short-term contraception by injection of antibodies with a high specificity against antigens of sexual hormones or gametes.

(3) Long-term contraception by passive application of antibodies in the form of a long-acting depot.

(4) Local immunological protection by application of antispermatocidal antibodies in the form of vaccinal ointments or gels.

Advantages of the application of human antibodies for passive immunization are:

(1) They are a cheap source of unlimited amounts of well-characterized and serologically very specific reagents.
(2) The action is short-lived and fully reversible.
(3) The degree of immunization is directly proportional to the amount of antibodies applied and does not depend on the individual variation of the immune response.
(4) As there are human proteins, a severe immunization against antibodies does not seem to be probable even if they are applied several times sequentially.

If the new contraceptive vaccines cause side-effects in some patients, they will nevertheless be applicable for other patient groups in which risk factors, when compared with the mortality of contraception and the normal regulatory process, are higher than this mode of contraception.

IMMUNIZATION AGAINST FEMALE SEXUAL HORMONES

LH Antibodies against human LH have been produced and it has been shown that they block ovulation. It has been suspected that immunological damage of the pituitary gland producing the hLH or of the kidney absorbing the hLH antibody can occur.

FSH Immunization against FSH may play a contraceptive role only in man. Even in man it is not yet clear whether a decrease in FSH level would cause a complete block of spermatogenesis.

GnRH GnRH also has been tested as a contraceptive vaccine. GnRH has a low molecular weight and has been fully synthesized. In female mice immunized with GnRH fixed to a carrier molecule, ovulation stopped and oestrogen levels fell. In male animals the immunization caused a decrease in testicular size, spermatogenesis ceased and a significant decrease in testosterone levels occurred (Carelli *et al.*, 1982).

Steroid hormones Steroid hormones involved in reproduction are not suitable as antigens for a contraceptive vaccine, because they are poor immunogens and cross-react among one another.

SPERMATOZOA ANTIGENS

Only a few sperm-specific antigens (protamine, lactate dehydrogenase C4, RSA-1, acrosin) have been characterized. In many laboratories monoclonal antibodies against a large number of spermatozoa antigens have been synthesized. Antibodies against hyaluronidase, a species-specific enzyme, has been found in some vasectomized men but an antifertility effect could not be shown (O'Rand, 1980). A significant decrease in fertility occurred in immunized rabbits (O'Rand, 1980) and sheep (Morton and McAnulty, 1979). Investigation of the acrosin and acrosomal antigens has been limited to date, owing to the poor availability and instability of the acrosin.

The sperm antigen which has been intensively characterized is lactate dehydrogenase C4 (LDH-C4), an isoenzyme of lactate dehydrogenase occurring only in male germinal cells (Goldberg, 1972). Recent studies are concerned with the development of a synthetic peptide causing an immune reaction with the native LDH-C4 protein (Wheat and Goldberg, 1981). Furthermore, monoclonal antibodies against LDH-C4 have been developed (Goldmann-Leikin and Goldberg, 1983).

Earlier studies have shown that active immunization of female rabbits and mice against LDH-C4 decreases the number of pregnancies significantly (Goldberg, 1973, 1975). Immunization of female baboons causes an antibody response and a decrease in fertility. The antifertility action occurs in the fallopian tubes, in which antisperm antibodies appear by serum transudation and cause a sperm agglutination or a complement-mediated cell lysis and therefore inhibit fertilization (Morton and McAnulty, 1979). These data in baboons are a preliminary hint that the LDH-C4 prevents fertilization in primates and that this effect is non-toxic and reversible (Goldberg et al., 1981).

Plasma membrane autoantigens seem to be the best target for antifertility agents. RSA-1 is a sperm-specific antigen occurring on pachyten spermatozoa and in the plasma membrane of rabbit sperm (O'Rand, 1977). The possibility of a local immune response in the female genital tract seems to exist, because a local production of IgA in the mucosa after antigen application could be shown. The production of immune globulins depends on a specific plasma cell in the lamina propria and in the secretory components of the epithelial cells (Austin, 1975). Both components join in the membrane and cytoplasma on the epithelial cells. The immune globulins IgA and IgG in the cervical mucus and in the cervical secretion are detectable in measurable concentrations. The IgM values are very low. Whereas the spermatozoa antigens could be detected in the cervical mucus by several groups of researchers, the immune competence of the endometrium and the mucosa of fallopian tubes is still doubtful. The development of an immune status in the female genital tract cannot be achieved by local antibody production, but by a general immunization. The transfer of circulating antibodies into the female genital tract depends on the permeability of the serum proteins, which, in general, is very low, but shows cycle-dependent variations.

Another possibility may be the production of antibody titres in the peritoneal fluid and in the follicular fluid, both of which contain already high immune globulin levels. Peritoneal fluid and follicular fluid can both be inserted with the oocyte in the fallopian tubes, where the specific antibodies can exercise a fertility-inhibiting action.

OOCYTE ANTIGENS

Development of a contraceptive vaccine According to Shivers (1975), the oocyte offers possibilities for immunological fertility control. The ovum is covered both in the ovary and after ovulation by fluid, cells and macromolecules possessing antigenic properties. The most important antigens around and in the oocyte are in the follicular fluid, the cumulus oophorus, the corona radiata, the zona pellucida, the membrana vitellina, the oocyte membrane and the oocyte cortex. The specific antibodies against the ovum can prevent oocyte maturation, ovulation, and loosening of the cumulus and the corona, and thereby prevent sperm penetration. Furthermore, they can influence negatively the fixation of the zona pellucida and the membrana vitellina, the passage of the oocyte and of the embryos through the genital tract, and, finally, the repulsion of the zona pellucida and the implantation. It seems to be important for the development of the oocyte and the embryo to take into consideration the time interval in which they are influenced by specific antibodies. The ovum may be exposed to this influence in the ovary for several days and after ovulation in the fallopian tubes for several hours, and the embryo for some days until implantation. Owing to the fact that immune globulins are already present in the follicular fluid and the fallopian tube fluid, low antibody titres are sufficient to damage the oocyte. The ovum and the surrounding medium are in contact for a relatively long period.

The initial phases of oogenesis occur during the fetal period, whereas the oocytes undergo their last maturation step in the female shortly before ovulation. This last maturation phase is linked to the production of specific antigen substances, which are the appropriate targets for immunological contraception in the female. The cumulus and the corona cells are unlikely to possess tissue-specific antigens (Shivers and Sieg, 1980), although little information is available concerning the surface antigens of the human oocyte.

Antigens To obtain an antiserum with a high titre against the oocyte, the presence of specific antibodies is necessary. To date, four or five specific antigens have been found in the follicular fluid of the human, some of them occurring also in the cervical mucus after ovulation.

According to recent reports, the cumulus and the corona radiata possess no tissue-specific antigens. It is important that the penetration of spermatozoa and the dispersion of the cumulus can be blocked by specific antibodies against spermic enzymes.

The antigens of the zona pellucida, a cell-free and gelatin-like layer around the ovum, has been predominantly analysed in animals. The antigens of the zona can be detected before and after fertilization in all embryonal phases. Antibodies against the zona pellucida change the surface of the ovum. This effect causes a disturbance of sperm attachment and sperm penetration.

The tissue specificity of zona antigens is well recognized. To date, they have not been demonstrated in any other tissue. Antibodies against other tissues (for instance, uterus, fallopian tubes and follicular fluid or serum) did not cross-react with the zona (Sacco and Shivers, 1973).

Sacco and Shivers (1973) have shown by means of a radio-immunoassay test that female mice hetero-immunized with a heat-solubilized zona pellucida substance from the pig reacted to these antigens with a high specific synthesis of antibodies. Fertility remained unchanged and they delivered normal infants. An investigation of the sera of young immunized mice by radio-immunoassay has demonstrated the occurrence of anti-zona pellucida activity, which means that the zona pellucida antibody has been transmitted passively by the placenta and the milk from the mother to the infant. Further immunofluorescent tests could show that the transmitted antibodies show a cross-reaction with the zona pellucida of the infants and are bound to these zona. These antibodies exhibit their biological activity in the infants, which could be demonstrated not only by the radio-immunoassay procedures, but also by *in vivo* binding to the zona pellucida of the female infants. All reports published to date show that zona pellucida antibodies, apart from the fertility inhibition, show no other physiological side-effect. *In vivo* investigations have shown that fertilization can be inhibited when oocytes are exposed to anti-zona antibodies before spermatozoa are added to the test. Oocytes isolated after passive immunization of the animals showed an immune precipitation at the external membrane of the zona, and an enhanced resistance to luteolytic compounds (Oikawa and Yanagimachi, 1975; Tsunoda and Chang, 1976a, b). Passive immunization can additionally prevent fertilization by contact between blastocyst and endometrium prior to implantation. This might be a new possibility for post-coital contraception.

Zhang and Liu in 1982 performed studies with zona pellucida material. Female rabbits were treated with several injections of fish zona pellucida material, by which the formation of antibodies against zona pellucida material could be induced. Forty days later various degrees of infertility occurred. After the anti-zona titre had reached a certain level, a significant increase in the anti-fertility effect could be observed. This effect could persist for a certain period of time if the antibody titre could be held on a high level. The possible role of the active immunization with zona pellucida material for contraception is the subject of further investigations (Zhang and Liu, 1982).

For longer-acting infertility action, active immunization against the zona antigen is possible. The zona pellucida antigen is an attractive vaccine: (a) zona antibodies can inhibit both fertilization and implantation; (b) a small number of mature oocytes are occurring at a different time period and only low antibody titres are necessary.

Study of antigens of the egg surface has so far been possible only in animals. Using rabbit antisera against mice oocytes, a surface antigen of the oocyte was identified, which could cross-react with SV-40 tumour viruses. The possibility that the egg antigens can be used for the production of contraceptive vaccines has not been investigated. The production of hetero-antibodies against the zona pellucida seems to be more successful.

SIDE-EFFECTS AND HAZARDS OF IMMUNIZATION

Possible hazards of immunological control of fertility depend on the development of cross-reactive auto-immunization. Cross-reactions of antibodies against seminal plasma components are well known. Of greater importance is the possibility that spermatozoa antigens, for example, cross-react with antigens of other tissues. In a patient with Addison's disease cross-reactions have been observed in the serum, both with spermatozoa and with cells of the adrenal cortex.

Sterilization

CURRENTLY AVAILABLE METHODS

The currently available methods of sterilization depend on a blockage of the fallopian tubes by either surgical dissection or laparoscopic electrocoagulation and dissection (Figure 33). These methods cannot essentially be

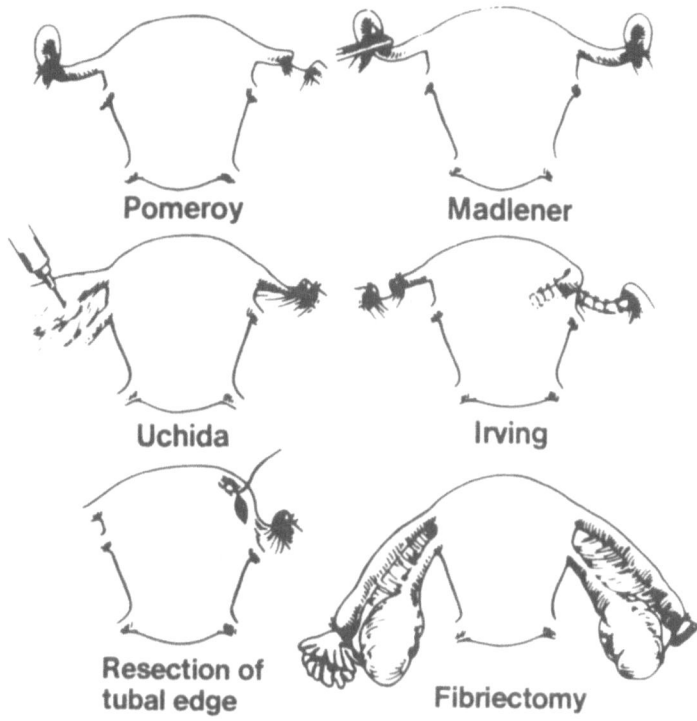

Figure 33 Different methods for surgical sterilization of the fallopian tubes (according to *Population Reports*, 1976)

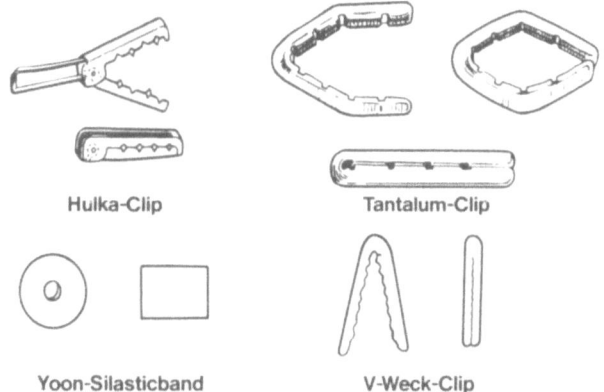

Figure 34 Different types of clip for tube sterilization (Rabe and Runnebaum, 1982)

improved in the foreseeable future. The carbon dioxide-laser technique induces a localized destruction of the tissue of the fallopian tube, which will permit a reanastomosis later, if another pregnancy is desired. The application of clips and ligatures (Figure 34) to the fallopian tubes is reversible. For surgical recanalization special skill in this field is required.

FUTURE DEVELOPMENTS

Chemical sterilization is performed by a specific substance causing a local inflammation and occlusion of the fallopian tubes; alternatively a substance is inserted, which polymerizes and thereby blocks the fallopian tube. The different compounds can be applied either blindly, by using special applicators, or under hysteroscopic control (Figure 35).

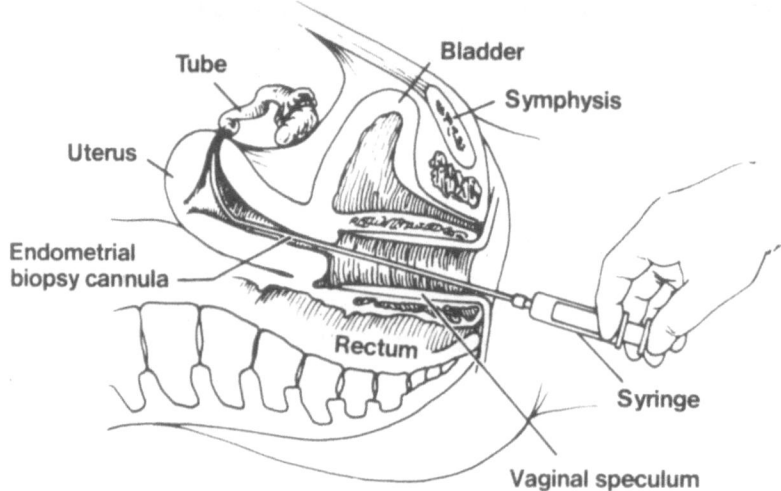

Figure 35   Chemical sterilization. Quinacrine is applied without visual contact, with a catheter or a needle

Methyl-2-cyanoacryl (MCA) is a liquid monomer, which polymerizes after contact with live tissue. MCA and Silastic cause a mechanical occlusion of the fallopian tubes after polymerization. For chemical sterilization by inflammation quinacrine can be used (Figure 35; Guzman-Serani, 1983). Zipper et al. (1975) performed a chemical sterilization with quinacrine in 638 patients and reported a Pearl Index of 4.1.

At the present time investigations are being carried out into covering the fimbria or the ovary with Silastic caps. Trials with Silastic showed a success rate of 86%. Although clinical studies are necessary to prove the applicability of this method in clinical routine, in the near future it may become of importance.

Hysteroscopic sterilization has been described extensively by Rimkus and Semm (1976). Reed and Erb (1982) report experience with 800 patients.

For tubal sterilization an intratubal device with a cylindrical hydrogel body (1.4 × 4 mm) fixed with a nylon thread can be placed by means of hysteroscopy (Brundin, 1983) (Figure 36).

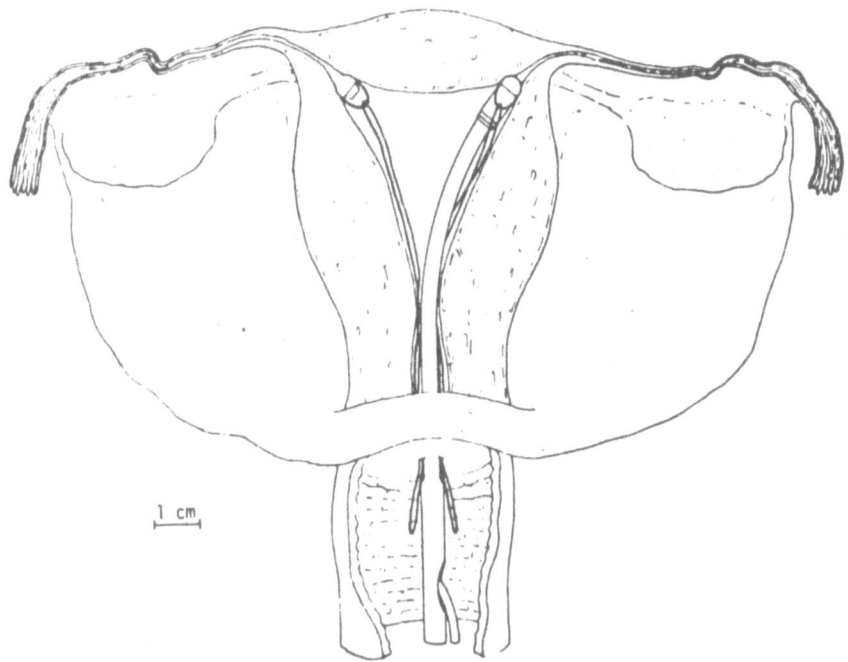

1 cm

Figure 36 Sterilization by hysteroscopic applied tubal blockage

Miscellaneous

DIBROMOCHLORPROPANE (DBCP)

DBCP is an effective nematotoxin suppressing spermatogenesis and causing infertility in man and animals. In a study by Sod-Moriah *et al.* (1983) this compound was given to mature rats. In low doses no effect was observed on ovulation, implantation, duration of pregnancy or number of young. [³H]-DBCP injected at day 14 of gestation was detected in the fetus, which implies that DBCP can pass the placenta barrier. At a dose of 80 mg/kg over a period of 8 days only undersized young had been delivered, which died immediately after birth.

PLANT EXTRACTS

Many plant extracts known in popular medicine decrease fertility in animals and man. Most of them are aqueous preparations (e.g. teas) or methanol or other solvent extracts. The major advantage of plant extracts in fertility control is that potentially new drugs can be extracted and detected for use in man as abortifacients.

Alcoholic extract of *Crotalaria juncea* Linn. showed an 83.3% antifertility effect in albino rats. The animals were treated with 300 mg/kg of the extract from day 1 to day 7 of pregnancy. An anti-implantation effect could only be observed in the early phase of pregnancy (Rao *et al.*, 1979).

One extract of the plant *Annona squamosa* Linn. showed a very good antifertility action of about 50% in a dosage of 200 mg/kg (Rao *et al.*, 1979).

Female rats had been fed from day 1 to day 7 of pregnancy and at day 10 a laparotomy was performed. The absence of an implanted fetus was taken as a parameter for the antifertility effect.

Rao *et al.* (1979) isolated an extract of the plant *Cuscuta reflexa*. In this extraction the total plant was used. At a dosage of 800 mg/kg an antifertility effect in 50% of the female albino rats could be observed.

p-Coumarine-3-(4-hydroxy phenyl)-2-propionic acid (PCA) has been extracted from the root of *Aristolochia indica*. PCA had a good antifertility action both in female and in male mice and rats. The contraceptive effect of PCA depends on the inhibition of prolactin secretion. No effect on oestrogens and progesterone could be achieved. The ovaries of the treated animals showed histologically a regression of the functional corpora lutea (Pakrasi and Pakrasi, 1980). PCA showed no effect when administered preimplantatorily, but only in days 4–8 of pregnancy. The results can be summarized as follows: (a) PCA needs an ovary for its antifertility activity; (b) PCA causes no contraceptive effect by intrinsic antiprogesterone activity; (c) PCA has no embryotoxic action.

Piper longum is widely used as a stimulant and as a menstruation-inducing drug. The dried fruits of *Piper longum* and its various extracts have been tested because of their antifertility effect in female rats. The benzene extract showed a contraceptive action in 57% of the treated rats, whereas the chloroform extract showed a 50% contraceptive action. The petrol ether and methanol extracts as well as the pulverized fruits had only a poor antifertility action. The most potent extracts have been mixed with the methanol extract of *Embelia ribes* berries. This mixture was given to female rats with the result that 80% of the animals did not become pregnant. The fruits, the methanol extract and the petroleum extract of *P. longum* had no effect on the oestrus cycle of female rats. Sixty per cent of the animals showed a prolongation of the oestrus cycle (of 5–10 days) after 2 weeks' treatment. Of the four extracts tested, the benzene extract had its maximal effect in a dose of 50 mg/day. In these studies it could be shown that pulverized *P. longum* and its extract had no potent antifertility action. It seems that this plant has not sufficient contraceptive action. It is possible that *P. longum* increases the contraceptive efficiency of other plant extracts.

Andrographis peniculata Nees. grows in Bangladesh. Studies by Shamsuzzoha and Ahmed (1979) demonstrated that the amount of the drug, the duration of application, the species, the age and the sex of the laboratory animals are important parameters for antifertility studies. Six-week-old male and female mice dieting were treated with 0.75% of pulverized *A. peniculata* Nees. The drug was given over time periods of 1, 2, 3 and 4 weeks. One control group consisted of animals which did not differ in nutrition and the general condition. A significant reduction of fertility could be achieved 4 weeks after nutrition tests, as well as a prolongation of the gestation period (Shamsuzzoha and Ahmed, 1979).

The alcoholic extract of *Butea monosperma* (100 mg/kg) reduced fertility significantly in animal tests (Garg *et al.*, 1978).

Alcoholic and aqueous extracts of the seeds of *Daucus longa* Linn. suppressed pregnancy by 66.6% and 60.0% in a dose of 500 or 100 mg/kg.

The petrol ether extract had only a 30% antifertility activity (Garg *et al.*, 1978).

Extracts of *Curcuma longa* Linn. inhibited the fertility of rats significantly when administered in a dosage of 100–200 mg/kg from day 1 to day 7 of pregnancy. The petrol ether extract and aqueous extracts (200 mg/kg) inhibited implantation in all rats (Garg *et al.*, 1978).

In a study by Garg *et al.* (1978) an alcoholic extract of the root of *Pelagonium hydropiper* Linn. had a 60% antifertility action in animal tests in a dose of 200 mg/kg.

The alcoholic extract of *Sapindus trifoliatus* Linn. prevented pregnancy in all tested animals in a dose of 500 mg/kg. In 80% of the animals a lower dose of 100 mg/kg was sufficient to prevent pregnancy (Garg *et al.*, 1978).
• The Mexican plant zoapatle (*Montañoa tomentosa*) has an antifertility effect in women and is used in popular medicine. It can be used as a tea for different gynaecological problems such as induction of menstruation and termination of early pregnancy. Hahn *et al.* (1981) were able to show that the administration of aqueous extracts similar to tea used in Mexican lay medicine as oral preparations had no antifertility action in the early stage of pregnancy. More concentrated preparations were more effective after oral or intraperitoneal application. The active compounds of this plant acting on uterine physiology have been isolated and identified (Figure 37). The montanol isolated from *M. tomentosa* is in a similar dose biologically less active than the zoapatanol, the activity of which could be demonstrated in almost all cases. Other authors, such as Landgren *et al.* (1979) and Gallegos and Cortes-Gallegos (1977), investigated the mode of action of this plant. Landgren *et al.* found that a freshly prepared concentrated tea of

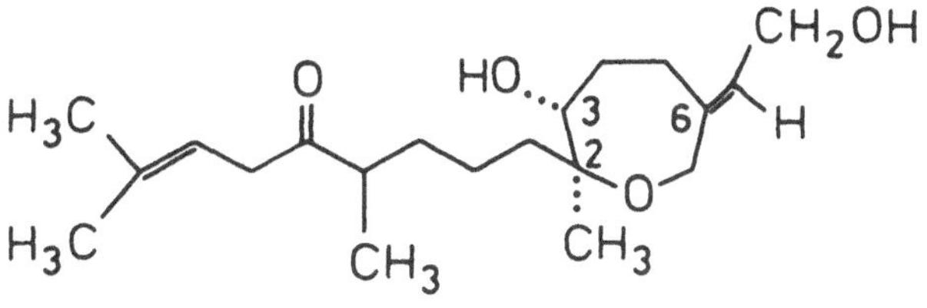

Zoapatanol

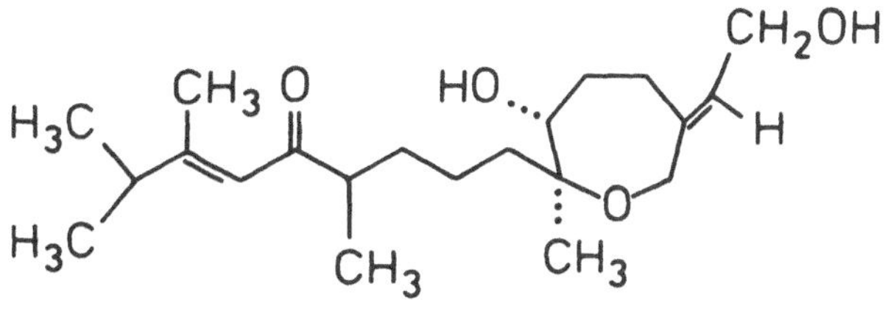

Montanol

Figure 37 Chemical structures of two components of *Montañoa tomentosa*

zoapatle had no luteolytic effect in the early stage of pregnancy in women. Gallegos and Cortes-Gallegos suggested that zoapatle has a luteolytic effect when administered early to women in the luteal phase of the normal menstrual cycle. Landgren *et al.* reported an induction of uterine contraction, cervical dilatation and uterine bleeding by concentrated *M. tomentosa* tea, which is in accordance with results from lay medicine in Mexico (Hahn *et al.*, 1981; Landgren *et al.*, 1979; Gallegos and Cortes-Gallegos, 1977).

The antifertility effect of *Embelia ribes* Burm. (Mysinaceae) in rats as well as in combination with *Piper longum* and borax is known in popular medicine. In a study by Pakrash (1979) 60–70% of the rats exhibited changes in vaginal cytology following the application of a 50% ethanolic extract in doses of 75 and 150 mg/kg over 18 or 12 days; furthermore a prolongation of the oestrus phase could be observed. In another study Pakrash investigated uterus weight under treatment with *E. ribes*. He treated ovariectomized juvenile rats with 50% ethanol and benzene extracts and found that both extracts induced a remarkable increase in uterus weight (Pakrash, 1979). Embelin (2,5-dihydroxy-3-undecyl-1,4-benzoquinone) is a crystalline substance isolated from the seeds of *E. ribes*. An antifertility effect of 83.3% was found in female rats in a dose of 120 mg/kg, when applied post-coitally between days 1 and 5 of pregnancy. Rathinam *et al.* (1976) were able to show that embelin in a dose of 10 mg/kg abolished fertility. Embelin induces a significant reduction of uterus weight and a reduction of glycogen and alanine-aminotransferase, which could be shown by group control studies. No change in total protein, alkaline phosphatase, acid phosphatase and lactic acid could be observed (Rathinam *et al.*, 1976; Seshardil *et al.*, 1978).

The blossoms of *Hibiscus rosa-sinensis* Linn. have a good antifertility effect in female albino rats (Bhatta and Santhakumari, 1979). This has also been proved by investigations of Kholkute and Udupa (1974). The benzene extract causes an interruption of the normal oestrus cycle in rats and a reduction of ovarian, uterine and pituitary weight (Kholkute *et al.*, 1976). Another action of *H. rosa-sinensis* Linn. depends on the increase in the protein concentration of the rat uterus and on the dosage and the duration of the administration. The optimal effect has been achieved by high dose and long-term treatment. The observed changes in the cycle and the uterus are due to the anti-oestrogenic effect of the extracts of *H. rosa-sinensis*.

Plant extracts used in Paraguay In Paraguay there are approximately 50 000 indians, who can be divided into five linguistic families. These indians belong to 17 tribes in two different geographic regions, separated by the Paraguay river (Figure 38). Arenas and Azorero (1977) investigated plants used in Paraguay for contraception, abortion and sterilization. The following data are concerned with information of natives, especially elder males and females possessing specific knowledge about medically potent drugs; in this connection especially shamans and priests were questioned.

The following abbreviations are used: G = inborn group; F = linguistic family; S = self-given name.

G: Angaite; F: Maskoy; S: 'Enslet'
Stylosanthes scabra Vog. (Leguminosae)
This plant can induce sterilization in the female. It has been reported that

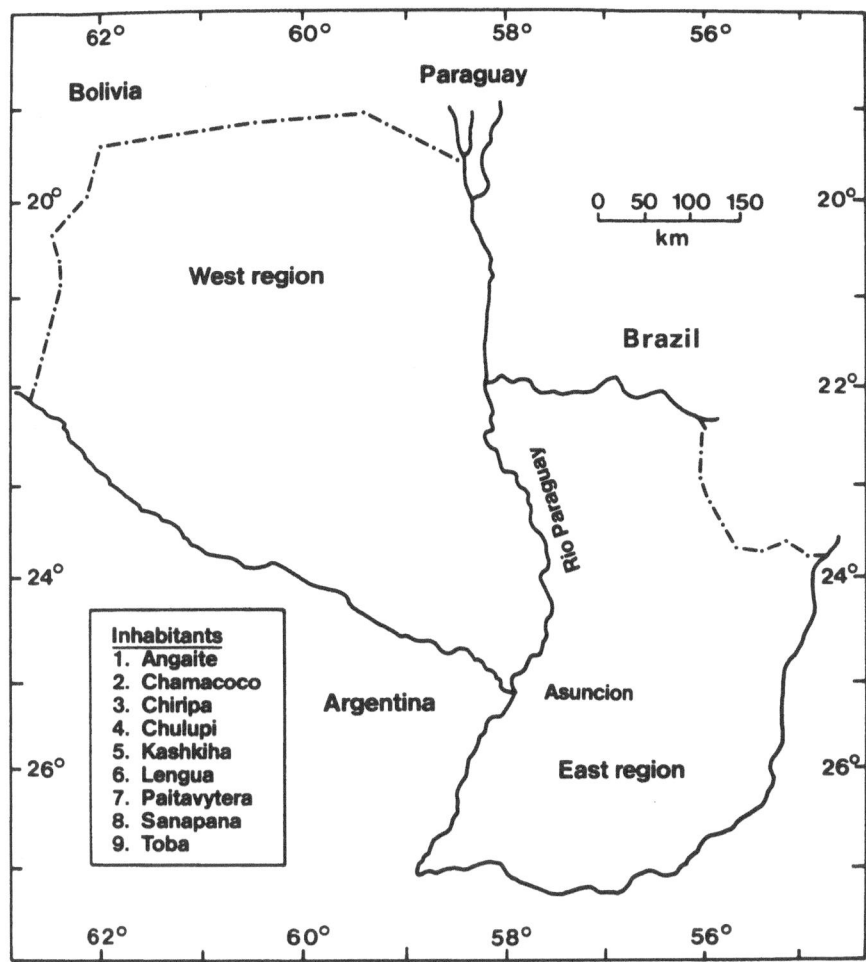

Figure 38 Geographical location of native tribes in Paraguay using plant extracts as abortifacients

after oral application of one preparation of *Stylosanthes scabra* Vog. menstruation did not occur from the time of application. For this purpose, a cold preparation of roots, branches and leaves must be prepared in the afternoon. The kettle is covered and put under the bed of the wife overnight. The next morning the wife must drink from the brew and is not allowed to breathe while drinking. The day after the treatment no further nutrition is allowed.

G: Chamacoco; F: Zamuvo; S: 'Xorshio'
Cienfuegegosia drummondii (A. Gray) Lewton (Malvaceae)
A drink is prepared from the roots of this plant which should be taken every month over some days and acts as a contraceptive.

G: Chirpipa
Maytenus ilicifolia Mart. (Celastraceae)
Maytenus ilicifolia Mart. is used as a long-term contraceptive. The patient drinks a preparation of leaves, branches and roots after the delivery and will not become pregnant again until the child is able to walk.
Xyris savanensis Miq. (Xyridaceae)
The sap of the soaked roots is drunk 2 weeks after the delivery of the child and induces sterilization. The rest of this preparation must be diluted and drunk on the following day.
Xyris jupicai L. C. Rich. (Xyridaceae)
A brew prepared from the whole plant can be used if *Xyris savanensis* is not available. This brew, too, causes sterility. Additionally, a small amount of *Maytenus ilicifolia* can be added.

G: Chulupi; F: Mataco; S: 'Nivaklé'
Camptosema paraguariense var. *parviflorum* Hassl. (Leguminosae)
The brew of the leaves, branches and roots must be drunk as a contraceptive every month. The literature provides no data about the brew's efficiency (Arenas and Azorero, 1977).
Crotalaria incana Linn. (Leguminosae)
The abortive action of this plant occurs after a small amount of the plant and the green fruits has been chewed and swallowed. It is then necessary to press with one's hand on the abdomen. This must be done two or three times a day.

G: Kashikiha; F: Maskoy; S: 'Kashikhá', 'Guaná'
Talinum sp. (Portulacaceae)
For use as a contraceptive, four or five plants are put in $\frac{1}{2}$ l of water. They must be left there until they begin to ferment. It may happen that the heat causes maggots to emerge. Nevertheless, the brew must be drunk before breakfast.

G: Lengua, F: Maskoy; S: 'Enthlet'
Cienfuegosia drummondii (A. Gray) Lewton (Malvaceae)
A brew prepared from the roots is drunk as a contraceptive.
Cyperus redolens Maury (Cyperaceae)
In order to achieve a contraceptive action, the sap of the roots must be drunk over 5 days unknown to others. Otherwise the drink is said to lose its contraceptive effect.
Euphorbia sp. (Euphorbiaceae)
In the evening the woman must drink a brew prepared from the whole plant, which is supposed to act as a contraceptive.
Melochia hermannioides Saint. Hill. (Sterculiaceae)
The sap of the roots must be drunk three times a day for 3 days and will then act as a contraceptive. On the first day of the treatment the woman is not allowed to eat. The contraceptive action lasts about 3 months.

G: Paitavytera; F: Tupl-Guarani; S: 'Pai tavyterá'
Catasetum fimbriatum (Morren) Lindl. (Orchidaceae)
In order to achieve sterilization 250 ml of the brew must be drunk at dawn. The following day the patient is not allowed to eat.

Typha latifolia Linn. (Typhaceae)
A brew made of pieces of the root is mixed with *Catasetum fimbriatum* and must be drunk. In this way sterilization is said to be achieved.

G: Toba; F: Guaicurú; S: 'Ntokowit'
Phaesolus bracteatus Nees. et Mart. (Leguminosae)
Only one dose of a brew made from the roots of the plant is sufficient to achieve sterilization.

Inhibition of implantation

General remarks

The group of implantation inhibitors consists of either intrauterine devices or compounds (steroids, plant extracts) which can be applied post-coitally

Table 13 Inhibitors of implantation: clinical methods and drugs used for inhibition of implantation

Site of action	Mechanism of action	Route	Substance	Assessment
Intrauterine devices	inhibition of implantation by mechanical stimulus or release of antifertility substances	intrauterine devices: 1. mechanical 2. devices releasing antifertility substances	plastics IUD metal salts copper silver alloy progestogens progesterone levonorgestrel antifibrinolytics: chloroquine histamine dimidine derivatives	world-wide use 15 m IUD users clinical use clinical use trial stage clinical use trial stage trial stage trial stage trial stage trial stage
Steroid hormones	effect on implantation by alteration of the endometrium, inhibition of tubal motility and corpus luteum function	oral, vaginal	oestrogens 17-oestradiol mestranol progestogens derivatives of 19- nortestosterone	clinical use clinical trial clinical use
Synthetic compounds	?	oral	chlortrianisene (TRACE)	trial stage
Immunological methods	immunization against placental antigens	parenteral immunization: active	hCG (C-terminal peptide) PL PP5 SP1	trial stage
		passive (monoclonal antibodies)		
Plant extracts	mainly unclear			use only in some developing countries

and which then influence the passage of the blastocysts through the fallopian tubes and the endometrium so that implantation is complicated or becomes impossible. One of the possible alterations of the passage of the blastocysts through the fallopian tubes is immunization of the patient against antigens of the placental tissue or placenta hormones (antibodies against hCG, hPL and SP1). The different possibilities for inhibition of implantation are summarized in Table 13.

Intrauterine devices

Intrauterine devices (IUDs) have been used for many years for contraception. In general, one distinguishes between two types of intrauterine device. The inert plastics devices obtain their contraceptive effect by a mechanical irritation of the endometrium, whereas the medicated IUDs release substances inhibiting fertilization. The major problem with IUDs consists of the side-effects, the disturbances of the menstrual cycle and the high expulsion rate. All attempts to reduce the side-effect rate of IUDs by a change in configuration or the addition of active substances have had only limited success. The expulsion of the IUD occurs during the first month of application after menstruation. If it is not inserted at the right place, cramps and pains can occur and thereby labour may be induced. The perforation of the

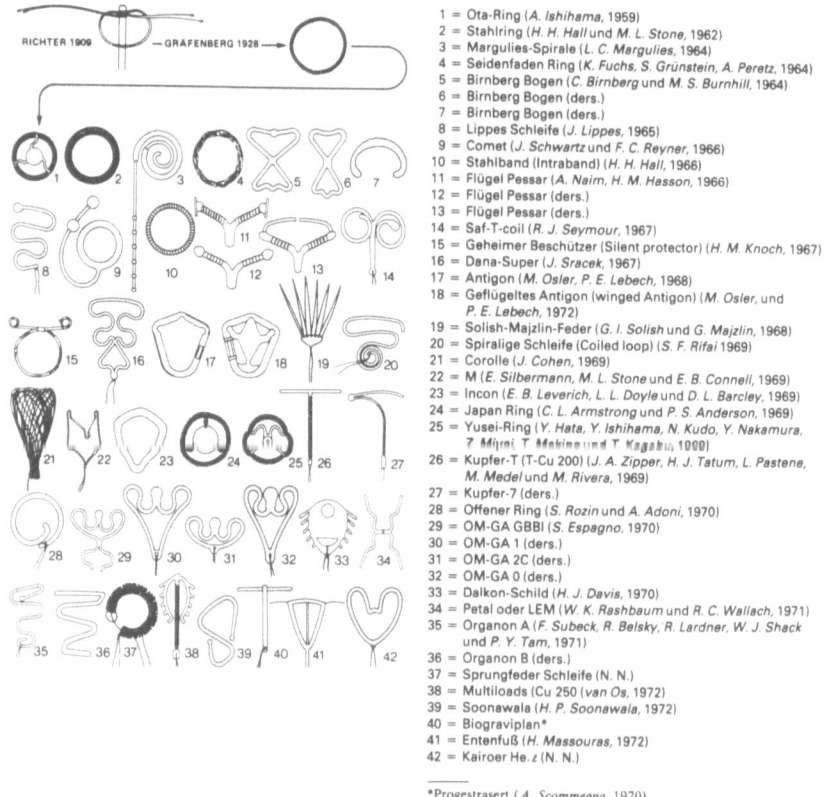

1 = Ota-Ring (*A. Ishihama*, 1959)
2 = Stahlring (*H. H. Hall* und *M. L. Stone*, 1962)
3 = Margulies-Spirale (*L. C. Margulies*, 1964)
4 = Seidenfaden Ring (*K. Fuchs, S. Grünstein, A. Peretz*, 1964)
5 = Birnberg Bogen (*C. Birnberg* und *M. S. Burnhill*, 1964)
6 = Birnberg Bogen (ders.)
7 = Birnberg Bogen (ders.)
8 = Lippes Schleife (*J. Lippes*, 1965)
9 = Comet (*J. Schwartz* und *F. C. Reyner*, 1966)
10 = Stahlband (Intraband) (*H. H. Hall*, 1966)
11 = Flügel Pessar (*A. Naim, H. M. Hasson*, 1966)
12 = Flügel Pessar (ders.)
13 = Flügel Pessar (ders.)
14 = Saf-T-coil (*R. J. Seymour*, 1967)
15 = Geheimer Beschützer (Silent protector) (*H. M. Knoch*, 1967)
16 = Dana-Super (*J. Sracek*, 1967)
17 = Antigon (*M. Osler, P. E. Lebech*, 1968)
18 = Geflügeltes Antigon (winged Antigon) (*M. Osler*, und *P. E. Lebech*, 1972)
19 = Solish-Majzlin-Feder (*G. I. Solish* und *G. Majzlin*, 1968)
20 = Spiralige Schleife (Coiled loop) (*S. F. Rifai* 1969)
21 = Corolle (*J. Cohen*, 1969)
22 = M (*E. Silbermann, M. L. Stone* und *E. B. Connell*, 1969)
23 = Incon (*E. B. Leverich, L. L. Doyle* und *D. L. Barclay*, 1969)
24 = Japan Ring (*C. L. Armstrong* und *P. S. Anderson*, 1969)
25 = Yusei-Ring (*Y. Hata, Y. Ishihama, N. Kudo, Y. Nakamura, T. Mijrei, T. Makina* und *T. Kagabu*, 1969)
26 = Kupfer-T (T-Cu 200) (*J. A. Zipper, H. J. Tatum, L. Pastene, M. Medel* und *M. Rivera*, 1969)
27 = Kupfer-7 (ders.)
28 = Offener Ring (*S. Rozin* und *A. Adoni*, 1970)
29 = OM-GA GBBI (*S. Espagno*, 1970)
30 = OM-GA 1 (ders.)
31 = OM-GA 2C (ders.)
32 = OM-GA 0 (ders.)
33 = Dalkon-Schild (*H. J. Davis*, 1970)
34 = Petal oder LEM (*W. K. Rashbaum* und *R. C. Wallach*, 1971)
35 = Organon A (*F. Subeck, R. Belsky, R. Lardner, W. J. Shack* und *P. Y. Tam*, 1971)
36 = Organon B (ders.)
37 = Sprungfeder Schleife (*N. N.*)
38 = Multiloads (Cu 250 (*van Os*, 1972)
39 = Soonawala (*H. P. Soonawala*, 1972)
40 = Biograviplan*
41 = Entenfuß (*H. Massouras*, 1972)
42 = Kairoer He.z (*N. N.*)

*Progestrasert (*A. Scommegna*, 1970)

Figure 39   Intrauterine devices (Semm and Giese, 1981)

device through the uterus is rare. The mode of action of the IUD depends on the local irritation of the endometrium, which causes changes of the mucosa and prevents the implantation of the fertilized oocyte.

In IUD-bearing females inflammations of the uterus, the fallopian tubes and the ovaries are 3.5-fold more frequent. Other side-effects are dysfunctional bleedings and a higher risk of ectopic pregnancies. The contraceptive safety of IUDs is about 1–3.6 pregnancies per 100 women per year.

CURRENTLY AVAILABLE IUDS

During the last 50 years numerous intrauterine devices have been developed and clinically tested. They can be divided into non-medicated and medicated IUDs (Table 14).

Table 14 Classification of IUDs (Mishell, 1982)

(1) Non-medicated IUDs
(a) Lippes Loop
(b) Saf-T-Coil
(c) Ota-Ring
(2) Medicated IUDs
(a) Copper IUDs
Tatum–Zipper Kupfer T
Copper 7
Multiload
Steryls
Nova
Latex leaf (copper or zinc)
Others
(b) Progestogen-loaded IUDs
Progestasert (progesterone)
Norgestrel T (levonorgestrel)

FUTURE DEVELOPMENTS

In new developments of intrauterine devices both the shape of the IUD as well as the material must be considered. The IUD consists of inert plastics holders, a wrapping in by copper wires or release of pharmacological compounds. Furthermore it must be considered whether the IUD possesses additional threads (e.g. chromic catgut threads) to prevent an expulsion. The advantages of the development of IUDs without threads must be investigated. The following aspects must be considered in the design of new IUDs.

The optimal length of the IUD is 1.2–1.5 cm shorter than the inner length of the uterine cavity, as the IUD is only inconvenient if it is situated in the upper part of the uterine cavity. IUDs that are too long lie in the uterine part of the isthmus, causing irritations and pains. The result would be uterine contractions, which are painful and also cause expulsion of the IUD. If the IUD is located in the cervical canal, no contraceptive safety is provided and the risk of pelvic inflammatory diseases increases. If the IUD is much shorter than the uterus, it slides down into the uterine cavity and under certain circumstances it may reach the isthmus. In all cases the IUD induces great pain similar to labour and can be expelled.

The width of the IUD is optimal if its maximal diameter is as large as the width of the uterine cavity just above the isthmus. It seems to be important that the IUD does not cause punctate trauma in the endometrium, which could lead to severe bleeding and also could serve as an ideal breeding place for anaerobes. IUDs with horizontal arms that are too wide can perforate the uterus wall.

Little information is available about the anteroposterior diameter. If the uterine cavity is overextended, the uterus will lose contractility; if the IUD is too flat, the pregnancy rate increases. The optimal ratio remains unknown.

The material of the IUD must be flexible and solid, to resist dynamic changes of the uterus.

Another important factor for the compatibility of an IUD is its shape. IUDs with thin low ends tend to slide into the cervix during menstruation, especially when they are not cranially fixed. With copper IUDs the diameter of the wire is also important. It was found that an enlargement of the diameter of the copper wire from 0.2 to 0.25 mm reduced the number of fractures. The corresponding copper fragments will be expelled out of the uterus shortly after fracture, as was shown in monkey studies. Fracture of the copper wire causes a decrease in contraceptive safety.

Furthermore, surface encrustation (calcium carbonate formation) plays an important role in contraceptive safety. Whether the diffusion of copper ions is influenced cannot yet be evaluated. Perhaps surface encrustation by calcium is related to the side-effects such as bleedings and pains, which can be mitigated by intrauterine contraception with copper medicated IUDs.

In the development of IUDs threads have been fixed at the arms of the pessary to avoid an expulsion—for instance, after insertion post partum (Figure 40). Thiery *et al.* (1983) investigated Laufe's hypothesis that the fixing of small catgut tapes at the upper side-arms of the Lippes IUD or at

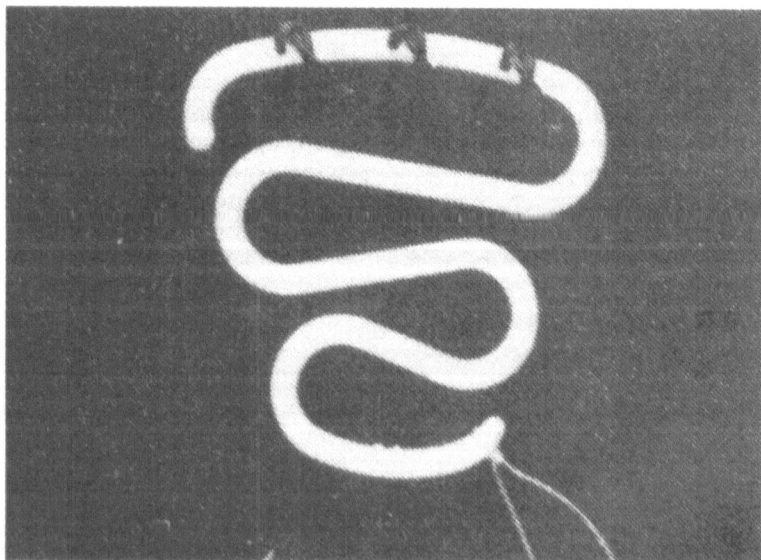

Figure 40   Intrauterine device with catgut threads

the horizontal arm of the T IUD would reduce the expulsion rate of post-placental insertion. This comparison study could show that the expulsion rates of Copper T IUDs with and without catgut threads were equal, a fact which is in opposition to the thesis. The marking threads of IUDs might be responsible for the increasing infection of the uterus. Whether threadless IUDs, the regular position of which is difficult to control during follow-up investigations, will achieve clinical importance cannot be evaluated. In opposition to the infection theory, it has been observed in electron microscopic surveys that the sperms are carrying bacteria in 'piggy-back' fashion into the uterus. With currently available IUDs the expulsion rate of the pessaries amounts to about 30% within the first months.

According to *Population Reports* (1979), research in the field of intrauterine contraception is mainly concentrated on four different aspects:

(1) Long-term investigation of side-effects of currently available IUDs, with specific evaluation of infrequent complications such as ectopic pregnancies and severe infections.
(2) Other clinical investigations with IUDs containing metal salts, steroid hormones and antifibrinolytic substances, with specific evaluation of the optimal amount of the active agent as well as of the action of the IUD.
(3) Improvement of the insertion technique, and development of sensors for the exact measurement of the uterine cavity and of insertion apparatus which allow of a precise localization of the IUD in the uterus with a minimal risk of perforation.
(4) Development of IUDs with biological degradable components preventing expulsion post partum and post abortum.

The development of new intrauterine devices is summarized in Table 15.

Copper IUDs Research in the field of copper IUDs is aimed at the development of a lower IUD-specific side-effect rate (e.g. inflammation, menstrual disturbances). The contraceptive efficiency of copper IUDs depends on the total surface of copper and the shape of the IUD. Enlarging of the copper surface in copper 380 A and T 220 increased the contraceptive efficiency (Sivin and Stern, 1978). Increasing the copper content prolongs the lifetime of the IUDs. In addition to the copper wire, a silver core has been applied. The copper T 220 model has a lifetime of approximately 5–10 years. The copper T 380 A model has a lifetime of approximately 6 years and the copper T 380 Ag model, with a silver core, has a predicted lifetime of approximately 6 years. Other investigations are concerned with the influence of the corrosion of the copper wire. Koch (1983) examined the loss of copper of an ML 250 (length of the copper wire 27 cm, diameter 300 μm, weight 172–180 mg, total surface 215 mm^2). The copper loss was 9.6 mg after the first year, 24.2 mg after 2 years, 29.7 mg after 3 years, 32.6 mg after 4 years and 34.6 mg after 5 years. The daily copper loss by corrosion reached a maximum of approximately 40 μg per day in the second year and decreased to 15 μg per day in the third year and to 5.4 μg per day in the fifth year (Koch, 1983). Compatible hydrogel-coated IUDs have been used to decrease the bleeding rate of the Spring coil IUD (Randic and Balogh, 1982).

Table 15   Strategies for the development of novel intrauterine devices

Aim	Site of action	Comments
No bleeding disorder	surface cover formal material changes: no traumatic end of branches	
No expulsion (including post partum or post abortum)	fixation of biologically digestible holding chests (anchor principle) on IUD to prevent expulsion fixation on uterine wall with spiral electrode	catgut threads ineffective up to now
No infections	threadless IUDs	infection develops by, e.g., sperms (bacterial transport) use of threadless IUDs requires ultrasound controls
Long period inside tube	prevention of surface corrosion by suitable metal alloy	
No dysmenorrhoea	changes in formal material drug-containing IUDs	
Inhibition of perforation	new methods for introduction with retreat— instead of release technique mechanical fixation of a suitable mobile IUD in the uterus	
No extrauterine pregnancies	IUD should not influence tubal passage	IUD effect should be limited to the uterus

Timonen *et al.* (1983) compared the Multiload-Cu 375, Fincoid and Nova-T models in a multicentre study. The pregnancy rate of patients with the Fincoid and the Nova-T was 1.1 and 2.0, respectively, and was higher than the rate of those with the Multiload-Cu 375 (0.4). Furthermore, the expulsion rates of both Copper Ts Fincoid and Nova-T were 1.1 and 1.7, respectively, higher than those of the Multiload, at 0.7 (complete expulsion rate).

Audebert (1983) performed a modification of both the shape and the consistency of the plastics frame to avoid specific side-effects and to lower the expulsion rate. The new copper IUD ('Ombrelle 250') has been clinically tested in 400 patients and showed a sufficient contraceptive safety.

Progesterone-loaded IUDs   Since 1973 intrauterine devices loaded with levonorgestrel have been investigated on the assumption that severe bleeding problems in IUD appliers could be solved. By use of these IUDs the blood loss could be reduced, but breakthrough bleedings could not be diminished.

At this time levonorgestrel-containing IUDs are still at a clinical trial stage. El Maghoub (1983) suggested the optimal release rate of 10 μg daily. In different studies the action of levonorgestrel on the bleeding pattern, the plasma concentration, the blood vessels and the side-effects after removal of the IUD have been analysed. The following paragraphs review the various investigations.

Nilsson *et al.* (1981) compared a levonorgestrel-loaded IUD with a copper Nova-T IUD. The clinical acceptability of the levonorgestrel IUD was similar to that of the copper T. A significantly lower menstrual blood loss was observed. The duration of menstruation was shortened and women suffering from dysmenorrhoea had a normal menstruation when bearing levonorgestrel IUDs. Only a slight fall in systolic and diastolic blood pressures occurred. No infections could be observed.

In a study by Heikkilä (1982), in which levonorgestrel IUDs with a levonorgestrel release rate of 30 μg and 10 μg per day were analysed, it could also be shown that the menstrual blood loss was diminished. The author observed no pregnancies during the application.

Kurunmäki et al. (1981) were able to show that 30 min after insertion of a levonorgestrel IUD with a release rate of 20 μg/day levonorgestrel could be detected in the peripheral plasma. The plasma level remained constant after an initial phase. Of 24 observed cycles, 19 were ovulatory. Only one patient had no ovulation. During the first 30 day period breakthrough bleedings occurred. The side-effects were low, and no patient became pregnant.

In another study by Shaw et al. (1981) the effect of progesterone-releasing IUDs on blood vessels was analysed. The microscopically detectable number of blood vessels in the endometrium was significantly lower in the progesterone-releasing IUDs than in the normal control group. This may explain the fact that patients with progesterone IUDs have a diminished menstrual blood loss. However, progesterone IUDs had in 35% of patients a higher rate of blood vessel defects.

The conception rate after removal of the levonorgestrel-releasing IUDs has been investigated by Nilsson et al. (1981). Eighteen patients (85.7%), of a group of 21 who had a levonorgestrel-releasing IUD removed in the hope of having a baby, became pregnant shortly after the removal. Apart from one pregnancy, all patients had a normal delivery at term.

In a study by El Maghoub (1983) the release rates of levonorgestrel-medicated IUDs were found to be 10–20 μg/day. The clinical efficiencies of the Cu T 200, Cu T 220 and Cu T 380 Ag models have been compared. The high efficiency of the levonorgestrel IUDs depends on the local effect on the endometrium and the cervical mucus combined with a reduction of the menstrual blood loss and the duration of menstruation. After a 3-year period of application no endometrial malignancy could be detected.

In the same year Nilsson et al. reported a study of two levonorgestrel IUDs compared with a copper IUD (Nova-T), with an observation period of 2 years. Clinical trials have been performed in Brasilia and in two Finnish clinics. Altogether, 100 patients were admitted to the trial and at its end 6000 cycles were observed with the levonorgestrel IUDs and 3000 cycles with the Nova-T IUD. The pregnancy rate in the group with the levonorgestrel IUDs was found to be 0.6 and was 3.2 for the Nova-T IUD. Removals of the pessary due to bleedings or pains occurred rarely and were found in 7.5%, 7.6% and 7.1%, respectively, during the first 24 months.

After 2 months' IUD application the length of menstrual bleedings in the levonorgestrel IUD group has been significantly shorter than in the patients with the Nova IUDs until the second year of application. No infections have been observed.

Immunization against placental antigens

GENERAL REMARKS

No acceptable post-coital drug for contraception is at present available. Substances preventing the normal implantation of the blastocysts in the uterine cavity or inducing a resorption of the embryo during the first days of pregnancy, and lacking any side-effects, would be ideal post-coital contraceptives.

ANTIBODIES AGAINST PLACENTAL ANTIGENS

Animal studies have shown that antibodies against placental proteins can be used for contraception. These antibodies induce an interruption of pregnancy without any cross-reactions. When animals are immunized with homogenates or crude extracts of placenta, fertility significantly decreases, but it could not be demonstrated whether reduced fertility is caused by antibodies against placental proteins or whether it occurs unspecifically. Fertility control in men by immunization with placental proteins is a possibility.

hCG ANTIBODIES

Immunization against hCG seems to be a hopeful approach for development of an antipregnancy vaccine. The pregnancy hormone, hCG, is an early product of the trophoblast. It is important for the support of steroidogenesis, without which pregnancy could not be maintained during the first trimester (until the 8th week of gestation). The hormone synthesized from the blastocysts is transported to the ovaries via the peripheral blood and stimulates the corpus luteum to maintain progesterone production. Implantation can be disturbed if antibodies against the trophoblast are applied actively or passively, causing damage of the trophoblast and inducing abortion.

In this regard attempts have been made to develop antibodies against the β-subunit of hCG and against specific placental proteins or sperm antigens. In general, each substance can be used as an antigen which is produced by the blastocyst and plays an important role in implantation and corpus luteum function. If the action of such substances is blocked, pregnancy can be interrupted at the time of implantation without disturbance of the menstrual cycle.

Among the hormonal trophoblast antigens, immunization against the β-hCG subunit has been studied. The hCG molecule consists, as do LH, FSH and TSH, of two subunits, of which the α-subunit is almost identical with those of LH, FSH and TSH. The smaller hormone-specific β-subunit of hCG possesses 30 amino acids which do not occur in the β-subunit of LH. After immunization against these 30 amino acids of the β-hCG subunit, one obtains antibodies which show no cross-reaction with LH.

The fertility-reducing action of hCG antibodies has already been described by Stevens (1975). In order to enlarge the molecular surface of the substance against which antibodies had been raised, the antibody has been linked to carriers to increase its antigenicity. To avoid expensive toxicological investigations, Talwar and Sharma (1976) have linked the β-subunit of hCG to the tetanus toxin.

The possibility cannot be excluded that such a vaccine causes unspecific side-effects which may be followed by long-acting disturbances and possible autoimmune reactions and eventually be carcinogenic.

SP1

One of the well-known placenta-specific proteins is SP1, which occurs during pregnancy in large amounts and can be isolated from the trophoblast membrane. In animal tests immunization against this substance showed an abortifacient action and also inhibition of fertility. Tests in female monkeys with pure and chemically modified SP1 either induced sterility or induced abortion in early pregnancy.

hPL

hPL (human placental lactogen), like hCG, is synthesized by the syncytio-trophoblast of the placenta. The antifertility action of hPL antisera has been investigated with the support of WHO. Gudson (1974) was able to show that after treatment of pregnant rats with an anti-hPL serum of rabbits an intrauterine expulsion reaction with intrauterine death of the fetus occurred.

Post-coital contraception

GENERAL REMARKS

Post-coital contraception would be ideal if it could be applied only once after intercourse and the patients did not need to take hormones continuously. If this method could be combined with a means of determining the ovulation data, this substance would only have to be taken once after intercourse in the preovulatory phase.

LUTEOLYTIC AGENTS

See under 'Abortifacients'.

STEROIDAL POST-COITAL CONTRACEPTION

A review of the different steroids used for post-coital contraception was given by Diczfalusy (1981) on the basis of studies in China (Table 16). This form of contraception can be used for population groups in which couples live together only for a limited time in a year, such as during the 2 weeks of vacation in China. In Germany as well as in the most industrialized nations post-coital contraception is only used in cases of emergency (e.g. unprotected intercourse, rapes or contraceptive failures).

Table 16 Clinical studies of the efficiency of post-coital contraception in China (Diczfalusy, 1981)

Steroid	Dose (mg)	Contraceptive safety (%)
Norethisterone	5.0	99.5
Megestrol acetate	2.0	99.6
D-Norgestrel	3.0	99.9
Norgestrienone (R 2323)	2.5	99.5
Norethisterone acetate-3-oxim	1.0	99.3
Anordrin	7.5	99.5
Quingestanol	80	99.8
Megestrol acetate + quingestanol	0.55 0.88	98.2
Chlormadinone acetate + quingestanol	0.25 0.85	98.2

STS-456 The steroid STS-456 (17β-($N'N'$-dimethyl-hydrazino-carbionxyl-oestra-1,3,5(10)-trien-3-ol) has been analysed by the Central Institute for Microbiology and Experimental Therapy in Jena (Goncharov *et al.*, 1978). Applied post-coitally, the compound inhibited fertility, which has been observed in female baboons after a 5-day post-coital application per os. A linear correlation between the efficiency of the substance and the side-effect and the applied dose could be observed. The hormone analytic investigations showed a luteolytic effect of the substance whereby ovarian steroidogenesis (not only of progesterone, but also of oestrogens) was inhibited.

STS-557 STS-557 (17α-cyanomethyl-17α-hydroxyoestra-4-9-(10)-dien-3-one) is a progestin-inhibiting implantation. The results of these investigations with STS-557 have been published by WHO (Ratnam and Prasad, 1983).

Anordrin Anordrin (Figure 41) has been studied intensively in China. It acts either by its anti-oestrogenic properties or by its effect on the motility of the fallopian tubes. A possible application of the substance for fertility control seems to be promising (Ratnam and Prasad, 1983).

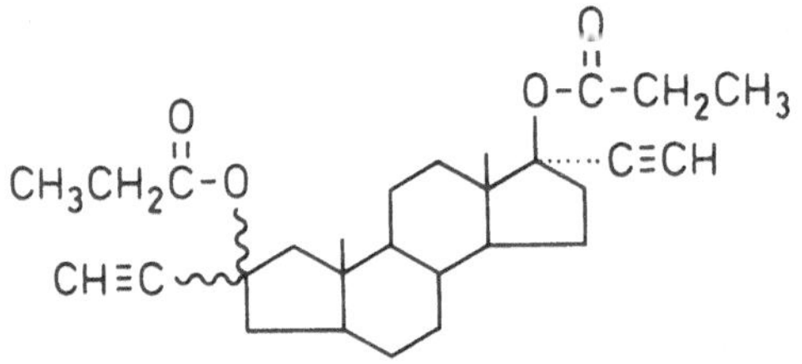

Figure 41 Anordrin

PROSTAGLANDINS

Little is known about post-coital application of prostaglandins in the female. Prostaglandins PGE_2 and $PGF_{2\alpha}$ can be absorbed in the vagina and induce menstruation in a short period of time. The plasma concentration of the prostaglandins 2–3 h after application reaches maximal values. The prostaglandins could be applied vaginally once a month at the time of expected menstruation. In patients with belated menstruation pregnancy could be terminated after instillation of 5 mg $PGF_{2\alpha}$ (Csapo, 1974). The mechanism of prostaglandins inducing menstruation has not yet been elucidated. It can be assumed that strong uterine contractions will be induced by prostaglandins, which may influence the endocrine function of the fetus and interrupt the corpus luteum.

MISCELLANEOUS

α-Difluoromethylornithine Ornithine decarboxylase (ODC, E.C.4.1.1.17) is an enzyme which regulates the biosynthesis of putrescine and polyamines. High ODC levels have been observed during the early pregnancy of rats. DL-α-difluoromethylornithine (RMI 71782) is an active inhibitor of ODC. In rats DFMO inhibits the ODC activity according to the dose given. DFMO suppresses embryogenesis in rats after intraperitoneal application in a dose of 200 mg/kg twice daily between day 4 and day 7 of gestation. DFMO has no effect on early pregnancy (days 1 to 3 of gestation). DFMO completely suppresses ornithine decarboxylase activity in the pregnant rat uterus. The action of DFMO seems to depend on a decrease in putrescine and polyamine levels during the critical phase of early embryonic development. Reddy and Rukmini (1981) believe that DFMO can be used effectively as a post-coital drug.

Plant extracts A special mixture (Ayush-47) consists of the plants *Sacara indica*, *Areca catechu*, *Cocculus lacca*, gold and sugar. In albino rats after oral application of 1.25–50 mg/kg an anti-implantation effect of 33.3–85.7% could be achieved. This compound does not change the oestrus cycle and has no significant oestrogenic, anti-oestrogenic, anti-ovulatory, gestogenic and androgenic or antigonadotrophic effect on the animals. An antiprogesterone effect could be demonstrated in rabbits. Furthermore, in rats no toxic action could be found after application of up to 800 mg per kg body weight. Also, in oral doses up to 10 mg/kg over a period of 6 months no significant changes in blood, liver and kidneys could be observed (Suganthan and Santhakumari, 1979).

Different tribes of the Madhya Pradesh use *Hyptis suaveolens* Poir. for family planning. It is also used against parasites and in the treatment of various dermatological conditions and respiratory infections. Saluja and Santani (1981) found that this plant reduced implantation in 20% and 40%, respectively, of the treated rats. The animals had been treated with 125 or 250 mg/kg over a time period of 1–7 days of pregnancy. This study also showed that this drug has no abortive action. The antifertility effect of the substance, especially the inhibition of implantation, may depend on its oestrogenic activity, because oestrogens can suppress pregnancy in rats by influencing the transport of the oocyte and the maturation of the endometrium. Furthermore, oestrogens can inhibit the luteal function (Saluja and Santani, 1981).

For a note on the use of *Curcuma longa* Linn. for contraception see p. 49.

Lygodium flexosum has frequently been used for contraception by the people of Adivase, in the north-west of the Indian state of Maharashtra. Plant extracts have been tested in three different animal species. The plant has been found to be post-coitally active. The alcoholic extract contained the pharmacologically active substance, whereas the petroleum ether extract was inactive. The aqueous extract had only low biological activity. It could be shown that in animals treated with the alcoholic extract in a dose of 500 mg/kg even at day 11 of pregnancy no implantation occurred. After withdrawal of the drug the animal showed a normal reproductive behaviour. The pregnancies which occurred afterwards showed that the action of this drug is reversible. The fetus did not show any malformations. Further studies are planned with the aim of analysing the active principle of *Lygodium flexosum* in detail (Gaitonde and Mahajan, 1980).

The alcoholic extract of the leaves of *Mentha arvensis* inhibits implantation in 80% of cases when given in 100 mg/kg dose. At a higher dose of 500 mg/kg no pregnancy occurred in the tested animals (Garg *et al.*, 1978). The antifertility action of the uterotonic fraction of *Mentha arvensis* has been tested in rats. After subcutaneous injections of the alcoholic extract in pregnant rats from day 1 to day 10 of pregnancy, pregnancies were terminated at a significant rate. The effective dose of the alcoholic extract showed no oestrogenic and antigonadotrophic activity. Female albino rats (150–200 g) with a normal menstrual cycle and male rats with proved fertility have been tested by Garg *et al.* (1978). The female rats have been treated from day 1 to day 10 of pregnancy with 5 and 10 mg/kg of the alcoholic extract or saline solutions. At day 10 laparotomy was performed; the uterus had been checked for implants, resorption of pregnancy, dead implants and the size and malformations of the fetus. At a dose of 10 mg/kg a good response was observed in the postimplantatory phase and to a lower degree during the phase of tubal transport and the implantation period.

In the Indian literature the oil of juniper fruits is said to possess a menstruation-regulating and abortifacient action. Agrawal *et al.* (1980) were able to show that the fruits induce fertility significantly. This plant inhibits implantation. The abortifacient action of *Juniperus communis* has been tested as an ethanol extract (50%) in albino rats. These animals were treated with 300 mg and 500 mg/kg from day 1 to day 7 of pregnancy. At day 10 laparatomy was performed and the anti-implantation action of the drug was analysed. Furthermore, the abortive action of the drug could be proved when the drug was given on days 14, 15 and 16 of the pregnancy. No teratogenic action or weight loss and other side-effects could be observed (Agrawal *et al.*, 1980).

Strumpfia maritima Jacq. is a low bush occurring in Southern Florida, in the Bahamas, in Venezuela and in Curacao. It has long been used as an antimosquito drug and as a contraceptive. The aqueous extract of the plant has been given to rats in a daily dose of 100 mg/kg. The number of implants and the corpora lutea decreased significantly. In a control group treated with the transport vehicle, 10% polysorbate 20, such a decrease in implants or corpora lutea did not occur (Hsu *et al.*, 1981).

The antifertility action of *Artabotrys odoratissimus* R. Br. (Anonaceae) was tested in rats. Pakrash *et al.* (1978) demonstrated that a 50% ethanol and benzene extraction of fresh, green leaves of the plant interrupts the normal oestrus cycle of adult albino rats and induces irregular cycles. Ethanol and benzene extracts (50%) possess an anti-oestrogenic activity in all doses tested. In tests with 75 and 150 mg/kg doses of the 50% ethanol extract and 300 mg/kg of the benzene extract, the weight of the uterus which is under oestrogen control of bilaterally ovariectomized, immature rats could be reduced. The activity depended on the doses. Pakrash (1979) believes that the anti-implantation effect of *A. odoratissimus* extracts depends on its anti-oestrogenic activity. Three mechanisms have been suggested: (1) the uterus reaches a stage in which implantation is not possible; (2) prolongation of the implantation of the ovum may occur; (3) a direct blastotoxic activity can exist.

The seeds of carrots have long been used in India to prevent undesired pregnancy. It is known that both oestrogens and progesterones are necessary for implantation. The application of antigonadotrophins, anti-oestrogens and high-dose oestrogens prevents implantation and induces the delay of implantation in rats (Prasad *et al.*, 1965). Alcoholic extracts of the carrot seeds prevent implantation in mice and rats (Sharma *et al.*, 1976; Garg and Garg, 1971). The alcoholic and the aqueous extracts can prevent implantation in both species (Garg and Garg, 1971). In a study by Kaliwal and Rao (1977) the petrol ether extract prevented implantation in rats also. This effect may depend on the disproportion between oestrogens and progesterones. This hypothesis could be proved by adding post-coitally 8 mg progesterone to extracts of carrot seeds. All animals treated in this manner showed normal implantation. No expulsion and no toxic reaction on the blastocyst could be shown. Seifert *et al.* (1968) have demonstrated that the oil of carrot seeds contains cumarin, which shows an oestrogenic effect.

The petrol ether extract as well as the alcoholic and the aqueous extracts of the nuts of *Areca catechu* Linn. prevent implantation in 60% of treated albino rats when given in a dose of 500 mg/kg. In the lower dose of 100 mg/kg implantation inhibition could be observed in 20% of the test animals. In a dose of 500 mg/kg the petrol ether extract induced abortion in two of the animals. The alcoholic and the aqueous extracts had no abortifacient activity (Garg and Garg, 1970).

A petrol ether extract prepared from a paste of the unripe fruits of *Carica carota* Linn. inhibited implantation in 60% of the treated rats when given in a dose of 500 mg/kg. In this dose a slight abortifacient activity could be shown (Garg and Garg, 1970).

Abortifacients

General remarks

The number of legal interruptions of pregnancies fell slightly between 1970 (40 million per year) and 1980 (30–40 million per year). One reason may be the more liberal use of oral contraceptives as well as their world-wide distribution. The frequency of legal and illegal abortions in different regions of the world is summarized in Figure 42.

The most efficient methods of contraception in the female inhibit ovula-

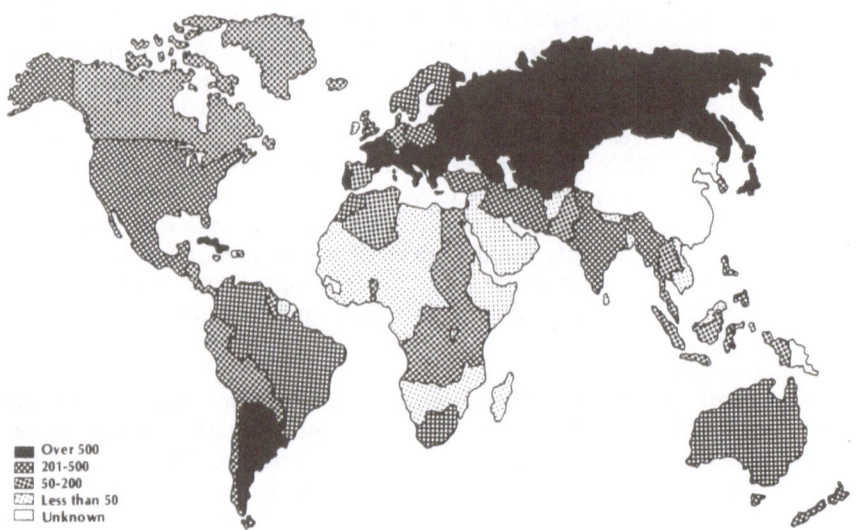

Over 500
201-500
50-200
Less than 50
Unknown

Figure 42 World-wide abortion rates (legal and illegal) per 1000 live births

tion by disturbing the endogenous endocrine regulation. All methods which do not suppress ovulation have a higher failure rate. In recent years the use of mechanical and chemical barrier methods has significantly increased. Therefore, the increased failure rate associated with use of this method has caused a higher number of unwanted pregnancies. As well as the

Table 17 Assessment of clinical methods and new approaches for termination of pregnancy

Site of action	Mechanism of action	Route	Substance	Assessment
Surgical techniques	mechanical removal of pregnancy product	surgical: suction menstrual regulation dilatation and curettage		world-wide use
Hormonal methods	inhibition of progesterone synthesis	oral	steroidogenic inhibitors: ergokornin cyclohexyliden mono-oxidase inhibitors	trial stage
	induction of labour	oral parenteral vaginal—intra-amnial vaginal—extra-amnial	prostaglandins prostaglandins prostaglandins	clinical use clinical use clinical use
	prevention of progesterone effect	oral	antiprogestins (R 2323)	trial stage
Plant extract	mainly unclear	oral	e.g. lithosperm acid, *m*-xylohydroqinone, rotterin	used world wide by aborigines

development of new contraceptive measures, there is also an urgent need for methods which inhibit or terminate early pregnancy. Investigation of these novel methods of fertility control has been partially supported by WHO. One research object is the specific interruption or inhibition of blastocyst nidation, which is dependent on the synchronized function of the endometrium, the ovaries and the embryo. The disturbance of this functional unit can inhibit nidation.

The contraceptive methods used at present rely on a constant level of active synthetic hormonal steroids in the human body during the entire menstrual cycle. This constant level can be achieved by daily intake or the use of long-acting depot injections. These methods combine a high efficacy with a relatively low rate of side-effects, but almost always cause an interruption of the normal cycle and therefore often give rise to fears as to what long-term side-effects these drugs may have. It seems likely that the use of new steroids may only slightly improve the safety of these drugs. However, it seems unrealistic to expect that new treatments which rely on the same principle should give dramatically improved results compared with those used at present. Safety would improve, however, if pharmacological interruption of the menstrual cycle could be reduced to one or two days of the cycle. Since the physiology of early pregnancy is dependent on progesterone in almost all mammal species (Csapo *et al.*, 1973a, b; 1974), specific antiprogestins control human fertility if these are applied at monthly intervals. Ideally antiprogestins given shortly prior to menstruation will induce menstruation by a short-term antagonism of progesterone. This event will occur with or without a fertilized ovum. Such an ideal compound would be rapidly excreted and the rest of the cycle would hardly be disturbed.

The interruption of early pregnancy should happen in the moment when the expected menstrual bleeding fails to occur. Two arguments are based on this. First, the woman will see a missed menstrual bleeding as a possible pregnancy. This signal will stimulate her wish to interrupt the suspected pregnancy. Second, coitus without contraception at mid-cycle will be followed by pregnancy only in 30 out of 100 women (Short, 1976). This means that interference with menstrual regulation at the time of the expected menstruation would help to avoid unnecessary long-term treatment in women.

Drugs which would cause an interruption of early human pregnancy may either cause a higher uterine motility (e.g. prostaglandins) or cause endogenous relaxation of the uterus. Since progesterone is required for inhibition of uterine motility, a block of progesterone synthesis in the corpus luteum or, later, in the human placenta could be achieved by steroidogenic blockers. Furthermore, the inhibition of the biological activity of progesterone may be also possible at the receptor site (e.g. by antiprogestins). A systematic summary of the various sites of action for the inhibition of early human pregnancy is shown in Table 18.

The mechanism of action of those substances used as abortifacients is still unknown (e.g. 5α-stigmastane-3β,5,6β-triol-3-monobenzoate). They can be classified either according to their site of action or according to the time of pregnancy at which they can be applied (either 7th/8th week or after 9th week of gestation). In the following paragraphs the abortifacients will be discussed according to gestational age.

Table 18 Different approaches for the induction of abortion during early human pregnancy

---

1. Corpus luteum
   1.1 Interception of the luteotrophic activity of the blastocyst, i.e. of hCG synthesis
   1.2 Blocking of steroid production of the corpus luteum

2. Target organ
   2.1 Blocking of the progesterone receptor in the endometrium by an inactive gestogen
   2.2 Induction of labour by prostaglandins
       2.2.1 Exogenous administration of prostaglandins
       2.2.2 Endogenous increase of prostaglandin level

IMPORTANCE OF PROGESTERONE FOR PREGNANCY

The steroid hormone progesterone is a C-21 steroid that is produced in the non-pregnant woman mainly by the corpus luteum of the ovary and, to some extent, by the adrenal glands. During pregnancy progesterone synthesis mainly occurs in the corpus luteum until the 7th or 8th week of gestation, and from the 9th week of gestation on, progesterone synthesis is taken over by the placenta (Csapo et al., 1974). During human pregnancy progesterone has two main functions. First, it causes the conversion of the endometrium to a secretory pattern, which is required by implantation: specific proteins (e.g. uteroglobin) are synthesized, their role in pregnancy still unclear. In addition, progesterone is required to protect the uterus from premature contractions.

Humans The monthly occurrence of menstrual bleeding in the female is a progesterone-withdrawal bleeding. If pregnancy occurs, the corpus luteum graviditatis produces progesterone to support pregnancy. This has been convincingly shown by Csapo et al. (1973a, b; 1974). The authors found that lute-ectomy during the first 50 days following conception caused a rapid decrease in serum progesterone, and rise in uterine contractility caused abortion. On the other hand, a sudden local increase of uterine motility, such as that caused by intrauterine applications of prostaglandins (Csapo, 1976), may cause a cyclic bleeding by suppression of placental progesterone synthesis. The explanation for this phenomenon lies in the shift of progesterone synthesis in the 7th–8th week of gestation to the human placenta.

Following lute-ectomy in early pregnancy (prior to the 9th week of gestation), a pregnancy can be supported by exogenous progesterone (e.g. progesterone vaginal suppositories).

In early pregnancy all mechanisms which inhibit the synthesis or the action of progesterone may cause an abortion. These include progesterone synthesis blockers which act on the corpus luteum or on the human placenta. They also include other substances which block the action of progesterone at the end organ—e.g. at the progesterone receptor in the myometrium. A further group of compounds cause direct contractions of the uterus. The first group of substances include compounds which inhibit certain enzyme systems of progesterone synthesis, whereas the compounds which block progesterone action on the myometrial receptor are called antiprogestins. Of all the substances which induce contractions as a direct mechanism of action on the uterine muscle cell, only the prostaglandins and oxytocin are known at present.

For the induction of abortion in early pregnancy, compounds with various sites of action have to be chosen according to gestational age. These include substances which inhibit progesterone production by the corpus luteum until the 8th or 9th week and thereby cause luteolysis. Following the 9th week of gestation, steroidogenic blockers of placental hormone production gain more importance. A further group of substances can be applied, independently of production, directly for the induction of contractions in the myometrium. Natural and synthetic prostaglandins can be used for this purpose.

Animals In all laboratory animals which have been investigated, progesterone seems to be required for the implantation of embryos in the endometrium and for the maintenance of pregnancy (Fraenkel, 1903; Bouin and Ancel, 1910; Butenandt *et al.*, 1934).

Induction of abortion up to 7th/8th week of gestation

LUTEOLYSIS

The normal life span of the corpus luteum is, without pregnancy, about 14 days; thereafter a decrease of progesterone synthesis follows for reasons unknown up to now and a progesterone withdrawal bleeding (menstrual bleeding) occurs in the endometrium. The stimulatory influence of the pregnancy hormone hCG, which is possibly secreted as early as during tubal passage by the contact of the blastocysts with the tubal walls by structures of the oviduct, increases the life span of the corpus luteum. This, however, is limited by time and, following the 7th/8th week of pregnancy, a luteolysis of the corpus luteum graviditatis occurs. At that point of time the progesterone synthesis is increasingly produced by the placenta for the maintenance of pregnancy.

The implantation of human blastocysts, as well as the later development of human early pregnancy in the 7th or 8th gestational week, can be inhibited at three sites (Aitken and Harper, 1977). One is the inhibition of early luteotrophic activity of the blastocyst—i.e. of hCG secretion. Thereby, the progesterone synthesis of the corpus luteum is indirectly inhibited. A second site of action is the depression of the corpus luteum which may be caused by either prostaglandins or steroids. A further possible action includes an inactive progestin at the progesterone receptor in the endometrium as well as in the myometrium and inhibits thereby the required progestin influence on both end organs.

Indirect site of action = inhibition of early luteotrophic activity of the blastocyst One of the early functions of pregnancy product in mammals is to prevent the regression of the corpus luteum at the end of oestrus and the menstrual cycle. In some animals which release a uterine luteolysin, such as guinea-pig, hamster, pig, rabbit, rat or sheep, the blastocyst has an anti-luteolytic effect (Anderson, 1972; Short, 1976). The role of this anti-luteolytic stimulus has not yet been clarified. Possibly the anti-luteolysin is identical with the pregnancy-specific antigen which has been demonstrated in the plasma, the myometrium, the corpus luteum and the ovine embryo as early as the 8th day of pregnancy (Cerini *et al.*, 1976). In the human and the monkey the early pregnancy product has a direct luteotrophic effect on the corpus luteum and has possibly also an anti-luteolytic action (Knobil, 1973). The luteotrophic factor could be hCG, which increases in the blood of pregnant women from the day of implantation onwards (Jaffe *et al.*, 1969; Saxena *et al.*, 1974). hCG causes a rapid increase in the plasma progesterone level (Hanson *et al.*, 1971; Niswender *et al.*, 1972). This increase in plasma progesterone following implantation (Reinius *et al.*, 1973) and the appearance of choriogonadotrophin in peripheral blood (Meyer, 1972) occurs in the rhesus monkey during early pregnancy. In other species, such as the rabbit (Fuchs and Beling, 1974), the rat (Haour, 1976) and the mouse (Beyer and Zeilmarker, 1974), there is some evidence that the feto-placental unity produces gonadotrophic hormones.

In principle, every substance produced by the blastocyst and having a vital function for implantation and the maintenance of the corpus luteum is a site of action for contraceptive compounds. If the effect of such factors is blocked, the pregnancy can be interrupted at the time of implantation without influencing the course of the menstrual cycle. Among those are antibodies against β-hCG.

Another site of action for the regulation of fertility is the development of antihormones which compete with hCG at the receptor side of the corpus luteum. Such compounds would have to be taken when menstruation does not occur or, possibly, once in the cycle at the time of expected menstruation, in order to guarantee the regression of the corpus luteum. Yang *et al.* (1976) have found an LH-receptor binding inhibitor (LHRBI) in the aqueous solution of luteinized rat ovaries. A similar LH/hCG-receptor binding inhibitor was identified in porcine corpus luteum extracts (Sakai *et al.*, 1977).

Finally, attempts have been made to enzymatically cleave carbohydrate moieties of the hCG molecule and to produce competitive inhibitors which lack the luteotrophic activities of the native molecule (Bahl, 1969). The removal of sugars and sialic acid (galactose, N-acetyl, glucose amine and mannose) does not influence the receptor binding activity of hCG *in vitro*; however, its ability to increase cyclic AMP, as in porcine granulosa cells, is lost (Channing *et al.*, 1976). The antigonadotrophic effect of such derivatives has shown that hCG-induced progesterone secretion in porcine and monkey granulosa cells is inhibited *in vitro* (Channing *et al.*, 1977, 1978). Several questions regarding the immunogenicity of such molecules and their biological half-lives are the subject of current research.

Direct site of action = luteodepression　　Fifty years ago the importance of the uterus for the control of the oestrus cycle was discovered. In some domestic and laboratory animals (cow, guinea-pig, hamster, pig, rabbit, rat, sheep) removal of the uterus prolongs the life of the corpus luteum (Anderson, 1972). This effect of hysterectomy has been claimed to prove the removal of a uterine luteolytic factor that is released at the end of the luteal phase and causes the regression of the corpus luteum. Today there are various indications that the uterine luteolytic factor is prostaglandin $PGF_{2\alpha}$ (Behrmann *et al.*, 1974). This prostaglandin causes luteolysis in the above-mentioned species (Anderson, 1972; Behrmann *et al.*, 1974). In position, however, a uterine luteolysin does not play an important role in the regulation of human luteal function. As human ovarian tissue is capable of synthesizing $PGF_{2\alpha}$ (Challis et al., 1976), it is conceivable that prostaglandins are involved in the luteoregression.

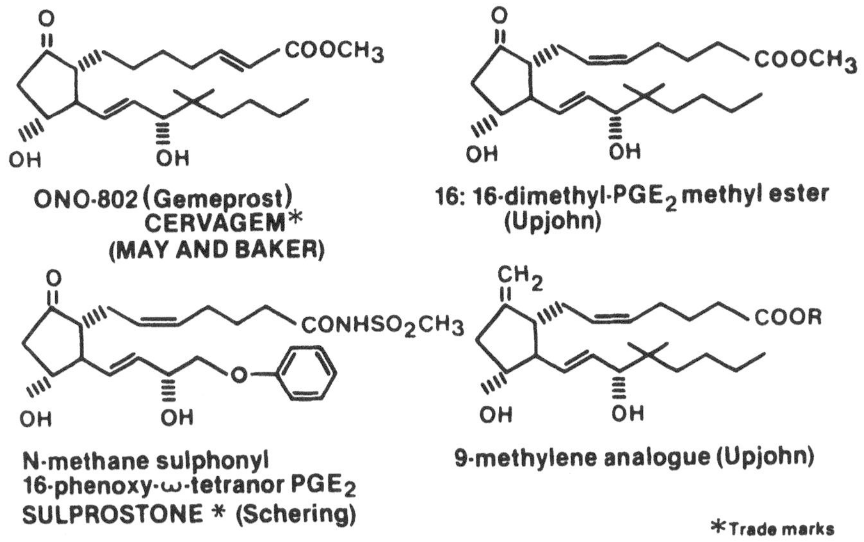

ONO-802 (Gemeprost)
CERVAGEM*
(MAY AND BAKER)

16: 16-dimethyl-PGE$_2$ methyl ester
(Upjohn)

N-methane sulphonyl
16-phenoxy-ω-tetranor PGE$_2$
SULPROSTONE * (Schering)

9-methylene analogue (Upjohn)

*Trade marks

Figure 43 Structure of prostaglandin E analogues undergoing clinical evaluation

Prostaglandins are able to stimulate the uterine muscle and to cause abortion in all gestational stages. This effect can be used therapeutically for premature termination of intact or disturbed pregnancies (Karim, 1975). The risk of systemic complication (bronchiospasm, cardiovascular failure, seizures) and the high rate of side-effects, especially gastrointestinal, reduce the spectrum of possible use of first-generation prostaglandin. In recent

Table 19 Prostaglandins and derivatives that are used for influencing fertility (e.g. induction of abortion). Prostaglandins are subdivided according to their stage of development: (1st generation, earliest development; 3rd generation, recent development). (Modified from Schmidt-Gollwitzer et al., 1981)

Stage of development	Prostaglandins	Assessment
1st generation	$PGF_{2\alpha}$ PGE_2	short half-life, high substance-specific risk
2nd generation	15-methyl $PGF_{2\alpha}$ 15-methyl $PGF_{2\alpha}$-methyl ester 16,16-dimethyl PGE_2	prolonged half-life
3rd generation	16,16-dimethyl-$trans\Delta^2$-PGE_1- methyl ester (ONO 802)	
	16-phenoxy-17,18,19,20-tetra- nor PGE_2-methyl-sulphonam- ide (sulprostone)	low substance-specific risk
	9-deoxo-16,16-dimethyl-9 methylene PGE_2 (Upjohn 46785)	

years prostaglandin derivatives have been developed with markedly reduced risks as compared with natural prostaglandins (Schmidt-Gollwitzer *et al.*, 1977).

The mechanisms of action of substances listed in Table 19 depend on the induction of uterine muscle contractions.

In various investigations the effect of 16-phenoxy-17,18,19,20-tetranor-PGE_2-methylsulphonamide (sulprostone; Nalador) was tested. Table 20 summarizes the fields of use and forms of application of sulprostone.

Table 20 Use of sulprostone (Nalador) for induction of abortion in early and late pregnancy (modified from Schmidt-Gollwitzer *et al.*, 1981)

Permitted use	Application
Intrauterine fetal death	i.m.
Induction of abortion in:	
hydatid mole	extra-amnial
1st trimester	
10 weeks' gestation	
softening 8 weeks' gestation	intracervical

Investigations by Schmidt-Gollwitzer *et al.* (1977) have demonstrated that the intravenous administration of sulprostone in disturbed as well as intact pregnancies for the induction of abortions has a high success rate. By this means a pregnancy can be terminated safely, rapidly, carefully. The average time for induction of abortion is approximately 10 h. A total dose of 1 mg sulprostone is sufficient. The success rate for therapeutically induced abortions was 98% with regard to the expulsion of the fetus, and in 92% of the cases abortion was complete.

The most frequent undesirable side-effects are nausea and vomiting. Analgesics are required for patients with contraction-induced pains. Other prostaglandin-related side-effects, such as diarrhoea, alteration of the blood pressure, increasing temperature, shivering, breathing complaints and pains in the infusion arm, are infrequent. Life-threatening complications have not been observed. Intramuscular application, as reported by Karim and Ratnam (1978), showed similar results.

The mechanism of action of sulprostone in early abortion—that is, at a time when the corpus luteum graviditatis is still essential for the maintenance of pregnancy—can primarily be explained by the stimulation of the uterine myometrium (Froewis, 1963). The decrease in the serum levels of oestradiol and progesterone secondarily causes a disturbance of the embryo and decreases hCG production. In favour of this mechanism is that 17α-hydroxyprogesterone formed in the corpus luteum remains almost unaltered during the treatment.

Wiechell (1981) reported that 328 women were treated by infiltration of $25\,\mu g$ sulprostone in the interior and posterior uterine wall. Directly following the injections, the single intramural dose caused contractions which lasted for 6–7 h on average. In 48% of the cases expulsion of the embryo occurred. In the other cases a suction curettage was performed after 7 h.

Apart from intravenous, intramuscular and intramural application, prostaglandins can be used locally (e.g. in the form of vaginal suppositories such as ONO-802). By 'softening' (cervical dilatation) it can be achieved that the cervix slowly opens and the interruption of pregnancy is largely simplified. Cervical tears, which may cause, especially in nulliparas, the formation of scars on the cervix and possibly lead to complications in later pregnancies, can thus be avoided.

With a combination of prostaglandins and steroidogenic blockers, anti-progestins and prostaglandins, the steroidogenic blockers would inhibit luteal progesterone synthesis, the antigestogens would block the gestational action on the endometrium and the prostaglandins could act luteolytically. This combination of drugs could inhibit the function of the corpus luteum in early pregnancy or possibly block placental steroidogenesis in the 8th/9th week of gestation, thereby inducing abortion.

Oestrogens can cause luteolysis in laboratory animals (guinea-pigs, hamsters, rabbits, rats) as well as in some domestic animals (cow, sheep, pig) (Anderson, 1972; Oriol-Bosch and Cortes, 1975). It has been demonstrated that high doses of oestrogens have a potent anti-fertility effect. There are indications that the post-coital administration of oestrogens at mid-cycle ($5 \mu g$ on five consecutive days) inhibits implantation in women and thus prevents pregnancy via the luteolytic mechanism of action (Gore *et al.*, 1973). This is supported by the fact that oestrogens cause a dose-dependent decrease in plasma progesterone concentration in the luteal phase as well as a shortening of the cycle (Gore *et al.*, 1973). Additionally, oestrogen crystals implanted in the corpus luteum cause a luteodepression (Hoffmann, 1960). No sign of luteodepression could be demonstrated by Oriol-Bosch and Cortes (1975) or by Board *et al.* (1973) following the administration of oestradiol benzoate and diethylstilboestrol. However, the dose and/or the potency of oestrogens that were used in experiments was lower than in the studies in which the so-called luteolytic or contraceptive effect was observed.

Progesterone production of the corpus luteum originates in cholesterol, either taken up from the maternal blood or synthesized *de novo* from acetate. For the conversion of cholesterol to progesterone two enzyme systems are required: first, the cholesterol side chain cleavage enzyme, and second, the 3β-hydroxysteroid dehydrogenase $\Delta^{4,5}$-isomerase (3β-HSDH). Both enzymes can be inhibited selectively. The cholesterol side chain cleavage enzyme, which is present in the mitochondria, is dependent on cytochrome P450 and its action is inhibited by compounds that act on cytochrome P450. One of those is *p*-aminoglutethimide. Another site of action is the inhibition of 3β-HSDH. These enzyme systems can be inhibited competitively or non-competitively by numerous steroids. The most potent blockers are androgen derivatives, such as cyanoketone, trilostane and azastene (Rabe *et al.*, 1983).

Aminoglutethimide (AG) is a derivative of a substance with hypnotic action, from which it differs only by an amino group attached to the benzene ring (Figure 44). In animal experiments by Glasser *et al.* (1972) AG was found to be a potent compound for the induction of abortion when used in the right dosage and at the right time. AG is not embryotoxic, and its action depends on the inhibition of luteal steroidogenesis and on diminishing serum progesterone levels. In 1970 Marek and Horky reported on a patient who had been treated for postural oedema with AG and frusemide (75 mg/day). The patient was given the drug until the third month of preg-

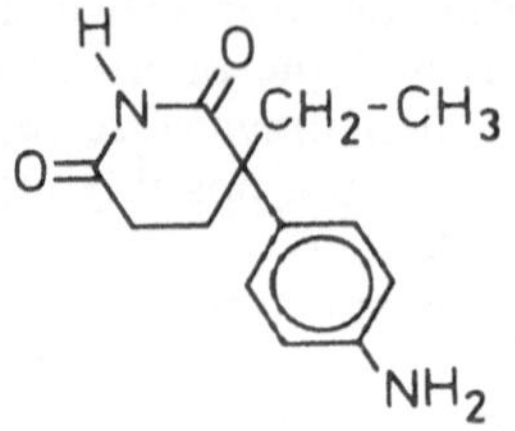

Figure 44 Aminoglutethimide

nancy. At this time, one was not aware of her pregnancy. The intake of the drug caused no disturbance of pregnancy nor did it cause an abortion.

The inhibitory action of synthetic steroids on enzyme systems *in vitro* was examined by Rabe *et al.* (1983). It was demonstrated that the cholesterol side chain cleavage enzyme is not inhibited by azastene (Figure 45) or trilostane (Figure 46). A 50% inhibition was achieved by cyanoketone.

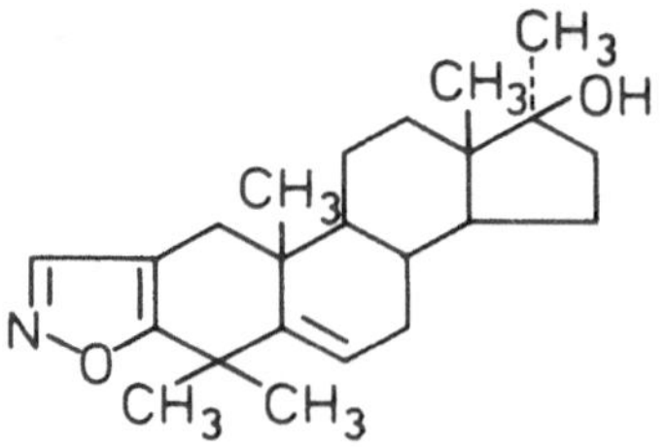

Figure 45 Azastene

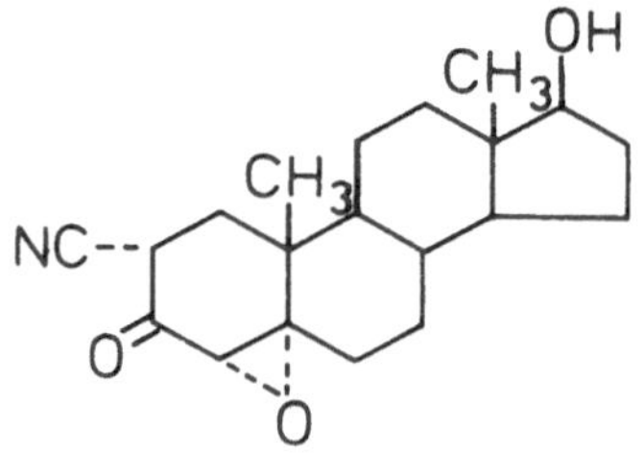

Figure 46 Trilostane

3β-HSDH was inhibited dose-dependently by azastene ($I_{50} = 1\,\mu M$), trilostane ($I_{50} = 4\,\mu M$) and cyanoketone ($I_{50} = 3\,\mu M$).

To what extent the inhibition of steroidogenesis in early pregnancy is applicable to the induction of abortions cannot be determined at the present time. Possibly, a combination of steroidogenic blockers with prostaglandins or antiprogestins is useful, since high concentrations at the same time inhibit adrenal steroidogenesis and cause adrenal failure.

5α-Stigmastane-$3\beta,5,6\beta$-triol-3-monobenzoate is a synthetic analogue of the steroidal compounds of the leaves of *Ananas comosus*. It was tested in mice at a dose of 14 mg/kg per day (Pakrashi and Chakrabarty, 1981). It had a significant antifertility effect with a single or a multiple oral dose during the preimplantation phase of pregnancy. In experiments on rabbits the interruption of pregnancy occurred with a single dose on the 8th day of pregnancy (Pakrashi and Chakrabarty, 1981). This compound has no oestrogenic or androgenic characteristics. In the McPhial tests a weak progestin effect was demonstrated.

Interference with the progestin receptor The transfer of hormone information from the extracellular space to the intracellular structures requires certain receptors. These special membrane proteins, too, are regulated by hormones. With extracellular overstimulation the receptor protein can briefly fuse with the membrane and only during receptor regeneration may it be formed again. The occupation of receptors by substances which do not have biological effect causes blockage of the transfer of information from the receptor to the intracellular substances. This can be compared with the key-lock theory. The right molecule, i.e. the right key, fits into the lock and can also open it, whereas the wrong key may well fit into the lock, but does not open the door. The changes in steroid receptors in the endometrium and the myometrium offer a promising approach for the development of new contraceptives.

The concentration of progesterone receptors in the uterus reflects the fluctuation of cyclic hormone production in the ovary. The number of receptors reaches a peak in the human myometrium and endometrium during the late proliferative phase, caused by a preovulatory rise in ovarian oestrogen secretion. In the second phase of the cycle the concentration of the receptors decreases, as oestrogen levels diminish and the corpus luteum produces progesterone.

The progesterone receptor can be influenced either by its occupation by an inactive gestogen (antiprogestin) or by substances which regulate the number of progesterone receptors.

The main use of antiprogestins lies in the pharmacological control of human fertility. The advantage of specific antiprogestins has long been known, and reports on substances with antiprogestin activity exist since 1962 (Banik and Pinkus, 1962). In spite of remarkable progress in this field, no compound with ideal characteristics of high potency with complete specificity could be found. This review does not try to summarize the literature on antiprogestins completely, but points out the current studies which lead to the development of new compounds that approach the ideal. Because of this knowledge, antiprogestins are searched for which compete with endogenous progestins at the specific receptors but at the same time do not have any premenstrual activity or progesterone action. The effect of antiprogestins on the human endometrium inhibits the implantation of the fertilized ovum at mid-cycle.

Various antiprogestins binding with the receptor irreversibly and covalently have been described but are not in use, because of their high toxicity. Meanwhile, the development of non-toxic substances seems to be possible. With these compounds the vacant progesterone receptors in the late proliferative phase could be saturated. Such a compound is 16α-bromoacetoxyprogesterone, an acylating substance which has the disadvantage of being a possible carcinogen. Recent studies using other substances such as R-2323 (13-ethyl-17α-hydroxy-18,19-dinor-17α-hydroxy-18,19-dinor-17-4,9,11-pregnantriene-20-yn-3-on) (Roussel-Uclaf) have demonstrated that the development of non-toxic antiprogestins is feasible (Raynaud *et al.*,

1975). These antiprogestins can be given during the cycle, by which the number of unoccupied receptor-binding sites in the endometrium could be occupied during the late proliferative phase and a secretory transformation of the endometrium could be prevented. The site of action of antiprogestins can be either in the endometrium or in the myometrium.

The efficiency of antiprogestins can be tested *in vivo* and *in vitro* by models listed in Table 21. The biological assessment of new steroid hormones includes the identification of the characteristic antiprogestin actions as well as the determination of specificity and studies of mechanisms of action. In general, the antiprogestin action of compounds *in vitro* can be determined by receptor studies (= competitive displacement of the compound specific for the receptor) and numerous biological essays (e.g. ACTH release in rat pituitary cell cultures). Among *in vivo* studies of antiprogestins using animal models, a distinction can be made between animal models in which the respective biological response is either progesterone-dependent or independent of progesterone at the site of the endometrium. With animal models, the maintenance of pregnancy, the support of decidualization in the rodent uterus as well as the endometrial proliferation in the rabbit can be determined. These effects can be achieved by exogenous as well as endogenous progesterone.

Table 21 Studies of the biological action of antiprogestins *in vivo* and *in vitro*

In vivo studies
  Interaction with exogenous progesterone and its action on implantation
    antiprogestomimetic effect (Pincus, 1965)
    antideciduogenic activity (Hisaw and Velardo, 1951)
    antiprogestin activity
  Interaction with endogenous progesterone
    abortion-inducing effect
  Effect on the endometrium at the time of implantation in various animal species
In vitro studies
  Receptor binding studies
  Bioassays (ACTH release) in rat pituitary cell cultures

The antiprogestins can be subdivided into those inhibiting progesterone production (= steroidogenic blockers) and those inhibiting its action. The first group inhibit the effect of endogenous progesterone, but is ineffective if exogenous progesterone is supplied, whereas the latter group inhibit both effects. In conclusion, studies of both sites of action of antiprogestins can be carried out using competitive displacement of endogenous progesterone at the receptor, and, following this, the exogenous progesterone model should be used. With the exogenous progesterone model, the distinction can be made as to whether the substances inhibit the action of progesterone or progesterone synthesis. In all animal experiments, the relation of oestrogens to progesterone has to be taken into consideration, as there is an interaction between the concentration of oestrogen and the number of progesterone receptors.

The specific biological response to steroid hormones is caused by the following sequence of actions. The hormone interacts with a specific receptor at the uterine cell, which is taken up as a steroid receptor complex in the nucleus, binds to chromatin and activates the chromatin complex, which process is followed by DNA and RNA synthesis. Thus a biologically inactive hormone may inhibit the biological response of an active hormone by binding to its receptor site. By use of the appropriate test models the activity of the antihormone may be assessed.

Steroids with antihormonal activity have been found among mineralocorticoids and oestrogens. In experiments *in vitro* and *in vivo* the antialdosterone spironolactone was found to bind with a relatively high-affinity constant to the cytoplasmic receptor, without the formation of a receptor complex in the nucleus (Marver *et al.*, 1974). Similar observations were reported for anti-oestrogens (Ruh and Ruh, 1974). According to this conception of the mechanism of action of steroidal antihormones, antigestogens should have a certain affinity to the progesterone receptor, but should inhibit the steps of action which cause biological response and result in no or little gestogenic effect.

The agonists of progesterone have been demonstrated to have a reason-

Table 22 Chemical nomenclature of various steroids with antigestogen activity evaluated in Table 21 and 23 (Raynaud *et al.*, 1981)

(1)	Progesterone	pregn-4-en-3,20-dione
(2)	16α-Methylprogesterone	16α-methyl-pregn-4-en-3,20-dione
(3)	6α,16α-Dimethylprogesterone	6α,16α-dimethyl-pregn-4-en-3,20-dione
(4)	RU 3163	19-nor-pregna-4,9-dien-3,20-dione
(5)	Demegestone (RU 2453)	17α-methyl-19-nor-pregna-4,9-dien-3,20-dione
(6)	Promegestone (RU 5020)	17α,21-dimethyl-19-nor-pregna-4,9-dien-3,20-dione
(7)	RU 25253	11β-ethinyl-17α-methyl-19-nor-pregna-4,9-dien-3,20-dione
(8)	Medroxyprogesterone acetate	17α-acetyloxy-6α-methyl-pregn-4-en-3,20-dione
(9)	Megestrol acetate	17α-acetyloxy-6-methyl-pregna-4,6-dien-3,20-dione
(10)	Chlormadinone acetate-20-dion	17α-acetyloxy-6-chloro-pregna-4,6-dien-3,20-dione
(11)	Cyproterone acetate	17α-acetyloxy-6-chloro-1,2-dihydro-(1β,2β)-3'H-cyclopropa(1,1)pregna-1,4,6-trien-3,20-dione
(12)	RU 22779	(17R) 2'oxido-spiro(oestr-4-en-17,5'(1,2)-oxathiolan)3-one
(13)	RU 23747	(17R)2'-oxido-spiro(oestra-4,9-dien-17,5'(1,2)-oxathiolan)3-one
(14)	RU 25051	(17R) 2'oxido-spiro(oestra-4,9,11-trien-17,5'(1,2)oxathiolan)3-one
(15)	Norethisterone	17β-hydroxy-19-nor-17α-pregn-4-en-20-yn-3-one
(16)	Norgestrienone (RU 2010)	17β-hydroxy-19-nor-17α-pregna-4,9,11-trien-20-yn-3-one
(17)	Norgestrel	13β-ethyl-17β-hydroxy-18,19-dinor-17α-pregn-4-en-20-yn-3-one
(18)	Gestrinone (RU 2323)	13-ethyl-17β-hydroxy-18,19-dinor-pregna-4,9,11-trien-20-yn-3-one
(19)	RU 25593	11β-(4-fluorphenyl)-17β-hydroxy-19-nor-17α-pregna-4,9-dien-20-yn-3-one
(20)	RU 25055	17β-hydroxy-11β-(2-thienyl)19-nor-17-pregna-4,9-dien-20-yn-3-one
(21)	Trenbolone (RU 2341)	17β-hydroxy-oestra-4,9,11-trien-3-one
(22)	Metribolone (RU 1881)	17β-hydroxy-17α-methyl-oestra-4,9,11-triene-3-one
(23)	RU 2999	17β-hydroxy-17α-methyl-2-oxy-oestra-4,9,11-trien-3-one
(24)	RU 2420	7α,17α-dimethyl-17β-hydroxy-oestra-4,9,11-trien-3-one
(25)	RU 4841	7α,17α-dimethyl-13β-ethyl-17β-hydroxy-gona-4,9,11-trien-3-one

able correlation between binding affinity to the uterine receptor protein in man, sheep and rabbit and the biological action (Kontula et al., 1975). It seems that pregnane and oestrane steroid skeletons that have a $\Delta^{4,3}$-keto group are required and that the most important bonds between the steroid and its receptor should be hydrophobic (Lee et al., 1975). It is most probable that the basic structure of a potent gestogen antagonist would be similar to that of the agonist. Table 22 gives the structural formulas of the various steroids tested for activity as progesterone agonists or antagonists listed in Table 23 and Figure 47.

Table 23 lists the receptor binding profiles of 25 tested steroids. The progestins most commonly used in clinics, such as medroxyprogesterone acetate, chlormadinone acetate and levonorgestrel, or the less well-known derivatives of progesterone such as promegestone, demegestone, the compounds RU 22779, RU 23474 and RU 25051 and the 11β-alkyl substituted compounds RU 24253, have a higher receptor binding activity for progesterone receptor, which increases with incubation time (binding activity > 300 after 24 h incubation), which indicates that a stable, slowly dissociating receptor complex has been achieved.

In most rodents or lagomorpha both the sensitivity to oestrogens and a continuous application of low oestrogen doses are a precondition for optimal gestogen response. It is known that oestrogens not only can enhance or reduce progestin response when administered in high doses, but also in rabbits they have an antiprogestational activity (Chambon, 1949) and can

Table 23 Binding of different steroids to the progesterone receptor (0°C) after 2 h and 24 h (Raynaud and Labrie, 1981)

	2 h	24 h
(1) Progesterone	100	100
(2) 16α-Methylprogesterone	65	60
(3) 6α,16α-Dimethylprogesterone	50	155
(4) RU 25253	200	245
(5) Demegestone	230	420
(6) Promegestone	220	535
(7) RU 25253	180	530
(8) Medroxyprogesterone acetate	125	305
(9) Megestrol acetate	150	120
(10) Chlormadinone acetate	175	320
(11) Cyproterone acetate	80	60
(12) RU 22779	205	335
(13) RU 23747	225	380
(14) RU 250051	330	870
(15) Norethisterone	155	265
(16) Norgestrienone	65	45
(17) Norgestrel	170	905
(18) Gestrinone	75	50
(19) RU 25593	40	35
(20) RU 25055	70	85
(21) Trenbolone	75	15
(22) Metribolone	210	190
(23) RU 2999	260	305
(24) RU 2420	280	330
(25) RU 4841	230	675

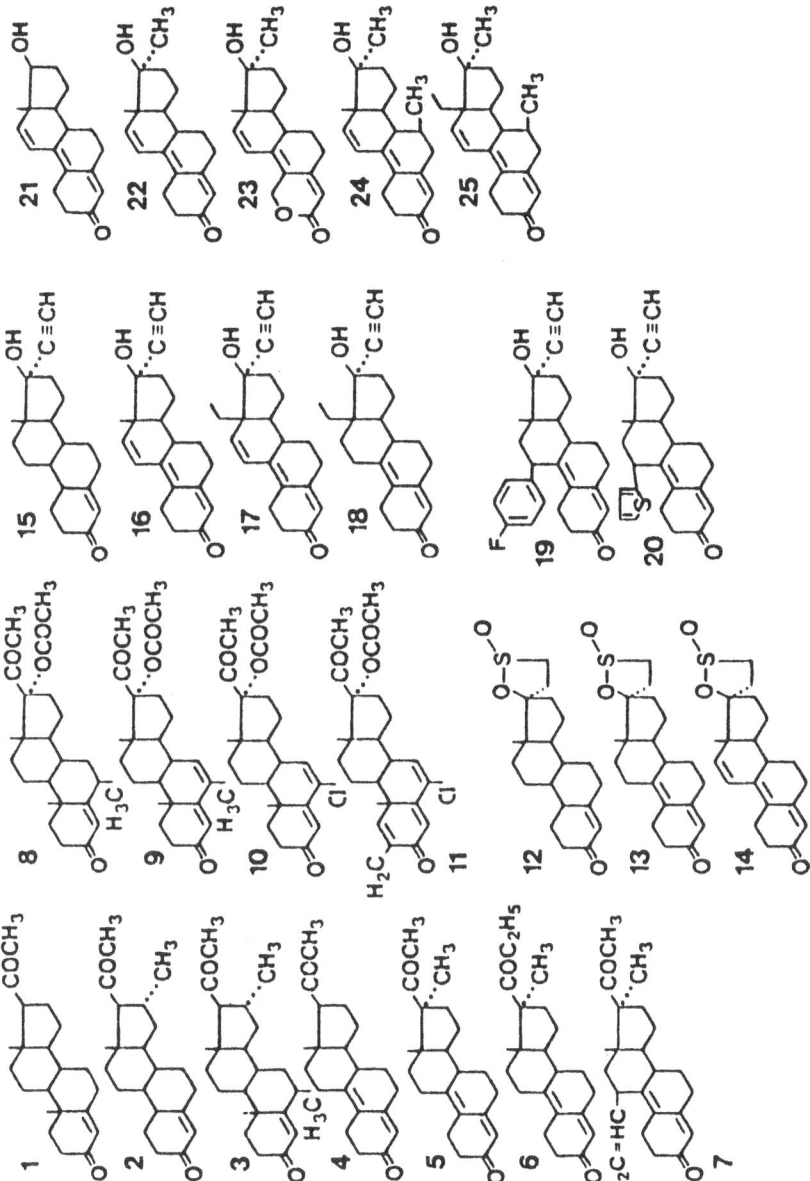

Figure 47 Structures of steroids tested. The respective compounds are numbered as in Table 22, with exact chemical names

inhibit peripheral antagonism by ovariectomized, progesterone-treated rats (Neumann and Elger, 1971). Receptor studies have partially explained these observations. The number of progesterone receptor sites in the rat uterus increases under oestradiol treatment (Rao *et al.*, 1973). It is obvious that high concentrations of progesterone are required for a biological response to result. The genetic point of view in oestrogen stimulation and the renewal of progesterone receptors have not yet been sufficiently investigated to provide a basis for a complete analysis of oestrogen–progestin interaction.

In rodents and lagomorpha the optimal progestin response is reached by a very large amount of progesterone in opposition to oestrogen. Comparably small amounts of oestradiol are sufficient for optimal conditions for the effect of progesterone, whereas high oestradiol doses cause an inhibition of progestin response. The inhibition of a certain dose can only be overcome by an increase of progesterone.

In primates little is known about the interaction between oestradiol and progesterone in the endometrium. In rhesus monkeys similar doses of progesterone per animal are required for optimal decidualization of the endometrium, but much higher doses of oestrogens are required (Good and Moyer, 1968). When compared with that of the rat, the endometrium of primates reacts more to progesterone and less to oestradiol.

It has long been known that the continuous administration of hCG from day 20 of the cycle to women will cause a prolongation of luteal function in the form of pseudopregnancy (Brown and Bradbury, 1947; Fried and Radoff, 1952). Daily doses of 5000 iu hCG and more are required to prolong the life of the corpus luteum over 13 days, which can be assessed by pregnandiol excretion and the length of the cycle.

In rhesus monkeys hCG treatment during the luteal phase has also caused a prolongation of the luteal function and thus of the length of the cycle. In women menstruation will occur in spite of continuous treatment over 20–25 days after ovulation—e.g. at the time when the corpus luteum is not required for the maintenance of pregnancy. Daily administration of 25–500 iu hCG will prolong the progesterone secretion of the corpus luteum in the monkey (Neill and Knobil, 1972). In addition, hCG treatment in the second part of the luteal phase will not only prolong the luteal function, but also increase progesterone levels as in early pregnancy.

hCG administration has also been used to investigate the abortifacient effect of steroids that interfere with the function of the human corpus luteum (i.e. luteolytic drugs). Oxymetholone, for example, which possesses luteolytic properties in the luteal phase without interrupting early pregnancy, is ineffective when given in an hCG-prolonged luteal phase (Henzl *et al.*, 1973). The authors remarked that compounds that are given for postconceptional fertility control should be investigated by an hCG test.

In primates little is known about the antiprogestational effect of high oestrogen doses which are given together with progesterone during the proliferative phase. It is well established that high doses of oestrogens (ethinyloestradiol up to 5 mg/day) are not able to interrupt early pregnancy in women (Bacic *et al.*, 1970).

In summary, the antigestational activity of a compound can be regarded as its oestrogenic activity in rabbits and rodents; since oestrogens are inactive as drugs to cause menstrual bleeding in women, these compounds have been investigated as regards their oestrogenic effect. The antiprogestational efficacy of oestrogens has been assessed in all applied experimental models.

In the development of antiprogestins attempts were made to synthesize alkylated derivatives of 17-acetoxyprogesterone in order to investigate the hypothesis that certain groups in certain positions of a steroid molecule may cause the conversion of the progestin into an antiprogestin. These groups change the binding of the molecule outside the area which is occupied by progestin itself. The compounds were investigated for competitive affinity to a receptor purified from rabbit uterine cytosol in comparison with radioactive tritiated progesterone. Because of the low affinity of these compounds, it is unlikely that they can be effective as antiprogestins (Beyer et al., 1980).

After intensive research the French company Roussel-Uclaf succeeded in developing a specific antigestogen, R 2323. The 'gestogen' inhibits the action of progesterone produced in the corpus luteum or in the placenta on the receptor of the endometrium or the myometrium. According to the manufacturers, no systemic side-effects were observed. R 2323 has an antiprogestational effect in relation to exogenous and endogenous progesterone (Sakiz and Azadian-Boulanger, 1971). The structural formula of the antiprogestin R 2323 is demonstrated in Figure 48.

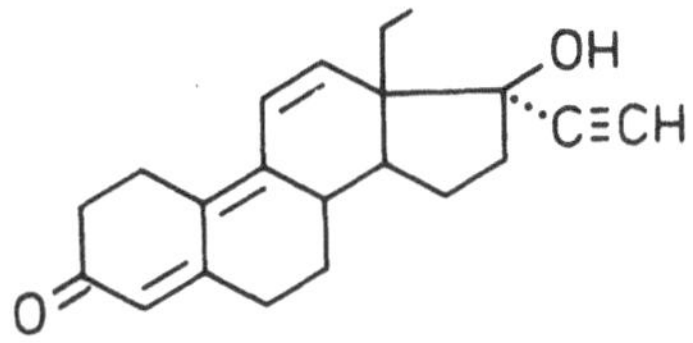

Figure 48 Antiprogestin R 2323 (13-ethyl-17-hydroxy-18,19-dinor-17α-pregna-4,9,11-triene-2-yn-3-one)

Following treatment with progesterone, this compound demonstrated antiproliferative activity in rabbits and antidecidual activity in rats. Termination of pregnancy in normal and ovariectomized rats, after treatment with exogenous progesterone, was achieved by R 2323. The antiprogestin action of this compound is partially oestrogenic, progestinic and androgenic. Ovulation was suppressed in mature rats with normal cycles, but not in premature gonadotrophin-treated rats. Transport of the ovum remained unaltered. The proliferative response in the rat uterus was counteracted by the administration of R 2323 or anti-oestrogens during the oestrogen period. R 2323 remained ineffective when used together with progesterone. In studies with cytosolic receptor proteins R 2323 displaced progesterone from the receptor, but not oestradiol (Philibert and Raynaud, 1974). These assumptions are the basis for the hypothesis that the occupation of progesterone binding sites by R 2323 at the beginning of the luteal phase, given after ovulation, inhibits progesterone-dependent changes and therefore also implantation.

In humans R 2323 used in various regimens was shown to be effective as an antifertility agent. In a trial with 181 women in 2971 cycles (Sakiz and Azadian-Boulanger, 1974) R 2323 administered in a dose of 2.5 mg at weekly intervals gave an index of 7.3% in endometrial biopsies, of which 4.4% was reported as drug failure.

Further studies were carried out to improve the efficacy of this antiprogestin (Sakiz and Azadian-Boulanger, 1974; Azadian-Boulanger *et al.*, 1976). At the time of ovulation the formation of progesterone receptors is induced by oestrogen secretion, at a time when progesterone levels are still low. This period represents the optimal time for antiprogestin activity, as the number of unoccupied progesterone receptors is maximal. A dose of 50 mg R 2323 was administered daily on days 5, 16 and 17 of the cycle. This amount of the compound represents the upper level of the tolerated dose. Nevertheless, a Pearl Index of 9.5% with a drug failure amounting to 5% in 2148 cycles of 160 women occurred. The use of antiprogestins gives good control of the cycle and only few menstrual irregularities occur. In some females 50 mg of the compound provoked vomiting and vertigo. Endometrial biopsies performed in the luteal phase showed only a weak secretory endometrium.

Apart from oral administration, R 2323 may be applied in the form of vaginal rings. In healthy volunteers (Viinikka *et al.*, 1975) vaginal rings with 10, 50 and 200 mg R 2323 were inserted on the first day of menstrual bleeding. This study was merely performed to investigate the pharmacokinetics of this drug and no clinical data are yet available.

RU 486 is a 19-nor steroid. In its substituents at positions C-17 and C-11 it resembles a progestin, but on the other hand its full structure is similar to that of anti-oestrogens of the triphenyl series. It binds with high affinity to the progesterone receptor, but lacks progestin-like activity. On the other hand, it acts as an antagonist to progesterone and thereby it can inhibit early pregnancy in the luteal phase.

The following observations were made in laboratory animals. The affinity of RU 486 is five times greater than that of progesterone for the progesterone receptor in the rat uterus and three times greater than that of dexamethasone for the glucocorticoid receptor of the rat thymus. On the other hand, the affinity for the androgen receptor is low, and is negligible for the oestrogen and mineralocorticoid receptors, as has been observed in conventional studies. At any stage of pregnancy RU 486 has an abortifacient effect. It has a strong antiglucocorticoid activity without agonistic effect, as demonstrated by *in vivo* and *in vitro* experiments with various species (Philibert *et al.*, 1981). There is no oestrogenic, anti-oestrogenic, mineralocorticoid or antimineralocorticoid activity at doses tested. The use of RU 486 over a period of 30 days in Sprague–Dawley rats and *Macaca fascicularis* monkeys produced no toxic effects, with the exception of symptoms which can primarily be attributed to the antiglucocorticoid effect at high doses (100 mg/kg per day and more) (Glomot, unpublished results).

In clinical trials RU 486 was found to have a high affinity for the uterine progesterone receptor. In women practically no affinity was observed for transcortin.

Herrmann *et al.* (1982) analysed the abortifacient effect of RU 486 in eleven woman volunteers (18–34 years of age), 6–8 weeks pregnant, who requested an abortion in conformity with the laws of the canton of Geneva. They were given complete information on the experiment before receiving 200 mg of RU 486 a day for 4 days, divided into two or four daily doses.

In seven cases vaginal bleeding occurred the day after administration of the first doses and in two cases the following day. There was an expulsion in two cases on the third day, in three cases on the fourth day, in three cases on the fifth day and in one case on the eighth day. Most of the patients experienced uterine cramps. Ovarian activity returned to normal in all cases where oral contraception was not administered immediately after treatment. In two patients, considered as failures in this experiment, pregnancy was not interrupted. They experienced only light bleeding of late onset and not followed by expulsion. No explanation has been found. Pregnancy was terminated by aspiration. Three further female volunteers aged 23-36 years with normal menstrual cycles (all with intrauterine devices) were given 50 mg RU 486 in the morning of day 22 of their menstrual cycle (7 days after ovulation). This dose was continued over 3 days. Forty-eight hours after the first dose bleedings occurred, which were comparable to but stronger than normal menstrual bleedings. Following the first dose of the compound, serum progesterone, oestrogen, FSH and LH levels were diminished and basal temperature decreased. The following cycle was normal, without any side-effects (Herrmann *et al.*, 1982).

RMI 12 936 (Figure 49), to which has been attributed a remarkable antiprogestin activity, is a $\Delta^{5,3}$ ketosteroid. Its antifertility effect is due to the enhanced transport of the ovum with the expulsion of the egg from the reproductive tract.

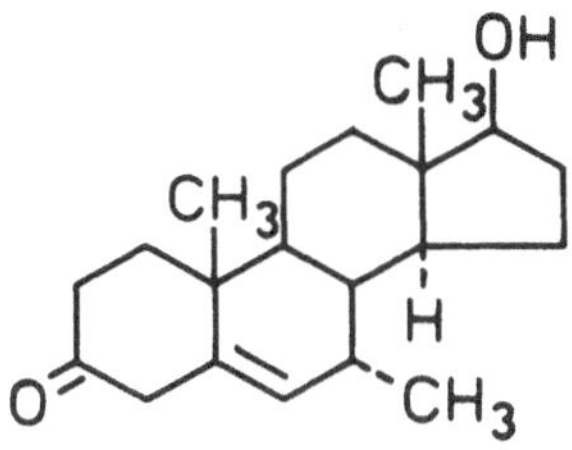

Figure 49 RMI 12 936 (17β-hydroxy-7α-methylandrost-5-en-one)

Preliminary experiments with animals showed that this compound was able to interrupt pregnancy in healthy rats when it was administered prior to implantation—i.e. on days 1-8 of pregnancy or shortly before delivery on day 19. RMI 12 936 had similar characteristics to those of the standard synthetic oestrogen ethinyloestradiol in functional tests. The termination of pregnancy following drug administration on day 1 of pregnancy was linked with a significant simultaneous reduction of ovarian weight, which was postulated to be a cause of corpus luteum regression. Experiments with the transport of the ovum demonstrated a reduced viability of the eggs following treatment with RMI 12 936 prior to implantation. A further important effect is the receptivity of the uterus for the ova.

When RMI 12 936 was given on day 8 of pregnancy, resorption of the fetus resulted. This effect was accompanied by a significant increase in weight, due to luteal hypertrophy. Even with progesterone implants capable of supporting pregnancy in ovariectomized rats, this effect was irreversible.

In studies to elucidate the mechanisms of antifertility activity in rats (Kendle, 1976) it is evident that luteal hypertrophy due to the use of RMI

12 936 occurred in pregnant, but not in pregnant and hysterectomized rats. A similar hypertrophy was achieved in pseudopregnant and immature, gonadotrophin-treated rats. Therefore it seems likely that a direct action on the functional corpus luteum is mediated via a luteotrophic factor of the uterus.

As RMI 12 936 is a $\Delta^{5,3}$ ketosteroid, it does not compete with labelled progesterone at the cytosolic receptor. One hypothesis concerning its mechanism of action is the suppression of progesterone biosynthesis. RMI 12 936 may thereby act as a competitive substrate of the $\Delta^{5,3}$-ketosteroid isomerase, decreasing the isomerization of pregn-5-en-3,20-dione and it is itself isomerized to 7α-methyltestosterone. 7α-Methyltestosterone either is a competitive inhibitor of progesterone on the receptor or is further metabolized. In experiments testing antifertility in rats, 7α-methyltestosterone had a similar effect and potency to those of RMI 12 936.

No data on clinical trials are available.

The results of the experiments with RMI 12 936 on the suppression of ovulation suggest that RMI 12 936 has long-term biological effects, following a single administration of the compound. RMI 12 936 can act as an anti-oestrogen as well as an antiprogestin.

Since the original aim of antiprogestin treatment was to influence the cycle for only a short period of time, the long-term effects of RMI 12 936 are undesirable. Further experiments are necessary to test whether this is due to a slow excretion of the mother substance, the formation of an active metabolite with a prolonged duration of action or the interruption of the sequence of events, which cannot be induced without an oxogenous stimulus.

In conclusion, antiprogestins may become useful compounds for contraception or for use as abortifacients. The respective substances may be administered at mid-cycle in the early luteal phase before or after the expected menstruation. The increased safety resulting from the use of antigestogens for contraception is ensured if the pharmacological interruption of the menstrual cycle can be reduced to a period of one or two days of the cycle. A method which depends on administration at a precisely determined time of the cycle will lose some of its high efficiency, since the interdependent events of the menstrual cycle vary among women and among cycles. Therefore the ideal compound must be sufficiently effective independent of the exact time of administration within the cycle. In spite of the difficulty in the development of such an ideal compound, this approach to finding an improved method in contraception seems very promising.

Influence of number of receptors   A recent review by members of the World Health Organization concluded that a manipulation of receptor function is very promising with a view to the development of new effective contraceptive compounds (Aitken and Harper, 1977). Various attempts had been made to synthesize alkylated receptor proteins (Clark *et al.*, 1968; Solo and Gardner, 1968, 1971). When diazoketone derivatives of 17-hydroxyprogesterone were used, it was observed that an alkylation of the receptor had not occurred. The initial success with the synthesis of antiprogestins (Beyer *et al.*, 1976) is based on the conversion of di-all-cylamino-acyl to alkylated derivatives of 17-hydroxyprogesterone (Beyer *et al.*, 1976). However, all derivatives had a low affinity for progesterone receptors, which made it unlikely that they would be active as antiprogestin compounds.

Structure–effect relationships demonstrated that full progestin activity was present with 1α- and 7α-substituted progesterone (Junkmann, 1954). Some of these derivatives even show a changed binding outside the site that is occupied by progesterone itself. The addition of several functional groups in the 1α- and 7α-positions may even enhance such binding sites outside the progesterone-binding site and may cause receptor blockade. Other laboratory investigations have shown that substituents in positions C-1 and C-7 have a high activity as inhibitors of oestrogen biosynthesis (Brueggemeier et al., 1978).

An alternative approach is the application of anti-oestrogens just before menstruation in order to inhibit the synthesis of progesterone receptors. The advantage is the availability of some anti-oestrogens such as RU 16117 (11α-methoxy-19-nor-17α-1,3,5(10)-pregnatriene-20-yn-3,17-diol: Roussel Uclaf) (Raynaud et al., 1975).

Inductional abortion after the 9th week of gestation

INHIBITION OF PLACENTAL PROGESTERONE SYNTHESIS

At present various groups are investigating steroidogenic blockers, especially inhibitors of 3β-hydroxydehydrogenase-Δ^{5,4}-isomerase (Shinada et al., 1978). It is obvious that inhibition of the enzyme systems will lead to inhibition of steroid production, for which progesterone and 17α-hydroxyprogesterone are precursors. The blockage of progesterone action at the cellular level in the uterus by compounds with antiprogestational activity would theoretically offer a method of high specificity. Investigators suggested that a progesterone antagonist, especially a compound with high affinity for progesterone receptors but without activity, would give effective antigestogens. The search for compounds with antiprogestational activity has been pursued by various groups for possible use as early abortifacients. Until now substances have been developed by affinity labelling (such as 16α-bromoacetoxyprogesterone) (Clark et al., 1975) or R 2323 (13-ethyl-17 ethinyl-17α-hydroxy-gona-4,9,11-trien-3-one) (Sakiz and Azadian-Boulanger, 1971). The first-named compound has been used only in animal experiments, whereas the other compound was administered to women as an early abortifacient and has been found ineffective (Mora et al., 1975).

DIRECT INFLUENCE ON THE CONTRACTILITY OF THE MYOMETRIUM

The induction of natural labour involves pituitary oxytocin. During human pregnancy an increase in oxytocin receptor numbers occurs and the response of the uterus to oxytocin changes. This receptability is highest in the second half of pregnancy. Although contractions can be brought about, only in few cases has abortion been induced. In general, the administration of prostaglandins prior to oxytocin is required. The concurrent administration of both compounds is regarded as unsafe.

Substances with unclassified mechanisms of action as abortifacients

PLANT EXTRACTS

Some plant extracts have been used for centuries as abortifacients in tribal medicine. There are many plants which, applied properly and at the right time, may inhibit fertilization or implantation of the fertilized egg and have bleeding-inducing characteristics. Most herbs with abortifacient effect contain ethereal oils. In addition, they contain amaroids and tannins. Some plants act as poisons, mostly alkaloids. Others inhibit cell division (e.g. *Colchicum*) or contain hormone-like substances, which can induce contractions (e.g. *Caulophyllum*). Nearly all herbs need to be administered very early, ideally prior to menstruation, but at the latest 5 days after the expected menstrual bleeding. A problem is the dose (e.g. with saffron and parsley). It has to be high enough to act, but should not cause health hazards. The limits differ from woman to woman. In addition, not every woman responds to each herb, and the most potent herbs are difficult to acquire. The efficacy of plant contraception has partially been investigated by modern, pharmacological methods and has been approved.

In order to cause abortion or increased perfusion, 5 g real saffron has to be boiled in ¾ l water and left to stand for 15 min. This solution has to be drunk within 8 h in small portions without reheating. Bleeding can occur up to 10 days later.

For the use of *Crotalaria juncea* Linn., see p. 47.

Abortion was caused by *Juniperus communis* if the drug was administered on days 14, 15 and 16 of pregnancy.

A mixture of 100 g of equal parts (1 part = 1 teaspoonful) of valerian or *Caulophyllum thalictroides* is prepared together with a part of rainfarn, two parts of wine root, one part of thyme, two parts of *Menta pulegium*, one part of mistletoe and one part of blue holy herb. The roots are cooked for 5 min, herbs are added and the tea is left to stand for 10 min. In all, ¾ l is

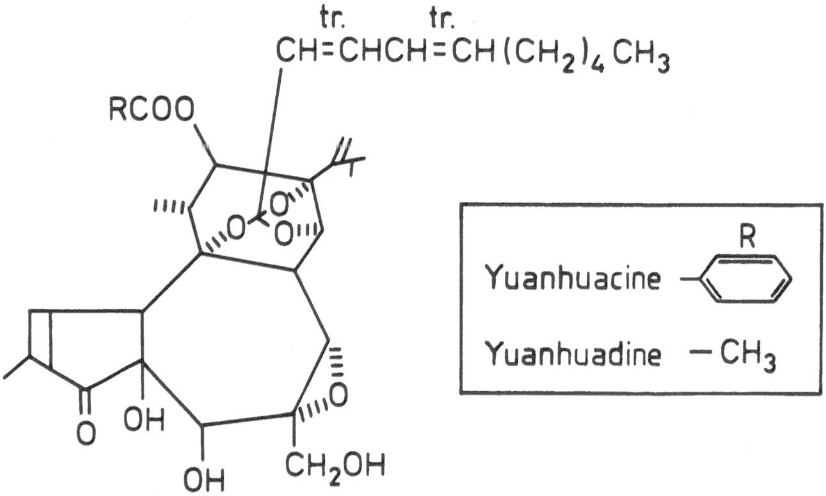

Figure 50   Structural formulas of yuanhuacine and yuanhuadine

drunk daily over a day. It is best to begin three or four days after the non-appearance of menstrual bleeding and to continue for 10 days or until bleeding occurs. Following the tea treatment one cup of nettle, shepherd's purse and lady's mantle is proposed to be drunk for several days.

Two diterpenoids have been isolated from the roots of *Daphne genkwa*— yuanhuacine and yuanhuadine (Figure 50). Yuanhuacine is administered in low doses of 60–80 µg intra- or extra-amniotically. The success rates are 98% and 84%, respectively. Serious side-effects are fever and strong pain due to uterine contractions; in some cases uterine tears have been observed. Analysis of the placenta shows necrosis in the area of the decidua but not of the trophoblast (Wang and Shuy, 1970). The abortifacient effect seems to be caused by a remarkable increase in prostaglandin synthesis. Unfortunately, adequate animal toxicological investigations into the long-term safety of yuanhuacine have not yet been carried out.

MALE CONTRACEPTION

General considerations

Male contraception consists generally of inhibition of spermatogenesis or prevention of fertilization. Different approaches for male contraception are summarized in Table 24.

The problem in male contraception is the fact that the individual drugs must not influence testicular testosterone production and secondary male characteristics. Furthermore, the substances should not have a mutagenic effect because by mutation of one spermatogonium the genetic defect will be reproduced many times. This is in contrast to female contraception, in which a mutation of one single oocyte seems not be so important statistically.

Ideal contraception for the male should induce azoospermia without any short- or long-term side-effects, and no more than one dose per day should be applied orally.

Under ideal conditions only a few or no spermatocytes should be detectable in the ejaculate. However, there is no consensus in the literature on the lowest sperm concentration inducing or causing infertility. It has to be taken into consideration that, even in healthy men, the sperm count varies from 10×10^6 to 250×10^6 per day (Smith *et al.*, 1977). In infertile couples a sperm count of less than 5×10^6 per ml has resulted in pregnancy.

Table 24 lists the different approaches for suppression of male reproductive function.

Inhibition of spermatogenesis and spermiogenesis

Substances blocking spermatogenesis and leading to infertility should fulfil the following conditions: (1) They should selectively block spermatogenesis without influencing the hypophyseal control of the testis (via gonadotrophin secretion and inhibiting testicular testosterone production). (2) They should have no influence on spermatogonia and spermatocytes, which would cause an irreversible loss of fertility and possible genetic mutations.

Table 24   Novel approaches to male contraception

Site of action	Mechanism of action	Route	Substance	Assessment
(a) testicular site of action = inhibition of spermatogenesis and spermiogenesis indirect site of action on testis = effect on incretoric testicular function				
Hypothalamus	inhibition of GnRH action on the hypothalamus: GnRH antagonist GnRH agonist	nasal spray, implantables, depot injections (e.g. with microcapsule)		clinical trial
Pituitary	inhibition of gonadotrophin secretion in the pituitary	implantables depot injections	oestrogens progestins androgens FSH inhibitors: inhibin	trial stage trial stage trial stage no experimental trials
Leydig cell	inhibition of gonadotrophin action in the Leydig cell			no experimental trials
	inhibition of testosterone biosynthesis in the testis	oral	steroidogenic blockers	trial stage
	inhibition of testosterone action in the testis	oral	antiprogestins: cyproterone acetate	clinical trial
	inhibition of testosterone transport by influence on androgen-binding proteins	oral, parenteral	testosterone and derivatives antiandrogenic synthetic steroids	clinical trial trial stage
	inhibition of testosterone action on androgen-dependent tubular cells	oral, parenteral	antiandrogens: cyproterone acetate	clinical trial
Influence in cell division	mitotic inhibitors	oral	alkylants: chlormethin derivatives alkansulphonic acid ester heterocyclic compounds antibiotics	trial stage
Sertoli cells	influence on Sertoli cell function	oral, parenteral	non-steroidal substances: glucose analogues steroids cyproterone acetate	trial stage

Site of action	Mechanism of action	Route	Substance	Assesment
Testicular tubuli	vascularization inhibited	oral	metal salts: cadmium salts other heavy metals	trial stage
Spermatogenesis	cytotoxicity heat damage ultrasound X-ray	oral local local local	gossypol	clinical trial trial stage trial stage trial stage
(b) post-testicular site of action				
Epididymis	disturbance of spermatic maturation		chlorohydrine	trial stage
Ductus deferens	spermatozoa transport: chemical mechanical	vasectomy: ligature extra- or intravasal blockage valve blockage	guanethidine	trial stage
Seminal plasma	liquefaction of sperms composition			no experimental trials
Sperms	motility and spermatic metabolism			trial stage
	capacitation	systemic immunization: sorbit dehydrogenase lactate dehydrogenase		trial stage
	inhibition of penetration enzymes	enzymatic inhibition: acrosine inhibitors protease inhibitors	NPGB (p-nitrophenyl guanidine benzoate) e.g. trypsinine inhibitor	trial stage

Testicular mode of action

INDIRECT INHIBITION OF INCRETORY TESTICULAR FUNCTION

Hypothalamus Continuous stimulation of the GnRH receptor (Figure 51) by superphysiological doses of the naturally occurring releasing hormone or its very potent releasing hormone agonists may cause sterility. The releasing hormones are secreted under the control of central nervous system neurons in the hypothalamus and transported to the pituitary by neurosecretion. At the pituitary level the specific trophic hormones LH, FSH,

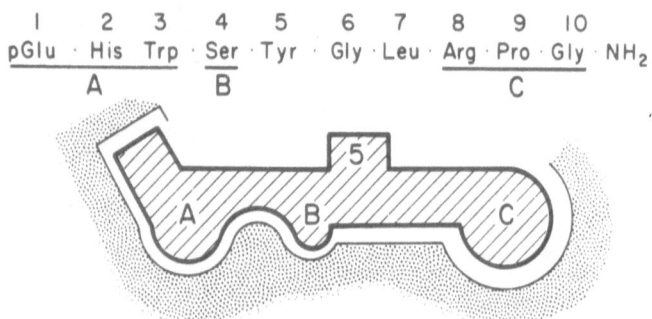

Figure 51   Schematic model of a GnRH receptor

TSH, ACTH and STH are secreted. The secretion of LH and FSH can be inhibited either by down-regulation of the pituitary GnRH receptor or by blockage with a non-biologically active GnRH molecule (GnRH antagonist), which prevents stimulation by endogenous GnRH.

It was suggested in 1971 that antagonists of GnRH can be used for contraception, while the agonists should be developed for the treatment of infertility. During clinical studies it could be proved that all the agonists have antifertility effects.

A large number of synthetic analogues with varying biological activity have been analysed for agonists and antagonists of GnRH. It could be shown that amino acids at both ends of the peptide chains are essential for both receptor binding and biological activity.

The central part of the GnRH molecule can be chemically modified without influencing receptor binding and biological activity. In tests with modified GnRH molecules, analogues have been found which are 150 times more potent than normal GnRH. Antagonists of the GnRH can be applied in female rats, in which they lead to prevention of ovulation; however, they were not effective in male rats. Chronic application of GnRH or GnRH analogues in animals led to an inhibition of gonadotrophin secretion and hypo-oestrogenism. The action was called 'paradoxical suppression of the activity of GnRH superagonists'.

By application of GnRH superagonists, the following biological effects could be obtained.

(1) Superagonists suppress the normal GnRH-dependent gonadotrophin synthesis and secretion; this leads to a diminished gonadotrophin secretion and, therefore, to a decrease in testicular steroidogenesis.

(2) GnRH superagonists stimulate gonadotrophin secretion, which induces initially an increase in gonadotrophin levels and testicular steroidogenesis but later suppresses gonadotrophin secretion by negative feedback on the level of hypothalamic–pituitary regulation. The result is a decrease in gonadotrophin and testicular steroidogenesis.

(3) Stimulation of gonadotrophin secretion. An increase in LH secretion and a decrease in LH receptor in the testes leading to a decrease in LH-dependent stimulation of the testis. In addition, a decrease in testicular androgen biosynthesis.

(4) Direct influence on testicular steroidogenesis. However, it has been suggested that only in the rat does the testis as well as the ovary possess specific GnRH receptors. These receptors are responsible for a blockage of testicular steroidogenesis.

During long-term application of GnRH analogues the question arose whether it is necessary to substitute testosterone simultaneously to prevent a decrease in testosterone and changes in the secondary male characteristics, including libido. According to this view it becomes necessary to combine GnRH analogues and testosterone in one treatment. By this combination, spermatogenesis would be suppressed, whereas androgen deficiency would be prevented. It remains unclear whether gonadotrophin secretion can be completely suppressed. It has to be considered that during incomplete suppression of gonadotrophin secretion a short-term increase in LH levels may stimulate spermatogenesis and result in fertility.

(D-Leu^6, des-Gly-NH$_2$^{10})-LHRH ethylamide is a GnRH analogue, in which the amino acid glycine in position 6 has been substituted by D-leucine; furthermore, it contains an N-terminal proline-CH$_2$-CH$_2$-NH$_2$ modification. Its mode of action has not yet been clarified. In rats, injections every three days led to a reduction in the testicular receptor levels, a loss of testicular weight and a fall in serum testosterone levels (Auclair *et al.*, 1977). In an experiment of Swerdloff *et al.* (1978) 60-day-old castrated rats were treated for 7 days with 20–200 ng/100 g body weight. A dose-dependent suppression of gonatrophin secretion was observed. The depression of LH was more marked than that of FSH.

Δ^9-Tetrahydrocannabinol (THC; Figure 52), an alkaloid, is the psychoactive moiety of marijuana. THC leads to the reduction of the male sexual function. This is combined with a depression of testosterone levels in man and various animal species. Furthermore, this compound inhibits rat testicular testosterone biosynthesis.

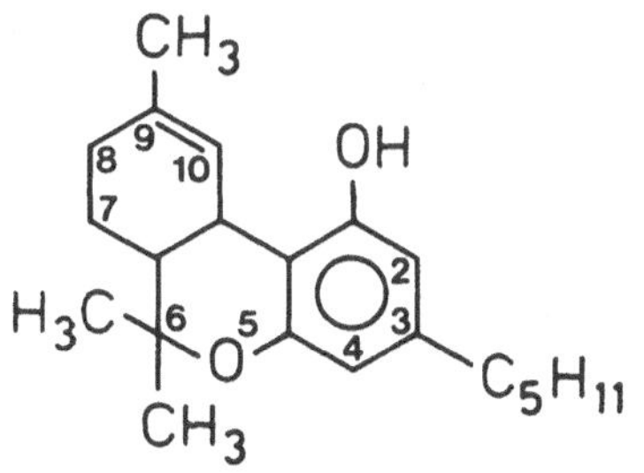

Figure 52 Δ^9-Tetrahydrocannabiol

Pituitary Inhibin is a peptide hormone with a molecular weight of 180 000, which is produced by the Sertoli cells and which selectively inhibits FSH secretion of the pituitary by negative feedback (Greep *et al.*, 1976). Germinal cells also secrete inhibin. As the function of the Sertoli cells is FSH-dependent, selective suppression of FSH secretion leads to a decrease in their function and a suppression of spermiogenesis. Theoretically, the advantage of inhibin would depend on a selective inhibition of spermatogenesis without influencing testosterone secretion, libido and function of the accessory sexual glands. Until now it has remained unclear whether inhibin can be used clinically, because no information on pharmacokinetics is available. In animal tests the half-life of inhibin is shorter in adult than in premature animals.

Observations of the action of N-methylthiocarbamoyl-N'-(1-methylallyl-thiocarbamoyl)hydrazine (methallibure) lead to the presumption that the suppressed gonadotrophin secretion depends on the effect of methallibure on the hypothalamus and on GnRH release. Side-effects are fatigue, lethargy, anorexia and nausea. Tests with rats show a reduction of the seminal vesicle, the ventral prostate and the testis. In contrast, the weight of the seminal vesicle did not change when methallibure was combined with postmenopausal gonadotrophin. In a dose of 10 mg given over a period of 6 days to male rats, methallibure suppresses the LH level. In similarly treated rats which were administered 100 ng synthetic GnRH, the plasma LH level was comparable with that of the GnRH-treated, castrated control group.

DL-6-(N-α-Pipecolinmethyl)-5-hydroxyindan maleate (Figure 53) (PMHI)

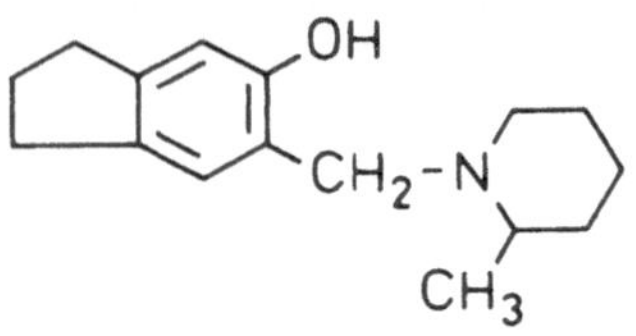

Figure 53   PMHI

acts by inhibition of androgen production in comparison with gonadotrophin secretion. The mode of action is not yet established. It may be of interest that zinc chlorides in drinking water prevent testicular atrophy in rats treated with PMHI. In rats treated with PMHI (1.5 mg/kg per day over 21 days) a significant reduction of the testicular and prostate weight was observed (Boris *et al.*, 1974). Comparable results could be obtained in rabbits, dogs, monkeys, hamsters and guinea-pigs. Daily oral doses of 6.25 mg/kg or an individual dose of 150 mg/kg induced permanent sterility (Boris *et al.*, 1974). Due to the irreversible sterility induced by PMHI this compound is of low interest for contraceptive purposes.

Leydig cell   Gonadal steroids can be used for male contraception, because of their inhibition of pituitary gonadotrophins, which leads to suppression of spermatogenesis with subsequent azoospermia. In this context, oestrogens, progestins and androgens can be administered; the disadvantage of the various compounds is that the individual doses of some substances are very high and, therefore, related to side-effects (e.g. feminizing side-effects), which limit the clinical application of these compounds. Of these compounds, the progestogens and androgens show the most potent contraceptive activity in man. Several studies are concerned with clinical efficiency of the compounds and various combinations. These investigations could show in good agreement that 200 mg testosterone enanthate (Figure 54), given at longer intervals of 10 days, leads to an interruption of spermatogenesis and thus to a decrease in the sperm count in the ejaculate of the test persons.

Clinical tests with testosterone enanthate (TE) showed that all volunteers

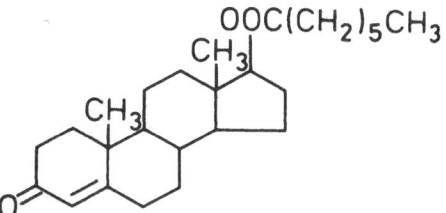

Figure 54   Testosterone enanthate

($n=7$) treated with 25 mg/day TE for 60 days developed azoospermia. This azoospermia improved 150 days after withdrawal of the drug (Reddy and Rao, 1972). Mauss *et al.* (1974) studied 7 men being given 250 mg TE per day for 21 weeks. However, azoospermia could not be detected in all cases: 4 men had a sperm count of less than 1×10^6/ml and the others counts lower than 5×10^6/ml. The FSH and LH levels were diminished, whereas the testosterone levels increased to twice the normal values. Six months after withdrawal of TE, normal sperm counts could be measured.

Paulsen *et al.* (1978) performed a clinical study with 42 men being given 200 mg TE per week over a period of 6 months. Sperm count was less than 5×10^6/ml in 39 men; 20 of 39 men showed azoospermia. In one of the test persons gynaecomasty could be detected. Five months after withdrawal of the drug, normal sperm count could be observed.

Clinical trials by Swerdloff *et al.* (1978) and Cunningham *et al.* (1979) also showed that 200 mg/week TE over 16 weeks and 200 mg/week over 12 weeks, respectively, caused azoospermia and recovery of normal sperm count after the withdrawal of the drug.

With these factors borne in mind, testosterone enanthate may be used as a male contraceptive if it is administered according to a fixed schedule. The following two-phase treatment should be performed: after a 4-week high-dose initial therapy, suppression of spermiogenesis can be maintained by injections of 200 mg TE every 10 days.

According to recent reports by Nieschlag *et al.* (1984), 19-nortestosterone can inhibit spermiogenesis without any remarkable side-effects. This anabolic drug has been tested in a group of sportsmen. Further clinical trials are yet to be performed. It has to be considered that this drug was admin-

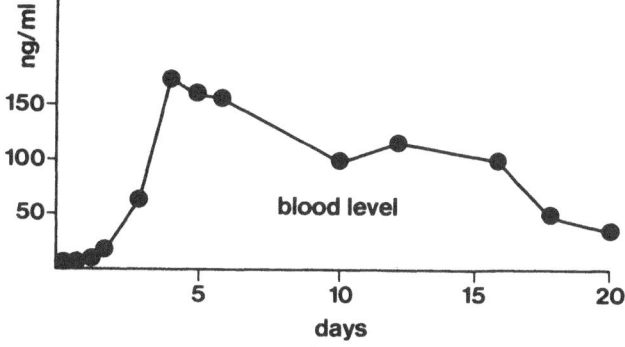

Figure 55   Blood levels of testosterone enanthate after i.m. injection of various doses (mg)

istered in a 200 or 300 mg dose every week; an oral application is impossible, owing to the toxic effect of the methylation of the compound. Blood levels of testosterone enanthate after i.m. injections are shown in Figure 55. The time course of testosterone propionate and testosterone enanthate (i.m. injection) is shown in Figure 56, and Figure 57 shows testosterone levels in blood and testis.

In conclusion, the prospects for the development of hormonal substances for safe and effective male contraception are good.

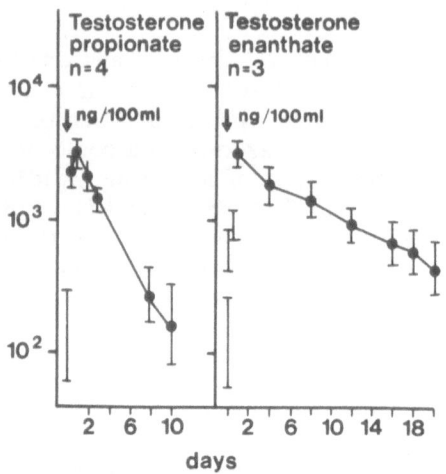

Figure 56 Serum levels of testosterone after i.m. injection of testosterone propionate (mg) or testosterone enanthate (mg)

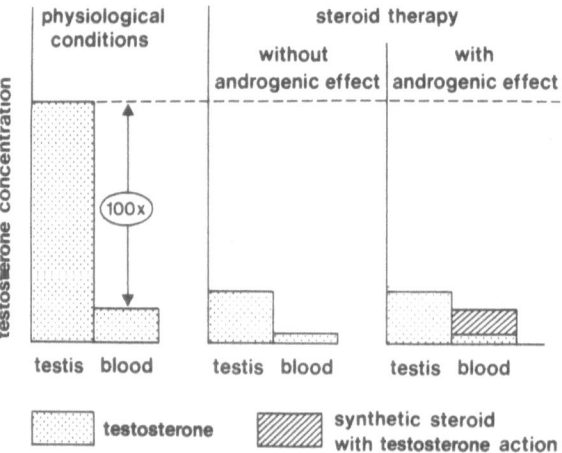

Figure 57 Testosterone levels in testis and blood. Under physiological conditions, testosterone concentration in the testicular tissue is approximately 100 times higher than in peripheral blood. After administration of an androgen without peripheral androgen action, a decrease in testosterone can be observed both in testis and in blood. Testicular androgen deficiency causes azoospermia, androgen deficiency in the peripheral blood, a loss of libido, and a disturbance of secondary male characteristics. Only an androgen with peripheral androgen action can inhibit testicular androgen biosynthesis and, thereby, cause a decrease in testicular testosterone production without influencing peripheral androgen action

Danazol (17α-pregna-2,4-dien-20 ino(2,3-*d*)isoxazol-17-ol) is a synthetic derivative of ethinyl testosterone (Figure 58). It possesses a strong antigonadotrophic effect (Neumann *et al.*, 1977); investigations were able to show that danazol also has a steroidogenic inhibiting action (Rabe *et al.* 1983/84).

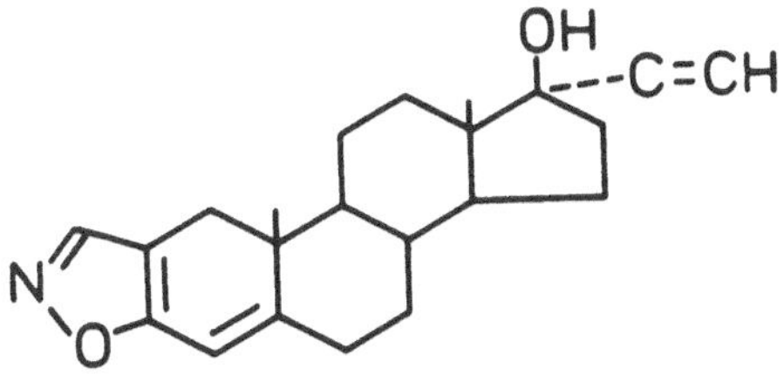

Figure 58   Danazol

Danazol (800 mg/day) was given to male volunteers receiving 200 mg testosterone enanthate monthly. Eight of 54 men showed a sperm count below 5×10^6/ml; in 19 men azoospermia could be observed; and gynaecomasty was found in 2 (Leonhard and Paulsen, 1978).

It could be shown that male rats treated with increasing amounts of androgens showed a decrease in testicular weight due to inhibition of LH. This induced an intratesticular androgen deficiency. In tests in which higher doses were applied, a sufficiently high concentration in the testis could be obtained, leading to an increase in testicular weight.

Cyproterone acetate (CPA: 1-methyl-6-chlor-α-⁶-progesterone-16-hydroxy acetate) is a strong anti-androgen which is a derivative of 16-hydroxy progesterone (Figure 59). It induces a decrease in serum testosterone and, furthermore, reduced spermatogenesis and sperm count in the male.

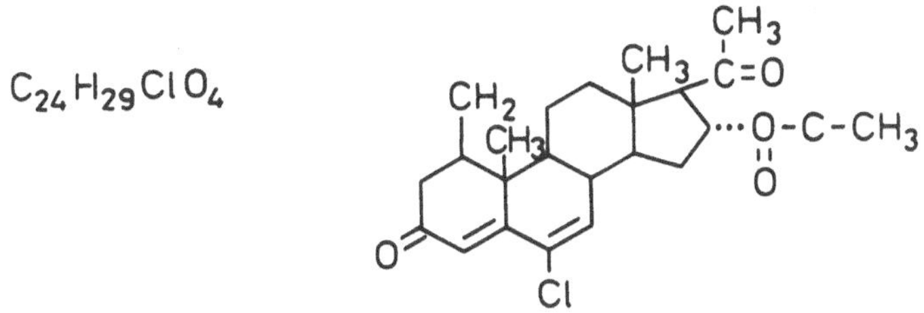

$C_{24}H_{29}ClO_4$

Figure 59   Cyproterone acetate

Toxicity of cyproterone acetate could be demonstrated in the male opossum (*Didelphia virginiana*) in a dose range of 22–28 mg/kg after i.m. administration. A decrease in spermatocytes in the epididymis occurred only 2 weeks after cyproterone acetate induced testicular degeneration (Heath *et al.*, 1983). The use of isomers 1-amino-3-chloro-2-propanol hydrochloride (CL 88 236 and CL 88 237) was tolerated up to a dosage of 30 mg/kg i.m. Eight days after the use of CL 88 236 and CL 88 237 an effect on the spermatocyte conjugation in the epididymis and in the semen-producing epithelium could be observed (Heath *et al.*, 1983).

Thirty fertile men were treated with CPA in a medium dose range over a period of 12–36 weeks. Sperm count and hormone measurements were performed before, during and after the treatment. CPA decreases sperm count, sperm concentration and motility. An increase in dead, pathologically changed and immature spermatocytes was observed. Glycerylphosphorylcholine and acid phosphatase were diminished in the seminal plasma; alkaline phosphatase was increased. Fructose concentration was normal. CPA led to a significant suppression of FSH and LH; furthermore, it led to a suppression of the pituitary response to GnRH. Peripheral testosterone and dihydrotestosterone levels were depressed. These metabolic changes occurred 15–18 weeks after CPA administration. All metabolic changes are fully reversible and no decrease in libido occurred. Conception occurred after a 12-week treatment.

The mode of the molecular contraceptive action of CPA has not been fully elucidated because the clinical studies described are Phase 1 studies. CPA administration inhibits in a high degree adrenocorticotrophic synthesis of steroids. This anti-androgen could also inhibit hypothalamic GnRH stimulation of pituitary LH secretion.

Fluoxymestrone (9-fluor-11-hydroxy-16-methyl-testosterone) is a synthetic anti-androgen (Figure 60). Studies in man have shown that it induces a fall in testosterone without changing LH or FSH secretion (Jones *et al.*, 1977). Only a medium-range decrease in sperm concentration could be observed.

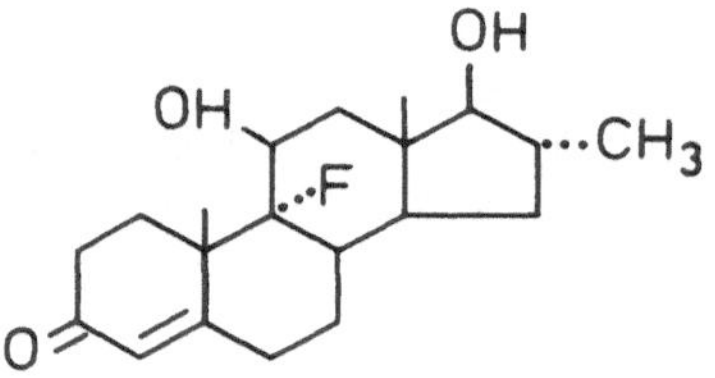

Figure 60   Fluoxymestrone

DIRECT INHIBITION OF SPERMATOGENESIS AND SPERMIOGENESIS

Influence on cell cleavage   Tretamin (TEM) belongs to the group of 1,3,5-triazines (Figure 61). It is an aziridine derivative, and is an alkylating substance which blocks irreversibly spermatogenesis by destruction of the spermatogonia.

In animal studies tretamin caused infertility in a dose of 0.05 mg/kg per day, which showed a recovery 2–4 weeks after withdrawal. TEM acts on

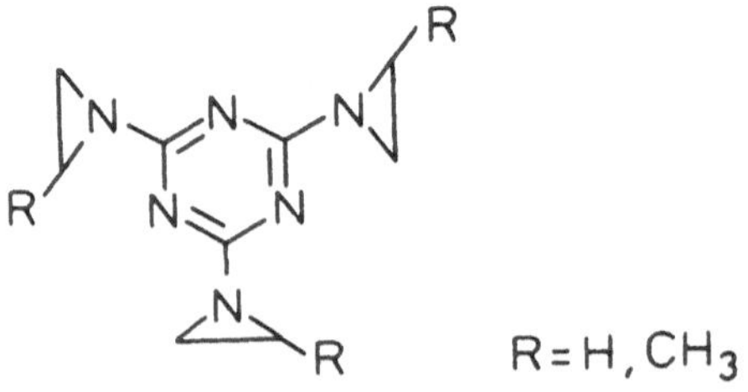

$R = H, CH_3$

Figure 61   Tretamin

cells in cleavage and on spermatocytes. It is not certain whether the drug has any effects on the embryo. It is assumed that TEM has a potentially mutagenic action and therefore would not be a good systemic antifertility drug (Jackson and Bock, 1955; Jackson *et al.*, 1959).

Another embryotoxic substance of this group is methyl sulphonate (MSS), which was found to react with DNA and RNA in ^{14}C-labelling experiments (Lawley and Brooks, 1963).

Busulphane (butane-dimethyl-sulphonester) is the first drug of the group of alkane sulphone esters to be used for the prevention of fertilization (Figure 62). In animal studies, after a single busulphane administration of 10 mg/kg, fertility remained normal for about 7 weeks; thereafter, the animals became sterile, which might depend on azoospermia. This suggests that busulphane inhibits the proliferation of the spermatogonia, whereas more mature cells can develop normally to spermatocytes. The duration of sterility after busulphane administration is dose-dependent (Neumann *et al.*, 1977).

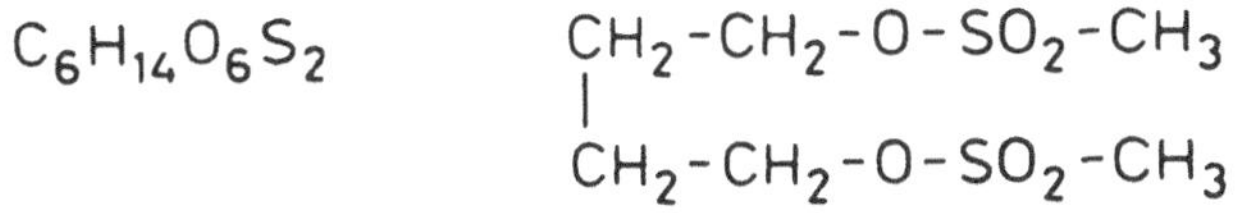

$$C_6H_{14}O_6S_2 \qquad \begin{array}{l} CH_2-CH_2-O-SO_2-CH_3 \\ | \\ CH_2-CH_2-O-SO_2-CH_3 \end{array}$$

Figure 62 Busulphane

Triethylenephosphoramide (TEPA; Figure 63) is an alkylating substance. The administration of 5×0.4 mg/kg allows fertilization, but owing to damage to the chromosomes, development of an embryo is inhibited (Epstein *et al.*, 1970; Joshi *et al.*, 1970).

Some heterocyclic compounds inhibit spermatogenesis without influencing the endocrine function of the testis. Figures 64, 65 and 66 show the molecular structures of the most important compounds of this group.

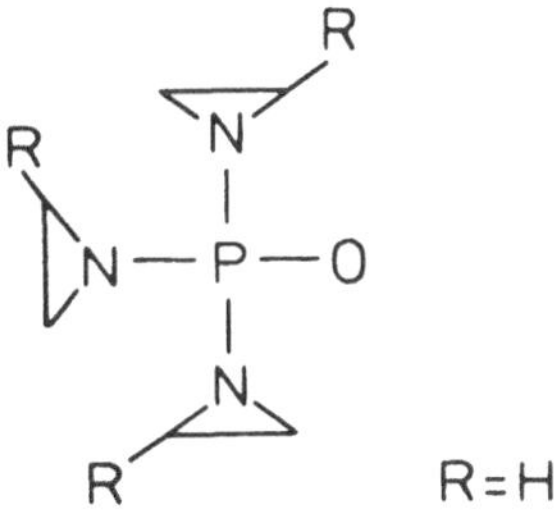

Figure 63 TEPA

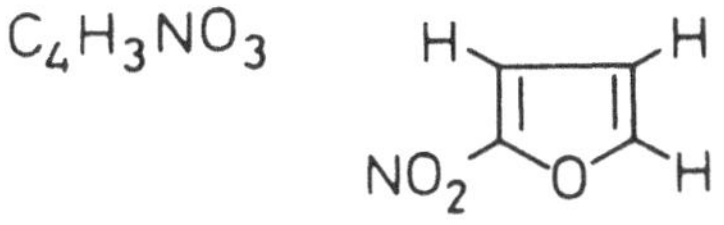

$$C_4H_3NO_3$$

Figure 64 Nitrofurane

$$C_4H_4S$$

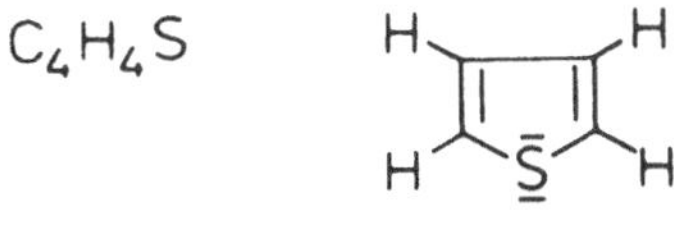

Figure 65 Thiophene

$$O_2N-\underset{N}{\langle\rangle}-NO_2$$

Figure 66   Dinitropyrrol

$$\underset{Cl}{\overset{Cl}{\diagdown}}CH-CO-\underset{\underset{C_2H_5}{|}}{N}-CH_2-\langle\rangle-CH_2-\underset{\underset{C_2H_5}{|}}{N}-CO-CH\overset{Cl}{\underset{Cl}{\diagup}}$$

Figure 67   WIN 13 099

$$\underset{Cl}{\overset{Cl}{\diagdown}}CH-CO-NH-(CH_2)_8-NH-CO-CH\overset{Cl}{\underset{Cl}{\diagup}}$$

Figure 68   WIN 18 446

Ditrooxyzone and nitrofurantoin also suppress spermatogenesis in the stage of early spermatocytes (Neumann *et al.*, 1978). Relevant clinical tests in men were able to show that these compounds lead to infertility; however, major toxic side-effects prohibit their use.

Inhibition of meiosis can also be achieved by suppression with other compounds with a heterocyclic 5-ring system—for instance, 5-chloro-2-acetylthiophene and 1-(*N,N*-diethylcarbamoyl-methyl)-2,5-dinitropyrrol (Neumann *et al.*, 1978). These compounds could not be used for contraception because of their toxic side-effects. Their antifertility mechanism has not yet been demonstrated.

Another group of compounds acts by direct destruction of the germinal epithelium. The two most effective drugs of this group are *N,N'*-bis-(dichloracetyl)-*N,N*-diethyl-1,4-xylenediamine (WIN 13 099) (Figure 67) and *N,N'*-bis(dichloracetyl)-1,8-octmethylenediamine (WIN 18 446) (Figure 68). The main effect of these compounds on the testis can be observed in the earliest phases of spermatogenesis. Electron microscopic examination has demonstrated that the Sertoli cells are the target cells for these compounds. Furthermore, these compounds do not interfere with the Leydig cells.

In animal tests with monkeys, rats, dogs, mice and guinea-pigs, a reversible antispermatogenetic action has been shown. Studies with guinea-pigs found an abnormal appearance of the nucleus and acrosome of mature spermatids, and, in addition, the occurrence of multiple large vacuoles in the Sertoli cells and a degeneration of the spermatocytes.

In human studies oligospermia and azoospermia occurred in men (Neumann *et al.*, 1978). However, clinical trials had to be stopped because aldehyde dehydrogenase and some liver enzymes had been suppressed. An examination of the mitochondria of the heart muscle showed that WIN 18 446 suppresses electron transport and oxidative phosphorylation. These biochemical effects allow one to suppose that WIN causes hypoxia in the tissue and exhaustion.

In conclusion, these compounds do not seem to be suitable for contraception.

Antineoplastic drugs (Figure 69) are used for the treatment of the nephrotic syndrome and for cancer treatment. These compounds can reduce fertility (Manson and Simons, 1979).

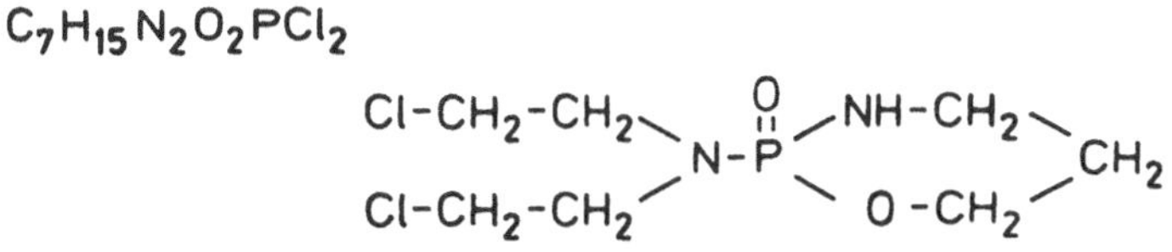

$C_7H_{15}N_2O_2PCl_2$

Cl-CH$_2$-CH$_2$
Cl-CH$_2$-CH$_2$
N-P
O
NH-CH$_2$
O-CH$_2$
CH$_2$

Figure 69 Cyclophosphamide

Adriamycin is successfully used for the treatment of leukaemia. In men and rats, testicular atrophy, destruction of the germinal epithelium, a decrease in the seminal vesicle weight and infertility occurred. FSH increased, as could be shown in studies by Bajpai and Anderson (1982). A correlation with the decreased number of spermatogonia could be demonstrated. The influence of adriamycin on the prostate has not been proved.

Drugs influencing the function of the Sertoli cells   AF 1312/TS, lonidamine and tolnidamine are analogues of a mother compound with the chemical structure 1-(4-chlorbenzyl)-3-carbo-benzyorzol (Figure 70). All three compounds act at the Sertoli cells and induce a morphological change in the epididymis.

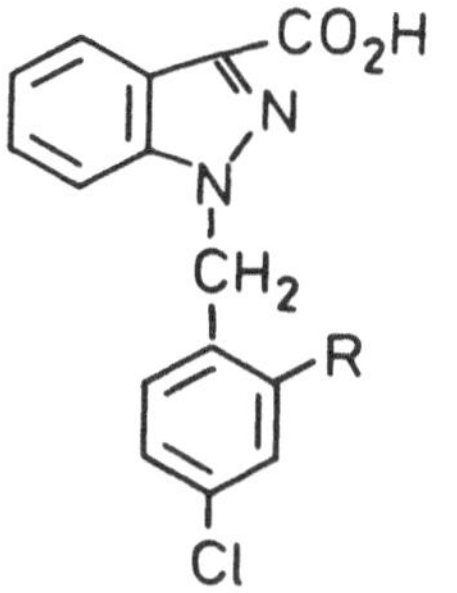

CO$_2$H
N
N
CH$_2$
R
Cl

Figure 70 Structural formula of the basic substance 1(4-chlorbenzyl)-3-carbo-benzyorzol (tolnidamine: R = CH$_3$; lonidamine: AF 1312/TS = R = H)

The mode of action of lonidamine is unknown. It is supposed that this compound acts at the Sertoli cells and not at the Leydig cells. Lonidamine causes a repulsion of immature germinal cells and a reduction in the testicular weight. No changes in the prostate and the seminal vesicles could be detected. In animal tests the LD_{50} in rats and mice was more than 1.7 g/kg (Lobl, 1979). Infertility in 10 of 12 rats occurred when this drug was applied once a month in a dose of 50 mg/kg. The same dose given only once a week caused infertility of 100% of the treated animals, but this was only reversible in 60% of these animals. In a dosage of 500 mg/kg an irreversible infertility occurred (Lobl *et al.*, 1979). FSH was increased 2 days after an application of 50 mg/kg and remained so at day 3 and day 7. No influence on LH and testosterone has been observed. In rhesus monkeys a dosage of 50 mg/kg per week caused a partial and a dosage of 500 mg/kg per week caused a complete suppression of spermatogenesis and no FSH increase (Lobl *et al.*, 1979). The 500 mg dosage was nephrotoxic; this effect, however, was reversible after withdrawal of lonidamine.

AF 1312/TS caused a reduction in testicular weight of adult rats after five oral doses of 200 mg/kg per day (Silversterini *et al.*, 1975). No effect on the accessory genital organs could be observed. Ultrastructural examinations showed various changes in the Sertoli cells, but no direct action in the germinal cells could be detected. The changes in the Sertoli cells consisted of vacuoles in the basal and the apical parts, swollen mitochondria and a large amount of phagocytosed material.

Tolnidamine is less nephrotoxic in action than lonidamine, but it is just as effective. The mode of action has not yet been fully investigated, but tolnidamine seems to have a similar antispermatogenic action to lonidamine. In a higher dosage of 500 mg/kg tolnidamine and 50 mg/kg lonidamine an FSH increase in rats can be observed.

The substances 6-chloro-deoxy-D-glucose and 5-thio-D-glucose belong to the class of chloride sugars.

In 6-chloro-deoxy-D-glucose (6-CDG) the hydroxyl group is substituted by chlorine (Figure 71). *In vitro* incubations of rat spermatocytes with 6-

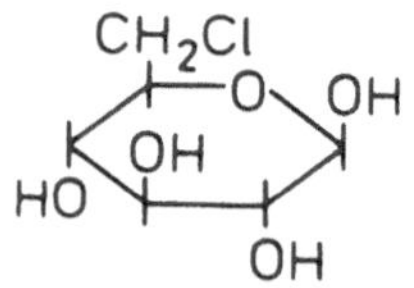

Figure 71   6-Chloro-deoxyglucose

CDG suppressed glucose oxidation (Ford and Waites, 1978a). After the spermatocytes had left the cauda epididymis, the ATP content of the spermatocytes of the animals treated with 6-CDG was 153% higher than in the control group. The specific mode of action needs further analysis.

Reversible infertility is caused in male rats by 6-CDG (Ford and Waites, 1978a, b). The effective dosage is 24–48 mg/kg per day, given once daily. Infertility occurred after 7 days of treatment. After withdrawal of the compound, fertility returned after 1 week. Warren *et al.* (1979) supposed that high doses of 6-CDG are necessary because of its short half-life.

6-CDG penetrates the blood–testis barrier in the rat and suppresses the transport of D-glucose. Owing to this influence on glucose transport, the possibility of using 6-CDG for male contraception is diminished. As glucose metabolism and ATP are necessary in all parts of the body, compounds such as 6-CDG do not seem to solve the problem of male contraception.

5-Thio-D-glucose (5-TG) is a glucose compound in which a sulphydryl residue is introduced at C-5. It is a competitive antagonist of active glucose

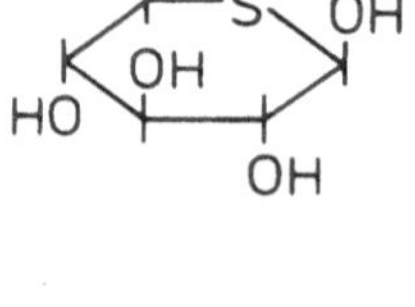

Figure 72   5-Thio-D-glucose

transport and causes sterility in mice by inhibition of spermatogenesis (Zysk et al., 1975; Neumann et al., 1977). Protein synthesis in mature and immature spermatids and spermatocytes was suppressed. However, this effect did not occur in the Sertoli cells and the Leydig cells. The exact mode of action has not yet been determined.

The first histological change in mice is the appearance of giant cells in the tubular lumen after 2 weeks of administration of 5-TG (Zysk et al., 1975). Furthermore, a progressive atrophy of the germinal epithelium occurred and after continuous treatment the testicular weight decreased after 3 weeks. After 7 weeks the tubuli seminiferi contained multinuclear giant cells with lumped nuclei. Some tubuli became atrophic and were filled with calcified debris (Lobl and Porteus, 1978). Following the withdrawal of the drug, fertility returned after 5–8 weeks. After the administration of 50 mg/ kg per day over a period of 49 days, infertility resulted which was not reversible in two-thirds of the animals after drug withdrawal (Lobl and Porteus, 1978). In rat tests, a dosage of 25 or 50 mg/kg per day was applied; fertility did not return after withdrawal. Capsules were implanted in hamsters with a daily release of 30 mg/kg per day. After 5 weeks only one animal of six was sterile; no effect on sperm motility could be observed (Das et al., 1978). In monkeys a suppression of spermatogenesis could be observed (Lobl et al., 1978). No human studies have so far been described in the literature.

5-TG does not seem to be suitable for contraception. It can be used, however, for a specific examination of mechanisms of spermatogenesis (Neumann et al., 1977).

Tubular milieu of the testis Cadmium salts and other metal salts which are, at the moment, in the investigatory stage, act at the tubular milieu by disturbing vascularization.

Dichlorvos (dimethyl-2,2-dichlor vinyl phosphate; Figure 73) is an organic phosphate and is used as an insecticide. Oral administration of dichlorvos leads in mice to degeneration of the tubuli seminiferi and to an interruption of spermatogenesis (Krause and Homola, 1974; Lucier et al., 1977).

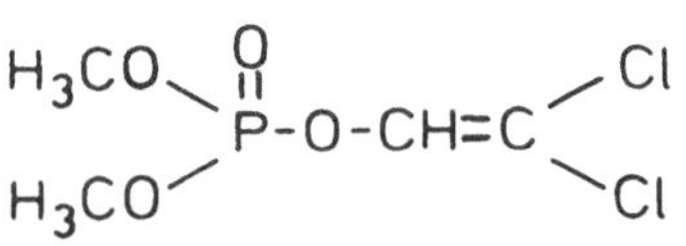

Figure 73 Dichlorvos

Polychlorpinene is a chlorified insecticide and belongs to the group of terpenes (Figure 74). In some animal species it induces change in the tubuli seminiferi (Lucier et al., 1977).

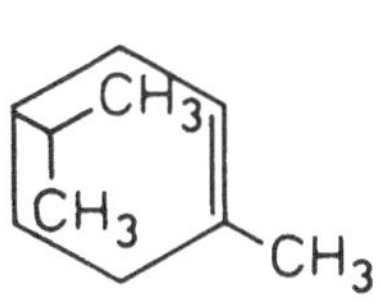

Figure 74 Pinene

Spermatogenesis   Among non-steroidal compounds, gossypol is the only one which in the near future has a realistic chance of being used as an oral contraceptive for males, as could be shown in large-scale clinical WHO trials in China. Clinical application of this compound might be possible, but not before 1990.

Gossypol is a polyphenolic compound with six hydroxyl and two alde-hyde residues; therefore, it is chemically stable (Figure 75). It occurs in three tautomer types: aldehyde, hemiacetal and ketone.

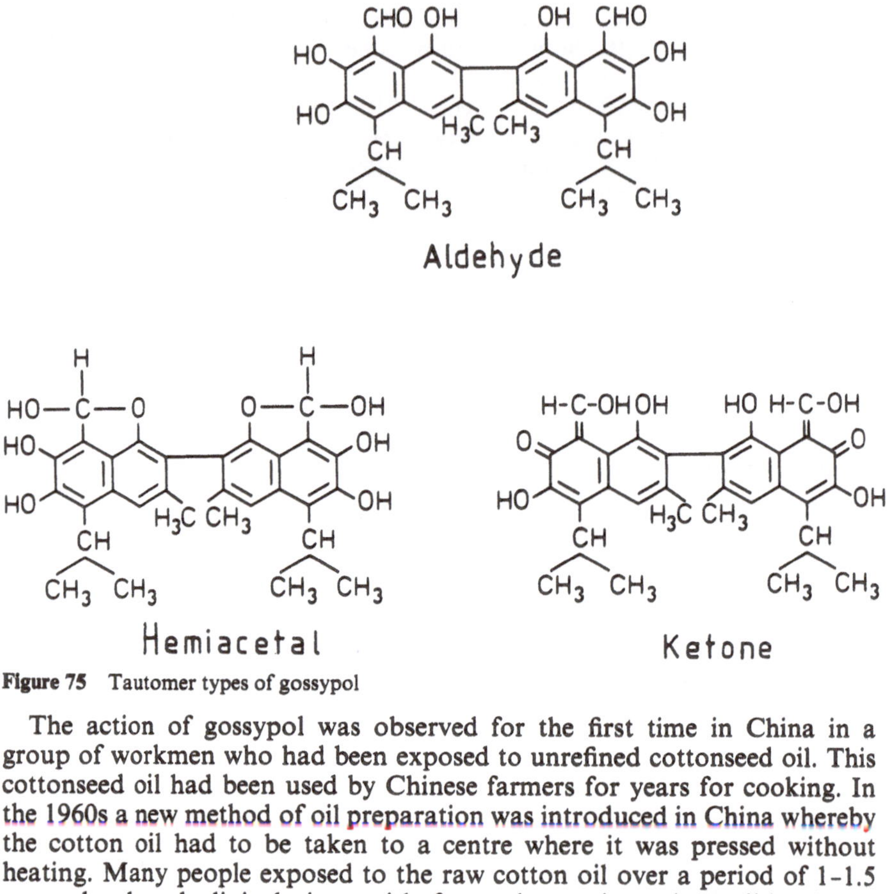

Figure 75   Tautomer types of gossypol

The action of gossypol was observed for the first time in China in a group of workmen who had been exposed to unrefined cottonseed oil. This cottonseed oil had been used by Chinese farmers for years for cooking. In the 1960s a new method of oil preparation was introduced in China whereby the cotton oil had to be taken to a centre where it was pressed without heating. Many people exposed to the raw cotton oil over a period of 1–1.5 years developed clinical signs with fever, dyspepsia and possible photo-phobia. In females amenorrhoea occurred, and males became infertile. Use of the method stopped when it could be shown that these symptoms were caused by the raw cottonseed oil. Normal cycles were restored in amenorrhoeic women, but many of the males remained infertile. Gossypol was isolated as the active compound in the cottonseed oil and was regarded as being responsible for the toxic effects and for the infertility of the Chinese farmers. All cottonseed products which had been used for human nutrition contained gossypol either in a free or in a bound form. The aldehyde groups of gossypol react with the free amino acids of proteins and form bound gossypol, which is less toxic than the free type.

Gossypol has a specific cytotoxic action on some spermatogenic cells, especially on spermatocytes and spermatids, but only a weak effect on steroid hormone production and libido in the male (Lee et al., 1982); furthermore, gossypol does not affect interstitial cells. Studies by Lee were able to show that gossypol selectively activates the testis and spermic lactate dehydrogenase (LDH-X) in vitro, and, furthermore, that some metabolites of gossypol had the same effect. In investigations using high-pressure liquid chromatography gossypol seemed to be stable in organic solvents and unstable in aqueous solvents. These in vitro observations suggest that for in vivo action the identification of gossypol metabolites could be important for its future application as a contraceptive.

Gossypol induces a hypokalaemic paralysis. This occurred in 66 persons of a group of 8806 in the study mentioned above. The occurrence of this paralysis showed regional differences and seems to be related to potassium uptake. At a dosage of 1.0 g potassium chloride/day this side-effect could be avoided. In studies with men in Brazil (Coutinho et al., 1975) no hypokalaemic paralysis occurred.

In hypokalaemic patients treated with gossypol the content of PGE_2 and metabolites in the urine was higher than in the control groups. By administration of indomethacin, a prostaglandin synthetase inhibitor, serum potassium and PGE_2 concentration in the urine were brought to a normal value. On the basis of animal studies with rats, it is supposed that gossypol activates the PG biosynthesis in the kidneys and other organs and tissues. This increase induces a release of potassium. In rats the antispermatogenic effect of gossypol could be partially reversed by aspirin (PG synthetase inhibitor) (Quain, 1982).

The development of possible analogues might lead to a reduction of side-effects and allow of development of substances with a higher drug safety.

In rats high doses of 15–40 mg/kg given over a longer period of time caused the death of the animals as a result of generalized oedema, necrosis of the liver and haemorrhages (Jones and Smith, 1977). Several of the studies showed that the correlation between toxicity and animal species and also the mode of administration, the mineral and the protein content of the food and the cumulative action of free gossypol might be important (Jones, 1977; Herman and Smith, 1973). The general phenomena associated with the toxicity of gossypol in the laboratory and in farm animals are lack of appetite, loss of weight and inefficient protein utilization (Mauss et al., 1975; Jones and Smith, 1977; Nieschlag et al., 1978). The mechanism of the toxic effects of this compound seems to depend on a disturbed iron metabolism and disturbed amino acid utilization. It is not certain that the toxic action of gossypol is related to its antifertility action.

In earlier studies in China male rats had been treated with gossypol acetic acid in a dosage of 40 mg/kg given orally five times daily over a period of 2–4 weeks. This treatment caused the development of headless spermatozoa. The animals became infertile, but showed normal reproductive behaviour. The majority of the animals became fertile again within 4 weeks after withdrawal of the drug (Dai et al., 1978). In this study, too, a dose-dependent action of gossypol could be demonstrated.

The metabolism of radioactive (^{14}C-labelled) gossypol was studied in

China. The intestinal half-life was 9.6 h and the half-life until elimination from the body was 60 h. It took 19 days to eliminate 97% of the labelled gossypol. The highest proportion of gossypol was found 5-48 h after oral administration to mice, rats, rabbits, dogs and monkeys. Large amounts could be detected in the muscle, kidneys and blood. The highest proportion was eliminated in the faeces and a smaller amount in the urine.

The mode of action of gossypol is supposed to be testicular action. Histological investigations showed a loss of germinal cells under chronic treatment. No morphological changes in other organs could be detected. By electron microscopical and autoradiographic studies it could be shown that the spermatocytes, spermatids and spermatocysts react to gossypol (Dai et al., 1978; Hsueh et al., 1979). The acrosomes of the spermatids were swollen and fragmented, and additionally the mitochondria in the middle parts of the spermatozoa showed morphological changes. Leydig cells and epididymal epithelium remained intact (Hsueh et al., 1979).

Since the beginning of the first clinical trials in 1972, 8806 men in 14 provinces of China have been treated with gossypol acetic acid. The doses applied were 20 mg/day over 60-70 days; thereafter a weekly administration of 60 mg was used. The antifertility effect (as defined by sperm concentration of less than 4×10^6/ml) could be demonstrated in more than 99% of the treated males within the first 3 months; the first changes which could be observed were loss of sperm motility, followed by severe oligospermia and azoospermia.

In a subsequent study by Liu (1980) it was shown that 1-4.5 years after the withdrawal of gossypol the sperm concentration exceeded 4×10^6/ml only in 75% of males and approximately 10% of males remained azoospermic.

Further studies showed that gossypol has a direct action on the spermatozoa. Human spermatozoa incubated with a micromolar concentration showed a suppression of motility and, in addition, a change in glucose and fructose metabolism.

In a recent study by Mori et al. (1983) volunteers were treated with gossypol tablets. The administration of gossypol tablets over 19 days in a daily dosage of 20 mg/day showed a falling tendency of sperm concentration and sperm count. No action on LH, FSH, prolactin and testosterone could be observed. The volunteers had no complaints and no side-effects could be detected in the laboratory tests. After the withdrawal of gossypol, the sperm concentration returned to its level prior to the medication. The results of this study showed that gossypol is effective as an oral contraceptive and has no acute side-effects.

In conclusion, gossypol seems to be a substance which might be valuable for male contraception. As it is new, toxicity, efficiency, reversibility and mode of action remain to be carefully analysed.

Investigations performed at the University of Missouri have shown that treatment of rats with ultrasound leads to azoospermia. Furthermore, direct radiation of the testes in men with prostate carcinoma was followed by testicular atrophy and a decrease in spermatogenesis. No details are available on the sperm count and the reversibility. Other investigators believe that this treatment might lead to radiation damage.

Studies performed at the University of Utah have shown that in rats high doses led to infertility and low doses had no effect. Therefore, it is doubtful whether the method is suitable.

Studies performed some years ago with rats proved that at 42 °C spermatogenesis was disrupted by treatment with ultrasound.

According to Djerassi (1980), man should become sterile after having taken a daily bath of 45 min duration at a temperature of 45 °C for 3 weeks. This sterility should persist for 6 months. In Japan, however, this observation could not be proved and, therefore, this method does not seem to be reliable.

Dixit (1982) investigated the occurrence of a reversible temporary sterility due to the following plant extracts: 3,4,7-trihydroxy-trimethoxy flavylium chloride, isolated from *Malavisus conzanitti* Greenm.; 2-hydroxy-2,3,7,8-tetra-methoxy flavon, isolated from the leaves of *Colebrookia oppositifolia*; dihydro-palmitinium hydroxide, $C_{21}H_{25}O_5N$, isolated from the roots of *Berberis chitria*; and gossypol acetic acid (1,1, 6,6, 7,7-dexahydroxy-3-3-dimethyl phenol). The substances were administered orally to monkeys over a period of 60–80 days in a dosage of 20 mg/kg per day. During this treatment an inhibition of spermatogenesis occurred on the level of spermatocyte formation. Therefore, no spermatine and no sperm was formed. The Sertoli cells were of normal shape; the size of the nuclei of the Leydig cells was significantly diminished. The inhibitory effect on steroidogenesis by the plants was evaluated by various biochemical parameters. A decrease in total protein and in the activity of acid phosphatase could be observed. Serum cholesterol rose; blood sugar, haemoglobin, transaminase, SGOT, SGPT, serum phospholipids and triglycerides remained unchanged. Normal spermatogenesis occurred 200 days after withdrawal of the compounds. Possible mechanisms by which the plant extracts inhibit steroidogenesis are being discussed.

Theophylline (methylxanthine (1,3-dimethylxanthine); Figure 76) is a drug used for the treatment of asthma patients. It belongs, as a methylxanthine, to a group of substances which inhibit phosphodiesterase and thus the decomposition of intracellularly formed cyclic adenosine monophosphate. Male rats treated with high doses of theophylline showed testicular atrophy and inhibition of spermatogenesis (Weinberger *et al.*, 1978).

Caffeine is a 1,3,7-trimethylxanthine (Figure 77). In high doses it causes severe testicular atrophy and inhibition of spermatogenesis in male rats (Weinberger *et al.*, 1978).

$C_7H_8N_4O_2$

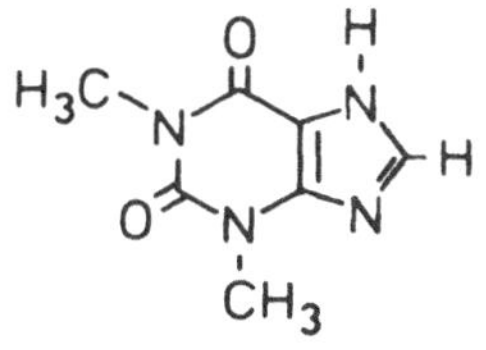

Figure 76 Theophylline

$C_8H_{10}O_2N_4$

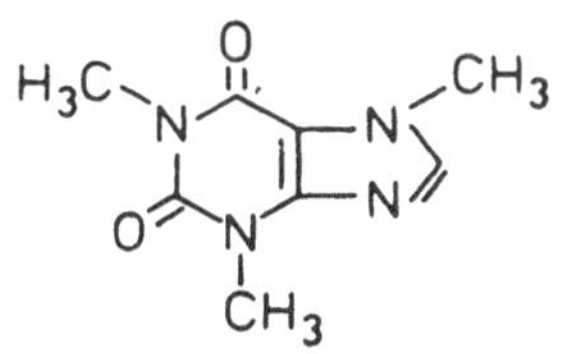

Figure 77 Caffeine

1,2-Dibromo-3-chloropropane (DBCP; Figure 78) seems to inhibit spermatogenesis. Tests in animals by Teramoto *et al.* (1980) showed dominant lethal mutation. In rats and mice the compound was carcinogenic (Powers *et al.*, 1975). Earlier studies showed that in men exposed to DBCP oligospermia or azoospermia occurred. Recent studies performed with 23

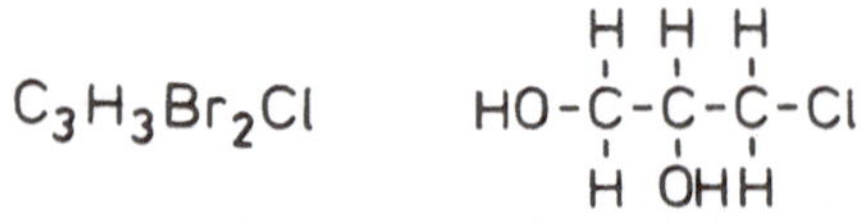

$$C_3H_3Br_2Cl$$

Figure 78   DBCP

workers in a firm who had been exposed there to DBCP showed severe suppression of spermatogenesis in 18 of these patients (78%). Azoospermia and an increased plasma FSH level were detected in 12 men who had been exposed to this substance for 100–6000 h. Oligospermia and normal FSH were found in 6 workers exposed to it for 34–95 h. Plasma LH, testosterone and thyroxine were normal. A testicular biopsy showed a selective atrophy of the germinal epithelium, intact Sertoli cells and a normal appearance of the Leydig cells (Potashnik *et al.*, 1978). Owing to its toxic effect, this compound is not suitable as a contraceptive (Teramoto *et al.*, 1980).

After administration on the skin of male rabbits tris(2,3-dibromopropyl) (TRIS; Figure 79) causes testicular atrophy (Osterberg *et al.*, 1977). Female animals did not show these side-effects.

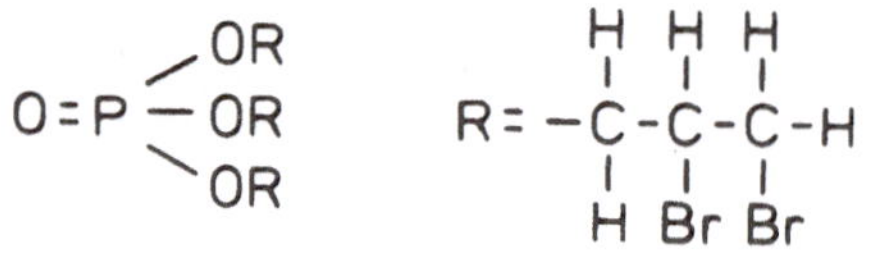

Figure 79   TRIS

Post-testicular contraception

The fertilization capacity of spermatocytes can be suppressed by compounds which cause the antifertility action to occur only when the spermatocytes have left the epididymis. In this context, there is a possibility of suppressing fertilization via the glycolytic enzymes of the spermatozoa, as well as by exerting influence on the acrosomal enzymes of the spermatozoa. This functional sterility has the following advantages: rapid occurrence of infertility; rapid reversibility; low mutagenic or teratogenic action (if any) during long-term use. Fertilization capacity can be modified by acrosin inhibitors, by immunization or by various compounds, the mode of action of which has not been established yet.

EPIDIDYMIS

In 1969 it was shown for the first time that small daily doses of α-chlorohydrine (glycerin-1-chlorohydrine; Figure 80) cause a reversible sterility. This action could be demonstrated in various animals. Although chlorohydrine is an alkylating agent, no mutagenic actions could be observed. It

$$C_3H_7Cl \qquad \begin{matrix} \text{H} & \text{Br} & \text{H} \\ | & | & | \\ \text{H-C-C-C-Cl} \\ | & | & | \\ \text{Br} & \text{H} & \text{H} \end{matrix}$$

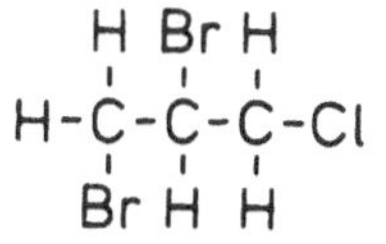

Figure 80 α-Chlorohydrine

is unclear whether α-chlorohydrine acts directly on the spermatozoa or indirectly, causing sterility due to testicular or epididymal dysfunction. *In vitro* incubation with α-chlorohydrine showed reduced spermatozoa cyclic AMP and reduced ATP concentrations in rats, mice and men. Furthermore, a diminished sperm mobility in the treated animals could be demonstrated, which might be due to reduced glycolysis, oxygen consumption and ATP concentration.

Reversible sterility was observed in rats, hamsters, rams, monkeys and wild boars. In rats sterility occurred a few days after the start of the treatment. Fertility returned one or two weeks after withdrawal of the compound (Neumann *et al.*, 1977). Libido and potency remained unchanged. The spermatozoa were able to reach the oocyte, but were not able to fertilize it. Low dosages (6.5 mg/kg administered over 9 days) caused no important histological changes in the testes and the epididymis, whereas high dosages led to degenerative damage (Guraya and Kaur, 1982). In rats spermatoceles could be induced this way.

In conclusion, α-chlorohydrine seems to be unsuitable for contraception, owing to its toxic effect on the bone marrow (Neumann *et al.*, 1977).

DUCTUS DEFERENS

Vasectomy In a vasectomy the ductus deferens is blocked by a ligature or a partial resection. The advantages are that no systemic side-effects occur and that it is only a minor operation. As it is an irreversible procedure (a later re-anastomosis is not possible in every case), psychological problems occur in the men. To avoid these problems, it has been rendered possible for some time to conserve sperm prior to a vasectomy and store it at sperm banks for later use.

Circumvasal Copper 200 wire Because of some morphological similarity to the male vas deferens, the contraceptive value of copper implants was tested in goats (Mahmoud *et al.*, 1982). Half the length of T Cu-200 B wire was wrapped around the vas deferens of goats and removed after 1 year. Seven days after wrapping, sperm mobility disappeared completely and sperm content was significantly diminished. Seven months later the occurrence of perivasal and epididymal sperm granulomata occurred. No changes in the testes, the seminal vesicles, the bulbourethral glands, the libido and the general condition of the animals could be observed. Furthermore, the serum levels of FSH, LH and testosterone and the fructose concentration in the semen remained normal. Six months after the removal of the wire, a high content of metal copper in the plasma, azoospermia and sperm granulomata remained. Reversibility might be achieved if lower dosages were used (Mahmoud *et al.*, 1982).

The possible mode of action of epididymal contraception in animals is summarized in Table 25.

Table 25　Possible mode of action of epididymal contraception in animals (Feghali and Feghali, 1983)

Compound	Mechanism and action on sperm	Toxicity and side-effects
Cyproterone acetate	anti-androgens interfere in small doses with the epididymis secretion without changing other androgen-dependent reproductive functions; diminishing of sperm count, no motility	no side-effects at low dosages decrease in ejaculate volume and libido at higher dosages
Methylmethane-sulphate	direct toxic action on the epididymis; decrease in implantation frequency in female animals matched with treated males	testicular disturbances
Chlorohydrine and related compounds	interference with the glycolytic activity of sperm and inhibition of the epididymal reabsorption of sodium and water causes immotility of sperm	high toxic epididymal necrosis, death
Chloro-desoxy sugar	reduces glycolytic activity of sperm and decreases ATP level; decrease in motility	none
N-(4-carboxy-3-hydroxy-phenyl)-maleimide (CPhM)	fluorescence probe for SH residues, impossible for penetration of membranes, binds only to exposed SH groups of intact sperms; inhibits epididymal maturation, sperm capacitation and fertilization of the oocytes	all studies have been performed in vitro only

SEMINAL PLASMA

Another approach for contraception in the male consists in the attempt to change the liquefaction of sperms. However, no reliable experimental clinical tests have so far been described.

SPERMS

Acrosin inhibitors　Acrosin is an enzymal system localized at the sperm head. It is necessary for the penetration of the zona pellucida of the oocyte and, therefore, necessary for the fertilization of the oocyte. The acrosin inhibitors are listed in Table 26. The problem with the clinical application of these compounds is the fact that, besides acrosin, other proteolytic enzymes of similar structure, such as thrombin and trypsin, might be suppressed.

Table 26 Acrosin inhibitors

Compound	Author
Peptidyl-arginyl-chloro-methane	Kettner *et al.* (1978)
Benamine derivatives	Parrish *et al.* (1978)
N-p-nitrophenyl-*p*-guanidinobenzoate	Bhattacharyya *et al.* (1976)

Contrasperm   A simple, effective, non-toxic, male oral contraceptive in the USA (Patent 4 148 892) and Europe (Patent Ap. 79300765.9) is Contrasperm. The active ingredient of the preparation of *Ecballium elaterium* Linn. is free of toxic chemicals, steroids, hormones and animal derivatives. *Ecballium elaterium* Linn. can be found in various countries—among others, in the USA, in the UK and in Greece. The active compound acts directly on sperm metabolism by inducing an acid milieu which inhibits sperm activity. By this, a reduction of sperm motility occurs within less than 30 min after oral application. It acts for 6–8 h, initial values being obtained after this period. Contrasperm is available in capsules or as a tablet. The decrease in the sperm count does not affect the morphology of the sperm (Nassar and Tierney, 1982). In animal tests no negative, toxic, histomorphological side-effects (Nassar and Tierney, 1982) could be observed.

In conclusion, Contrasperm might be an alternative to commonly used contraceptives for male contraception.

Factor VII of scorpion poison   Of seven fractions isolated from the poison of the scorpion *Hirus quinquetriatus*, only fraction VII blocks the motility of human sperm. After mixing human sperm and factor VII, akinesia of the sperm occurs, which might be used as a method of contraception (Hafez *et al.*, 1982).

Immunization   On the experimental basis of auto-immunorchitis in animals, which is an organospecific immune syndrome that can be induced by injection of autologous or homologous testes or spermatozoa in combination with Freund's adjuvant, inhibition of fertilization in the male might be obtained by an immunological approach. In immunized animals damage to the testes with destruction of the germinal epithelium and azoospermia occurs. After the development of an auto-immunorchitis, the physiological blood–testes barrier is disrupted, especially in the region of the rete testis and the efferent tubuli, in which lymphocytes induce the initial disruption (Jones *et al.*, 1975).

The alteration and blockade of the efferent system leads to a secondary, immunologically caused lesion in the sperm canals. Immune response in this form of the orchitis induces the formation of circulating and cell-bound antibodies and hypersensitivity reactions of the immediate and the late type can develop. Only a minor local correlation exists between the occurrence and the degree of testicular lesion and immune reaction. Auto-immunorchitis can be transferred passively by immune cells, but rarely and incompletely by serum (Dondero and Isidori, 1972).

The application of the experimentally induced auto-immunorchitis for the regulation of male fertility has been quite promising. Although testicular tissue is destroyed by this method to some extent, a hormonal depression does not occur and fertility returns within 6 months after the injections.

In a clinical trial in men, patients with prostate carcinomas were immunized prior to orchidectomy by testicular extract and adjuvant. Some of the men developed the classical but weakened type of allergic orchitis with low antibody titres, positive skin reaction and localized destruction of the germinal epithelium.

Miscellaneous

TCDD

2,3,7,8-Tetrachlorodibenzo-*p*-dioxin (TCDD; Figure 81) is a herbicide and was used in Vietnam as a chemical weapon. The precise mode of action has not yet been elucidated.

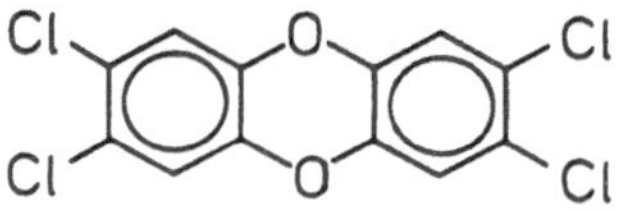

Figure 81 TCDD

Birth defects could be detected in the children of Vietnam veterans, with a decrease in libido and diminished fertility. Other side-effects are hepatic dysfunction and neurological disturbances.

High doses caused in rats and mice diminished fertility and spermatogenesis. Low doses did not induce these changes and did not change the testicular weight, sperm count, sperm mobility or morphology, nor could any influence on the plasma testosterone level be shown.

ALDRINE

Aldrine is an organochloride pesticide (Figure 82). It causes a decrease in fertilizing capacity and libido in beagle dogs (Lucier *et al.*, 1977).

$$C_{12}H_8Cl_6$$

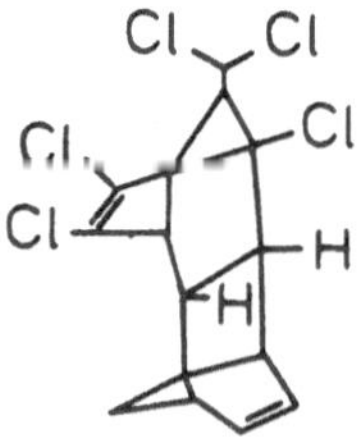

Figure 82 Aldrine

ALKYL ETHER OF ETHYLENE GLYCOL

The alkyl ether derivatives of ethylene, diethylene and triethylene glycol are very often used as solvents in various industrial products. The National Institute of Occupational Safety and Health (NIOSH) believes that approximately 200 000–2 000 000 persons occasionally are in contact with at least eight different glycols and glycol ethers. Degenerative testicular changes have been observed in animals treated with alkyl ethers of ethylene glycol. As early as 1938 this observation was made for the first time, but it was not then considered to be important. In studies of NIOSH, rats became reversibly sterile and mice showed a significant increase in the number of abnormal sperms after inhalation of ethylene glycol monomethyl ether or diethylene glycol dimethyl ether (Hardin, 1982). Haematological, CNS, liver and nephritic toxicity were described for human and animal experiments (Hardin, 1982). Monomethyl ether and monoethyl ether of ethylene glycol are embryotoxic and teratogenic.

CONCLUSIONS

Overpopulation and increasing depletion of resources have urged the optimal use of currently available as well as the development of new contraceptive measures to suppress the explosion of world population. The World Health Organization aims at the development of contraceptives which are more secure and easier to handle. In addition, these methods should be acceptable to patients of various religious, ethical and cultural backgrounds and their long-term use should be without health risk. The methods should also require neither complicated distribution systems nor frequent clinical check-ups in order to promote their application in developing countries.

Female oral contraception

Inhibition of ovulation

Oral contraception is currently used by 60–80 million women all over the world. Altogether, 150 million women have already used it. The amount of the two components (oestrogen and progestogen) has been reduced in recent years, since they have been found to cause cardiovascular side-effects. The limitation of the reduction of the dose is set by the control of the cycle as well as by a definite inhibition of ovulation. The development of the triphasic pill has provided the lowest steroid dose of the cycle. A novel approach to the route of administration has been offered by steroids administered on cellulose acetate paper, especially to reduce expensive packaging. The further improvement of galenic release has been achieved by microencapsulation. The use of natural oestrogens as well as the development of new progestogens will show to what extent side-effects will be avoidable. Large-scale clinical studies will elucidate the risks of the pill for the health of the women and demonstrate advantages (such as prevention of certain diseases, including certain carcinomas). A new development in contraception is the application of GnRH analogues (agonists and antagonists). Although these compounds still cause some disorders of the menstrual cycle, their combination with gestogens in the second half of the cycle will help to avoid this side-effect. These steroid-free compounds will have to be tested for effect on control of the cycle and inhibition of ovulation, as well as possible side-effects on other organs. Besides affecting the pituitary, they also block steroidogenesis in the ovary, prostate and testis and have a beneficial effect on endometriosis.

Inhibition of fertilization

Inhibition of fertilization includes new behavioural methods, locally applicable methods and hormonal methods which influence the cervical mucus or inhibit tubal motility. Recently progress was made in the field of sympto-thermal methods, since the microprocessor technique has enabled an automatic continuous registration of the temperature and visualization on screens. In developing countries a prolonged period of lactation (up to 3 years in Africa) has still remained of world-wide importance. Among the locally applicable methods, condoms and diaphragms will be of further importance in the future, once the medical personnel have been instructed. Apart from spermicides, creams, etc., vaginal sponges and vaginal rings will be used in future. In addition to local influence by the minipill on the cervical mucus, direct release of progestogens around the cervix (i.e. vaginal rings) is also promising, especially because systemic side-effects could be avoided.

Inhibition of implantation

Implantation can be inhibited by intrauterine devices, steroid hormones and synthetic compounds as well as immunological methods. In the field of intrauterine devices, various developments occurred recently with the aim of reducing side-effects, including the expulsion of IUDs. One of these approaches was the development of an IUD with progesterone or levonorgestrel release which decreases uterine motility occurring with IUDs *in situ* and prevents an increased rate of salpingitis. Immunological methods have been further developed and antigens to spermatozoa such as LDH-X, isoenzyme of lactate dehydrogenase, acrosomal hyaluronidase, as well as acrosin can be used as possible targets for contraception. In addition, immunization against special peptides such as hCG have been carried out. The results indicate, however, that contraception is partially irreversible and possible auto-immune diseases may occur.

Interruption of pregnancy

Pregnancy can be interrupted by surgical and hormonal methods, or by plant extracts as well as antihormones. No new approach has been developed in the field of surgical methods. Hormones can inhibit progesterone synthesis of the corpus luteum (luteolysis) or of the placenta by inhibiting steroidogenic enzymes. On the other hand, progesterone effect can be inhibited in the endometrium by the use of antiprogestins. These compounds are hormone antagonists and they can be applied either as a mid-cycle pill, as menstrual regulators or for interruption of pregnancy. A direct induction of uterine contraction can be achieved by prostaglandins. A possible new approach has been suggested by the use of antiprogestins as well as prostaglandins. In various developing countries, plant extracts have been used as abortifacients, but no extensive data are yet available.

Male contraception

Fertility in the male can be inhibited by substances which block spermato-genesis or fertilization ability. Various steroids can inhibit spermatogenesis, which, however, cause a decrease in peripheral testosterone levels. A new approach consists in a decrease in testicular testosterone synthesis and in keeping the peripheral level of testosterone at normal concentration in order to enable the development of secondary sexual characteristics. One approach is the inhibition of testosterone production by GnRH analogues and the substitution of this loss by exogenous testosterone. Another new aspect of male contraception has been developed in China using gossypol to cause azoospermia. This phenolic extract of cottonseed oil can selectively inhibit spermatogenesis and sterility has been found in more than 98% of the cases. Several side-effects of this compound, including irreversible oligo-asthenazoospermia, should be reduced by the development of gossypol metabolites. An inhibition of fertilization capacity can be achieved by immunization against spermatozoa or by the use of various pharmacologi-cal compounds. A reversible blockade of the ductus deferens by vasectomy in combination with sperm banks may enable men to opt for this contra-ceptive method.

The development of secure contraceptives is a precondition for control of overpopulation. In developing countries governmental control (e.g. China) has demonstrated good results and the explosion of population can thereby be controlled. Although governmental influence on the personal sphere of individuals is not to be promoted, the achievement of voluntary self-control of the world population is of great importance.

ACKNOWLEDGEMENT

The authors wish to thank Mrs Diemel for reviewing the literature and for her help in preparing the German manuscript.

REFERENCES

Agrawal, O.P., Bharadwaj, S. and Mathur, R. (1980). Antifertility effects of fruits of *Juniperus communis*. *Planta Med.*, **6**, 98

Ahren, T., Lithell, H., Victor, A., Vessby, B. and Johansson, E.D.B. (1981). Comparison of the metabolic effects of two hormonal contraceptive methods: An oral formulation and a vaginal ring. II. Serum lipoproteins and apolipoproteins. *Contraception*, **24**, 451

Ahren, T., Victor, A., Lithell, H. and Johansson, E.D.B. (1981). Comparison of the metabolic effects of two hormonal contraceptive methods: An oral formulation and a vaginal ring. I. Carbohydrate metabolism and liver function. *Contraception*, **24**, 415

Aitken, R.J. and Harper, M.J.K. (1977) New methods for the regulation of implantation. *Contraception*, **16**, 227

Allen, W.M. (1930). Physiology of the corpus luteum. *J. Physiol. Lond.*, **92**, 174

Anderson, L.L. (1972). In Moghissi, K.S. and Hafez, E.S.E. (eds.) *Biology of Mammalian Fertilization and Implantation*, pp. 379–421. (Springfield, Ill.: Thomas)

Arenas, P. and Azorero, R. (1977). Plants used as means of abortion, contraception, sterili-zation and fecundation by Paraguayan indigenous people. *Econ. Bot.*, **31**, 302

Asch, R., Greenblatt, R.B. and Virendra, B. (1978). Pure crystalline estradiol pellet implantation for contraception. *Int. J. Fertil.*, **23**, 100

Auclair, C., Kelly, P.A., Coy, D.H., Schally, A.V. and Labrie, F. (1977). Potent inhibitory activity of (D-Leu⁶,des-Gly-NH₂10) LHRH ethylamide on LH/hCG and PRL testicular receptor levels in the rat. *Endocrinology*, **101**, 1890

Audebert, A.J.M. (1983). A French Copper IUD: Preliminary results. In *Proceedings of the International Symposium on Reproductive Health Care: Contraceptive Delivery Systems*, Maui, Hawaii. Vol. 3, Abstract no. 243

Austin, C.R. (1975). Fate of spermatozoa in the female genital tract and the problem of induction of local anti-sperm immunity in women. Presented at *Third International Symposium on Immunology in Reproduction*, Varna

Azadian-Boulanger, G., Secchi, J., Laraque, F., Raynaud, J.P. and Sakiz, E. (1976). Action of a midcycle contraceptive (R 2323) on the human endometrium. *Am. J. Obstet. Gynecol.*, **125**, 1049

Azadian-Boulanger, G., Secchi, J. and Sakiz, E. (1973). In *Proceedings of the VIIth World Congress on Fertility and Sterility*, Tokyo, 1971. Amsterdam: Excerpta Medica

Bacic, M., Wesselius de Casparis, A. and Diczfalusy, E. (1970). Failure of large doses of ethinyl estradiol to interfere with early embryonic development in the human species. *Am. J. Obstet. Gynecol.*, **107**, 531

Bacic, M., Wesselius de Casparis, A. and Diczfalusy, E. (1979). Failure of large doses of ethinyl estradiol to interfere with early embryonic development in the human species. *Am. J. Obstet. Gynecol.*, **107**, 531

Badr, F.M., Bartke, D., Dalterio, S. and Bulger, W. (1977). Suppression of testosterone production by ethyl alcohol. Possible mode of action. *Steroids*, **30**, 647

Bahl, O.P. (1969). Human chorionic gonadotrophin. II. Nature of the carbohydrate units. *J. Biol. Chem.*, **244**, 575

Bajpai, P.K. and Anderson, K.J. (1982). Effect of adriamycin on reproductive system of male rats. In *Proceedings of the International Symposium on Reproductive Health Care: Contraceptive Delivery Systems*, Maui, Hawaii. Vol. 3, Abstract no. 291

Banik, U.D. and Pincus, G. (1962). Effect of steroidal anti-progestins on implantation of fertilized eggs of rats and mice. *Proc. Soc. Exp. Biol. Med.*, **111**, 595

Barwin, B. (1983). Benzalkonium chloride—a new contraceptive. In Proceedings of the First Annual Meeting of the Society of the Advancement of Contraception, Cairo, Egypt: *Contraceptive Delivery Systems*. Vol. 4, Abstract no. 58

Baskin, J.M. (1932). Temporary sterilization by the injection of human spermatozoa. *Am. J. Obstet. Gynecol.*, **24**, 892

Beck, L.R. (1983a). Clinical evaluation of an injectable microcapsule contraceptive system. In Proceedings of the First Annual Meeting of the Society of the Advancement of Contraception, Cairo, Egypt: *Contraceptive Delivery Systems*. Vol. 4, Abstract no. 14

Beck, L.R. (1983b). Long-acting steroidal contraceptives. In *Proceedings of the International Symposium on Reproductive Health Care: Contraceptive Delivery Systems*, Maui, Hawaii. Vol. 3, Abstract no. 85

Beck, L.R., Ramos, R.A., Flowers, C.E., Lopez, G.Z., Lewis, D.H. and Cowsar, D.R. (1981). Clinical evaluation of injectable biodegradable contraceptive system. *Am. J. Obstet. Gynecol.*, **140**, 799

Behrmann, H.R. and Caldwell, B.W. (1974). In Greep, R.O. (ed.) *Reproductive Physiology*, Vol. 8, pp. 633-694. (London: Butterworths)

Behrmann, H.R., Ng, T.S. and Orczyk, G.P. (1974). In Moudgal, N.R. (ed.) *Gonadotropins and Gonadal Function*, pp. 332-344. (New York: Academic Press)

Bergquist, C., Nillius, S.J. and Wide, L. (1979). Inhibition of ovulation in women by intranasal treatment with a luteinizing hormone-releasing hormone (LRH) agonist. *Acta Endocrinol. (Copenh.)* (*Suppl.*), **225**, 135

Beyer, B., Terenius, L., Brueggemeier, R.W., Ranade, V.V. and Counsell, R.E. (1976). Synthesis of potential antiprogestigens. *Steroids*, **27**, 123

Beyer, G. and Zeilmarker, G.H. (1974). Prolonged pseudo-pregnancy in mice bearing ectopic trophoblastic tissue. *J. Endocrinol.* **61**, 509

Bhatta, S.K. and Santhakumari, G. (1971). The antifertility effect of *Ocinum sanctum* and *Hibiscus-rosa sinensis*. *Indian J. Med. Res.*, **590**, 717

Bhattacharyya, A.K. and Zaneveld, L.J.D. (1976). Kinetic studies on the interaction and specificity of synthetic proteinase inhibitors towards human acrosin. *Andrologia*, **8** (Suppl. 1)

Bhattacharyya, A.L., Zaneveld, L.J.D., Pragoje, B., Schuhmacher, G.F.B. and Travis, J. (1976). Inhibition of human sperm acrosin by synthetic agents. *J. Reprod. Fertil.*, **47**, 577

Board, J.A., Bhatnagar, A.S. and Bush, C.W. (1973). Effect of oral diethylstilbestrol on plasma progesterone. *Fertil. Steril.*, **24**, 95

Boris, A., Ng, C. and Hurley, R. (1974). Antitesticular and antifertility activity of a pipecolinomethylhydroxyindane in rats. *J. Reprod. Fertil.*, **38**, 387

Bouin, P. and Ancel, P. (1910). Recherches sur les fonctions du corps jaune gestatif. I. Sur le déterminisme de la préparation de l'utérus à la fixation de l'oeuf. *J. Physiol. Path. Gen.*, **12**, 1

Boyarsky, G.P. and Polakoski, K. (1981). *Goals in Male Reproductive Research*. (Oxford, New York: Pergamon Press)

Bradley, M.P. and Forrester, I.T. (1982). Calsemin: a novel Ca^{2+}-dependent regulator of mammalian sperm functions. In *Proceedings of the International Symposium on Reproductive Health Care: Contraceptive Delivery Systems*, Vol. 3, No. 3/4, Abstract no. 267, Maui, Hawaii

Brown, W.E. and Bradbury, J.T. (1947). A study of the physiologic action of human chorionic hormone. *Am. J. Obstet. Gynecol.*, **53**, 749

Brueggemeier, R.W., Floyd, E.E. and Counsell, R.E. (1978). Synthesis and biochemical evaluation of inhibitors of estrogen biosynthesis. *Med. Chem.*, **21**, 1007

Brundin, J. (1983). A hydrogelic intratubal occlusive device: The P-block. In *Proceedings of the International Symposium on Reproductive Health Care: Contraceptive Delivery Systems*, Maui, Hawaii. Vol. 3, Abstract no. 247

Butenandt, A., Westphal, U. and Hohlweg, W. (1934). Über das Corpus luteum. *Z. Physiol.*, **227**, 84

Carelli, C., Audibert, F., Gaillard, J. and Chedid, L. (1982). Immunological castration of male mice by a totally synthetic vaccine administered in saline. *Proc. Natl. Acad. Sci. USA*, **79**, 5392

Cerini, M., Findlay, J.K. and Lawson, R.A.S. (1976). Pregnancy-specific antigens in the sheep: Application to the diagnosis of pregnancy. *J. Reprod.*, **46**, 65

Challis, J.R.G., Calder, A.A., Dilley, S., Forster, C.S., Hillier, K., Hunter, O.J.S., MacKenzie, I.Z. and Thorburn, G.D. (1976). Production of prostaglandins E and F by corpora lutea, corpora albicantes and stroma from the human ovary. *J. Endocrinol.*, **68**, 401

Chamboon, Y. (1949). Besoins endocriniens qualitatifs et quantitatifs de l'ovoimplantation chez la lapine. *C.R. Soc. Biol. (Paris)*, **143**, 1172

Chang, C.C. and Kinel, F.A. (1979). Sustained release of hormone preparations. 4. Biological effectiveness of steroid hormones. *Fertil. Steril.*, **21**, 134

Channing, C.P., Engel, B. and Bahl, O.P. (1978). Role of carbohydrate residues of human chorionic gonadotropin in stimulation of luteinization of monkey granulosa cell cultures. *Biol. Reprod.*, **18**, 707

Channing, C.P., Sakai, C. and Bahl, O.P. (1976). Role of the carbohydrate residues of human chorionic gonadotropin (hCG) on its ability to bind and stimulate cyclic AMP accumulation in porcine granulosa cells. [Abstract No. 3268.] *Fed. Proc.*, **35**, 798

Channing, C.P., Sakai, C. and Bahl, O.P. (1977). Role of carbohydrate residues of human chorionic gonadotropin in binding and stimulation of cyclic AMP and progesterone secretion by porcine granulosa cells. *Endocrinology*, **103**, 341

Chulavatnatol, M., Hasibuan, I., Yindepit, S. and Esittikult, T. (1977). Lack of effect of α-chlorohydrin on the ATP content of rat, mouse and human spermatozoa. *J. Reprod. Fertil.*, **50**, 137

Cicero, T.R., Bell, R.D., Meyer, E.R. and Schweitzer, J. (1977). Narcotics and the hypothalamic-pituitary-gonadal axis: acute effects on LH, testosterone and androgen-dependent systems. *J. Pharmacol. Exp. Ther.*, **201**, 76

Clark, S.W., Sweet, F. and Warren, J.C. (1975). Synthesis and use of affinity-labeling steroids for interceptive purposes. *Am. J. Obstet. Gynecol.*, **121**, 864

Clayton, R.N. and Catt, K.J. (1981). Gonadotrophin hormone releasing hormone receptors: characterization, physiological regulation and relationship to reproductive function. *Endocr. Rev.*, **2**, 186

Cochrane, R.L. and Meyer, R.K. (1957). Delayed nidation in the rat induced by progesteron (23418). *Proc. Soc. Exp. Biol.*, **5**, 155

Cohen, J. (1975). Gametic diversity within an ejaculate. In *WHO Workshop: Immunological Response of the Female Reproductive Tract*, Genoa, 1975 (Copenhagen: Scriptor)

Coutinho, M.D. (1978). Clinical experience with implant contraception. *Contraception*, **18**, 411

Coutinho, E.M., Da Silva, A.R., Carreira, C.M., Chaves, M.C. and Adeodato-Filho, J. (1975). Contraceptive effectiveness of Silastic implants containing the progestin R-2323. *Contraception*, **11**, 625

Coutinho, E.M., Da Silva, A.R. and Kraft, H.G. (1976). Fertility control with subdermal capsules containing a new progestin (ST-1435). *Int. J. Fertil.*, **21**, 103

Coutinho, E.M., Mattos, C.E.R., Sant'Anna, A.R.S., Adeodato Filho, J., Silva, M.C. and Tatum, H.J. (1970). Long term contraception by subcutaneous Silastic capsules containing megestrol acetate. *Contraception*, **2**, 313

Coutinho, E.M., Mattos, C.E.R., Sant'Anna, A.R.S., Adeodato Filho, J., Silva, M.C. and Tatum, H.J. (1972). Further studies on long-term contraception by subcutaneous Silastic capsules containing megestrol acetate. *Contraception*, **5**, 389

Cremer, J.E. and Cunningham, V.J. (1979). Effects of some chlorinated sugar derivates on the hexose transport system of the blood/brain barrier. *Biochem. J.*, **180**, 677

Csapo, A.I. (1974). 'Prostaglandin Impact' for menstrual induction. *Popul. Rep. G*, **4**, 33

Csapo, A.I. (1976). Prostaglandin impact. In *Advances in Prostaglandin and Thromboxane Research*. Vol. 2, pp. 705-718. (eds.) Samuelsson, B. and Paoletti, R. (New York: Raven Press)

Csapo, A.I., Pulkkinen, M.P. and Kaihola, H.L. (1973). The effect of estradiol replacement therapy on early pregnant luteectomized patients. *Am. J. Obstet. Gynecol.*, **117**, 987

Csapo, A.I., Pulkkinen, M.P. and Kaihola, H.L. (1974). The relationship between timing of luteectomy and the incidence of complete abortions. *Am. J. Obstet. Gynecol.*, **118**, 985

Csapo, A.I., Pulkkinen, M.O. and Wiest, W.G. (1973). Effects of luteectomy and progesterone replacement therapy in early pregnancy patients. *Am. J. Obstet. Gynecol.*, **115**, 759

Cullberg, G., Eriksson, O., Knutsson, F. and Steffensen, K. (1982). Desogestrel, a new pro-gestational compound. *Acta Obstet. Gynecol. Scand., Suppl.*, **111**, 13

Cullberg, G., Lindstedt, G., Lundberg, P.A. and Stennensen, K. (1982). Central and peripheral effects of desogestrel 15-60 μg daily for 21 days in healthy female volunteers. *Acta Obstet. Gynecol. Scand., Suppl.*, **111**, 13

Cunningham, G.R., Silverman, V.E., Thornby, I. and Kohler, P.O. (1979). The potential for an androgen male contraceptive. *J. Clin. Endocrinol. Metab.*, **49**, 295

Dai, R.X., Pang, S.N., Lann, X.K., Ke, Y.B. and Liu, Z.L. (1978). Studies on the antifertility of cottonseed. *Acta Biol. Exp. Sinica*, **11**, 1

Dalterio, S., Bartke, A. and Burstein, S. (1977). Cannabinoids inhibit testosterone secretion by mouse testes in vitro. *Science, N.Y.*, **196**, 1472

Damm, R.R. (1979). Use and acceptance of the 'paper pill'. A novel approach to oral contraception. *Contraception*, **19**, 273

Daniel, J.W. (1978). Toxicity and metabolism of phthalate esters. *Clin. Toxicol.*, **13**, 257

Das, R.P. and Yanagimachi, R. (1978). Effects of monothioglycerol, α-chlorohydrin and 5-thio-D-glucose on the fertility of male hamster. *Contraception*, **17**, 413

Davies, T.F., Gomez-Pan, A., Watson, M.J., Mountjoy, C.Q., Hanber, J.P., Besser, G.M. and Hall, R. (1977). Reduced gonadotropin response to releasing hormone after chronic administration to impotent men. *Clin. Endocrinol.*, **6**, 213

De Visser, J., de Jager, E., Ylikorkala, O., Nummi, S., Virkkunen, P., Ranta, T., Alapiessa, U. and Vihko, R. (1977). Ovulation inhibition by a new low-dose progestagen. *Contraception*, **16**, 51

Di Raddo, J. and Wardell, W.W. (1981). Research activity on systemic contraceptive drugs by the US pharmaceutical industry, 1963-1979. *Contraception*, **23**, 345

Dixit, V.I. (1982). Contraception-like properties of certain plant materials in male presbytis monkeys. In *Proceedings of the International Symposium on Reproductive Health Care: Contraceptive Delivery Systems*, Maui, Hawaii. Vol. 3, no. 3/4, Abstract no. 300

Djerassi, C. (1980). *The Politics in Contraception*. (New York, London: Norton)

Donat, H. (1979). Stand und Entwicklung immunologischer Kontrazeptionsmethoden. *Zbl. Gynakol.*, **101**, 433

Dondero, F. and Isidori, A. (1972). Autoimmunisation antitesticulaire chez l'homme. *Ann. Endocrinol.*, **33**, 417

El Maghoub, S. (1983). The levonorgestrel contraceptive effect. In *Eleventh World Congress on Fertility and Sterility*, Dublin. Abstract no. 150

Emperaire, J.C. and Greenblatt, R.B. (1969). L'implantation de pellets d'oestradiol dans la contraception. *Gynecol. Prat.*, **5**, 327

Epel, D. (1982). Novel modes of contraception based on a molecular comprehension of fertilization. In *Proceedings of the International Symposium on Reproductive Health Care: Contraceptive Delivery Systems*, Maui, Hawaii. Vol. 3, no. 3/4, Abstract no. 255

Epstein, S.S., Arnold, E., Steinberg, K., Mackintosh, D., Shafner, H. and Bishop, Y. (1970). Mutagenic and antifertility effects of TEPA and METEPA in mice. *Toxicol. Appl. Pharmacol.*, 17, 23

Epstein, S.S., Joshi, S.R., Arnold, E., Page, E.C. and Bishop, Y. (1970). Abnormal zygote development in mice after paternal exposure to a chemical mutagen. *Nature (London)*, **225**, 1260

Erny, R., Rouit, S. and Moulias, M. (1983). The effects of benzalkonium chloride on human spermatozoa. In Proceedings of the First Annual Meeting of the Society of the Advancement of Contraception, Cairo, Egypt: *Contraceptive Delivery Systems*. Vol. 4, Abstract no. 61

Fan, M.M. (1980). Studies on long-acting oral contraceptives. In Chang, C.F. (ed.) *Recent Advances in Fertility Regulation*. Proc. Symp. in Beijing, September 1980

Feghali, G. and Feghali, V. (1983). Interference with epididymal function and male contraception. In *Proceedings of the International Symposium on Reproductive Health Care: Contraceptive Delivery Systems*, Maui, Hawaii. Vol. 3, Abstract no. 282

Ferin, J. (1971). The effects of progesterone on the human uterovaginal tract. In Tausk, M. (ed.) Pharmacology of the Endocrine System and Related Drugs: Progesterone, Progestational Drugs and Antifertility Agents, pp. 441–456. (Oxford: Pergamon Press)

Ford, W.C.L. and Waites, G.M.H. (1978a). A reversible contraceptive action of some 6-chloro-6-deoxy sugars in the male rat. *J. Reprod. Fertil.*, **52**, 153

Ford, W.C.L. and Waites, G.M.H. (1978b). Chlorinated sugars: a biochemical approach to the control of male fertility. *Int. J. Androl.*, **2** (Suppl.), 541

Fraenkel, S. (1903). Die Funktion des Corpus luteum. *Arch. Gynakol.*, **68**, 438

Fraser, H.M. (1982). New prospects for luteinising hormone releasing as a contraceptive and therapeutic agent. *Br. Med. J.*, **285**, 990

Freese, U.E. and Goepp, R.A. (1983). The custom fitted cervical cap. In Proceedings of the First Annual Meeting of the Society of the Advancement of Contraception, Cairo, Egypt: *Contraceptive Delivery Systems*. Vol. 4, Abstract no. 63

Fried, P.H. and Rakoff, A.E. (1952). The effects of chorionic gonadotropin and prolactin on the maintenance of corpus luteum function. *Eur. J. Clin. Endocrinol. Metab.*, **12**, 321

Froewis, J. (1963). Wann erfolgt die ausreichende Umschaltung der schwangerschaftserhaltenden Hormonproduktion des Corpus luteum gravidatatis auf die Plazenta. *Wien. Klin. Wochenschr.*, **75**, 368

Fuchs, A.R. and Beling, C.G. (1974). Evidence of early ovarian recognition of blastocysts in rabbits. *Endocrinology*, **95**, 1054

Gaitonde, B.B. and Mahajan, R.T. (1980). Antifertility activity of *Lygodium flexosum*. *Indian J. Med. Res.*, **72**, 597

Gallegos, A.J. and Cortes-Gallegos, V. (1977). U.S. Patent, 4,006,227

Garg, S.K. and Garg, G.P. (1970). Antifertility screening of plants. Part VII. Effect of five indigenous plants on early pregnancy in albino rats. *Indian J. Med. Res.*, **59**, 302

Garg, S.K., Mathur, V.S. and Chaudhury, R.R. (1978). Screening of indian plants for antifertility activity. *Indian J. Exp. Biol.*, **16**, 1077

Gillman, J. and Stein, H.B. (1942). Quantitative study of antagonism of estrogen and progesterone in castrate rabbit. *Endocrinologia*, **31**, 167

Glasser, S.R., Northcutt, R.C., Chatil, F. and Strott, C.A. (1972). The influence of an anti-steroidogenic drug (aminogluthethimide phosphate) on the pregnancy maintenance. *Endocrinology*, **90**, 1363

Goldberg, E. (1972). Amino acid composition and properties of crystalline lactate dehydrogenase-X from mouse testes. *J. Biol. Chem.*, **247**, 2044

Goldberg, E. (1973). Infertility in female rabbits immunized with lactate dehydrogenase X. *Science, N.Y.*, **181**, 458

Goldberg, E. (1974). Effects of immunisation with LDH-x on fertility. In Diczfalusy, E. (ed.) *Immunological Approaches to Fertility Control: Seventh Karolinska Symposium on Research Methods in Reproductive Endocrinology*, pp. 202–222

Goldberg, E. (1975). Effects of immunization with LDH-X on fertility. *Acta Endocrinol. (Copenh.) (Suppl.)*, **78**, 202

Goldberg, E., Wheat, T.E., Powell, J.E. and Stevens, V.C. (1981). Reduction of fertility in female baboons immunized with lactate dehydrogenase C4. *Fertil. Steril.*, **35**, 214

Goldmann-Leikin, R.E. and Goldberg, E. (1983). Immunology characterization of monoclonal antibodies to the sperm-specific lactate dehydrogenase isoenzyme. *Proc. Natl. Acad. Sci. USA*, **80**, 3774

Goncharov, N.P., Komor, A., Pachalia, A.I., Simarina, K., Ponsold, K. Grosse, P., Oettel, M., Strecke, J. and Schubert, K. (1978). Postkoitale Kontrazeption bei Primaten. *Zbl. Gynäkol.*, **100**, 263

Good, R.G. and Moyer, D.L. (1968). Estrogen–progesterone relationships in the development of secretory endometrium. *Fertil. Steril.*, **19**, 37

Gore, B.Z., Caldwell, B.V. and Speroff, L. (1973). Estrogen-induced human luteolysis. *J. Clin. Endocrinol. Metab.*, **36**, 615

Gould, K.G. and Ansari, A.H. (1983). Non-hormonal modification of cervical mucus. In *Proceedings of the International Symposium on Reproductive Health Care: Contraceptive Delivery Systems*, Maui, Hawaii. Vol. 3, Abstract no. 40

Greenblatt, R.B. (1967). One-pill-a-month contraceptive. *Fertil. Steril.*, **18**, 207

Greep, R.O. (1976). *Reproduction and Human Welfare: A Challenge to Research.* (Cambridge, Mass.: MIT Press)

Griffin, B.F. and Bajpai, K. (1982). Effect of adriamycin on the testes and seminal vesicles of the prepubertal rats. In *Proceedings of the International Symposium on Reproductive Health Care: Contraceptive Delivery Systems*, Maui, Hawaii. Vol. 3, no. 3/4, Abstract no. 288

Gudson, J.P. (1974). A long term follow-up of passively immunologically sterilized rats. *Am. J. Obstet. Gynecol.*, **118**, 1145

Guraya, S.S. and Kaur, S. (1982). Effect of low dose of chlorohydrin on histochemical and biochemical characteristics in rat testis and epididymis. In *Proceedings of the International Symposium on Reproductive Health Care: Contraceptive Delivery Systems*, Maui, Hawaii. Vol. 3, no. 3/4, Abstract no. 294

Hafez, E.S.E. (1980a). *Human Reproduction.* (Hagerstown, Md.: Harper and Row)

Hafez, E.S.E. (1980b). *Medicated Intrauterine Devices.* Development in Obstetrics and Gynecology, Vol. 5. (The Hague, Boston, London: Martinus Nijhoff)

Hafiez, A.R.A., Mahoud, K., El-Asmar, M.F., Safouri, L.S.A. and Halwa, F.A. (1982). Andrological evaluation of scorpion venom fraction inducing akinesia of human spermatozoa. In *Proceedings of the International Symposium on Reproductive Health Care: Contraceptive Delivery Systems*, Maui, Hawaii. Vol. 3, no. 3/4, Abstract no. 298

Hahn, D.W., Ericson, E.W., Lai, M.T. and Probst, A. (1983). Antifertility activity of *Montanoa tomentosa* (zoapatle). *Contraception*, **23**, 133

Hahn, D.W., McConnell, R.F. and McGuire, J.L. (1981). Prototype for a new class of antifertility agents, 3,5-bis (dimethylamino)-1.2.4-dithiazolium chloride. *Contraception*, **21**, 529

Hanson, F.W., Powell, J.E. and Stevens, V.C. (1971). Effects of hCG and human pituitary LH on steroid secretion and functional life span of the human corpus luteum. *J. Endocrinol. Metab.*, **32**, 211

Hanson, V. (1976). Regelmechanismen männlicher Fertilität. *Sexualmedizin*, **5**, 91

Haour, F. (1976). Rat chorionic gonadotropin (rCG): radioreceptor assay and correlation with corpus luteum function during gestation. In *Fifth International Congress of Endocrinology*. p. 321 (Abstract 777)

Happ, J., Scholz, P., Weber, T., Cordes, U., Schramm, P. Neubauer, M. and Beyer, J. (1978). Gonadotropin secretion in eugonadotropic human males and postmenopausal females under long-term application of a potent analog of gonadotropin-releasing hormone. *Fertil. Steril.*, **30**, 30

Hardin, B.D. (1982). Antifertility effects in rodents following treatment with alkyl ethers of ethylene glycol. In *Proceedings of the International Symposium on Reproductive Health Care: Contraceptive Delivery Systems*, Maui, Hawaii. Vol. 3, no. 3/4, Abstract no. 295

Heath, E., Olusanya, S. and Pijanowki, L.P. (1983). Initial experiments with cyproterone acetate and 1-amino-3-chloro-propanol hydrochloride in the male virginiana opposum (*Didelphis virginiana*). *Andrologia*, **15**, 50

Heber, D. and Swerdloff, R.S. (1980). Brain peptides and fertility control in the male. In Zatuchni, G.I., Labbok, M.H. and Sciarra, J.J. (eds.) *Research Frontiers in Fertility Regulation*, pp. 176-186. (Hagerstown, Md.: Harper and Row)

Heckel, N.J. (1939). Production of oligospermia in a man by the use of testosterone propionate. *Proc. Soc. Exp. Biol. Med.*, **40**, 640

Heikkilä, M. (1982). Puerperal insertion of a copper-releasing and a levornorgestrel-releasing intrauterine contraceptive device. *Contraception*, **25**, 561

Heitfeld, F., McRae, G. and Vickery, B. (1979). Antifertility effects of 6-chloro-6-deoxyglucose in the male rat. *Contraception*, **19**, 543

Heller, J., Penhale, D.W.H., Helwing, R.F. and Fritzinger, B.K. (1983). In vitro and in vivo delivery of contraceptive steroids from poly(ortho ester) matrices. In *Proceedings of the International Symposium on Reproductive Health Care: Contraceptive Delivery Systems*, Maui, Hawaii. Vol. 3, Abstract no. 57

Henzl, M.R., Segre, E.J. and Nakamura, R.M. (1973). The influence of oxymetholone on the HCG-stimulated corpus luteum. *Contraception*, **8**, 515

Herman, D.L. and Smith, F.H. (1973). Effect of bound gossypol on the absorption of iron by rats. *J. Nutr.*, **103**, 882

Hermann, W.L. (1984). Personal communication

Herrmann, W., Wyss, R., Riondel, A., Philibert, D., Teutsch, G., Sakiz, E. and Baulieu, E.-E. (1982). Effect of an antiprogesterone in women: interruption of the menstrual cycle and of early pregnancy. *C.R. Acad. Sci. (Paris)*, **294**, 933

Hicks, J.J. and Guzman-Gonzalez, A.M. (1979). Inhibition of implantation by intraluminal administration of concanavalin A in mice. *Contraception*, **20**, 129

Hisaw, F.L. and Velardo, J.T. (1951). Inhibition of progesterone in decidual development by steroid compounds. *Endocrinology*, **49**, 732

Hoffmann, F. (1960). Untersuchungen über die hormonale Beeinflussung und Lebensdauer des Corpus luteum im Zyklus der Frau. *Geburtsh. Frauenheilk.*, **20**, 1153

Houck, R.M. and Cooper, J.M. (1982). Hysteroscopic tubal occlusion with formed-in-place silicone plugs: A clinical study. *Obstet. Gynaecol.* (In press)

Hsu, C.C., Dobberstein, R.H., Bingel, A.S., Fong, H.H.S., Farnsworth, N.R. and Morton, J.F. (1981). Biological and phytochemical investigation of plants. XVI. *Strumpfia maritima* (Rubiaceae). *J. Pharm. Sci.*, **70**, 682

Hsueh, S.P., Tsong, S.T., Su, S.Y., Wu, Y.W., Chou, T.H. and Ma, H.H. (1979). Cytological, radioautographic and ultrastructural observations on the antispermatogenesis action of gossypol in the rat. *Sci. Sinica*, **9**, 915

Irvine, W.J., Chan, M.M. and Scarth, L. (1969). The further characterisation of autoantibodies reactive with extra adrenal steroid-producing cells in the adrenal cortex. *Clin. Exp. Immunol.*, **4**, 489

Jackanicz, T.M. (1981). Levonorgestrel and estradiol release from an improved contraceptive vaginal ring. *Contraception*, **24**, 323

Jackson, H. and Bock, M. (1955). Effect of triethylene melamine on the fertility of rats. *Nature (London)*, **175**, 1037

Jackson, H., Fox, B.W. and Craig, A.W. (1959). The effect of alkylating agents on male rat fertility. *Br. J. Pharmacol.*, **14**, 149

Jaffe, R.B., Lee, P.A. and Midgley, A.R. (1969). Serum gonadotropins before, at the inception of, and following human pregnancy. *J. Clin. Endocrinol. Metab.*, **29**, 1281

Jain, G.K., Pal, R. and Khanna, N.M. (1980). Spermicidal saponins from *Pittosporum nilghrense* Wight et Apnott. *Indian J. Pharm. Sci.*, January/February, 12

Johnson, A.D. and Gomes, W.R. (1977). *The Testis*, pp. 605-628. (New York: Academic Press)

Jones, L.A. and Smith, F.H. (1977a). Effect of bound gossypol and amino acid supplementation of glandless cottonseed meal on the growth of weanling rats. *J. Anim. Sci.*, **44**, 401

Jones, L.A. and Smith, F.H. (1977b). Effect of gossypol on the removal of nitrogen and amino acids from feed in digestion by the rat. *J. Anim. Sci.*, **44**, 410

Jones, T.M., Fang, V.S.D., Landau, R.L. and Rosenfield, R.L. (1977). The effects of fluooxymestrone administration on testicular function. *J. Clin. Endocrinol. Metab.*, **44**, 121

Jones, W.R., Ing, R.M.Y. and Hobbin, E.R. (1975). Approaches and perspectives in the development of anti-sperm immunity as a contraceptive principle. Presented at Third *Int. Symp. Imm. Reprod.*, Varna

Joshi, S.R., Page, E.C., Arnold, E., Bishop, Y. and Epstein, S.S. (1977). Fertilization and early embryonic development subsequent to mating with TEPA-treated male mice. *Genetics*, **65**, 483

Junkmann, K. (1954). Über protrahiert wirksame Gestagene. *Arch. Exp. Pathol. Pharmacol.*, **223**, 244

Kaiser, R. (1981). *Global 2000: Bericht an den Präsidenten*, p. 43. (Frankfurt: Zweitausendeins)

Kaliwal, B.B. and Rao, M.A. (1977). Inhibition of implantation by carrot seed extract and its rectification by progesterone in albino rats. *J. Karnatak Univ.-Sci.*, **22**, 167

Karim, S.M.M. (1975). *Prostaglandins and reproduction*. (Lancaster: MTP)

Karim, S.M.M. (1979). Prostaglandins in fertility control. *Lancet*, **ii**, 610

Karim, S.M.M. and Ratnam, S.S. (1978). Termination of second trimester pregnancy with intramuscular administration of 16-phenoxy-ω-tetranor PGE_2-methylsulfonamide (SHB 286). *Obstet. Gynecol.*, **16,** 146

Kasper, K.C., White, R.J., Redrick-Highberg, G. and Lankford, J.C. (1984). Performance characteristics of the OvuSTICK urine LH test. In *III World Congress of in vitro Fertilization and Embryo Transfer*, Helsinki, Finland. Abstract no. 222

Kendle, K.E. (1979). Current investigations of antiprogestational steroids. In Agrawal, M.K. (ed.) *Antihormones*, pp. 293-305. (Amsterdam, New York, Oxford: Elsevier/North-Holland Biomedical Press)

Kent, J.S., Sanders, L.M., McRae, G.I., Vickery, B.H., Tice, T.R. and Lewis, D.H. (1983). In vivo controlled release of an LH-RH analog from injected polymeric microcapsules. In *Proceedings of the International Symposium on Reproductive Health Care: Contraceptive Delivery Systems*, Maui, Hawaii. Vol. 3, Abstract no. 58

Kettner, C.S., Springhorn, S., Shawn, W., Muller, A. and Fritz, H. (1978). Inactivation of boaracrosin by peptidyl-arginal-chloromethane, comparison of the reactivity of acrosin, trypsin and thrombin. *Hoppe-Seyler's Z. Physiol. Chem.*, **359,** 1183

Kholkute, S.D., Chatterjee, S. and Udupa, K.N. (1976). Effect of *Hibiscus-rosa sinensis* Linn. on oestrus cycle and reproductive organs in rats. *Indian J. Exp. Biol.*, **14,** 703

Kholkute, S.D., Kekare, M.B. and Munshi, S. (1979). Antifertility effects of the fruits of *Piper longum* in female rats. *Indian J. Exp. Biol.*, **17,** 289

Kholkute, S.D. and Udupa, K.N. (1977). Studies on the antifertility potentiality of *Hibiscus rosa-sinensis*. *Planta Med.*, **31,** 35

Knobil, E. (1973). On the regulation of the primate corpus luteum. *Biol. Reprod.*, **8,** 246

Koch, U.J. (1983). Corrosion of copper in utero: Longterm investigations with the IUD ML 250. In Proceedings of the First Annual Meeting of the Society of the Advancement of Contraception, Cairo, Egypt: *Contraceptive Delivery Systems*. Vol. 4, Abstract no. 43

Kontula, K., Jänne, O., Vihko, R., de Jager, E., de Visser, J. and Zeelen, F. (1975). Progesterone-binding proteins: in vitro binding and biological activity of different steroidal ligands. *Acta Endocrinol. (Copenh.)*, **78,** 574

Korda, A.R., Shutt, D.A., Smith, I.D., Shearman, R.P. and Leyneham, R.C. (1975). Assessment of possible luteolytic effect of intraovarian injection of PGF_2 in the human. *Prostaglandins*, **9,** 443

Krause, W. and Homola, S. (1974). Alterations on the seminiferous epithelium and the Leydig cells of the rat testis after the application of dichlorvos (DDVP). *Bull. Environ. Contam. Toxicol.*, **11,** 429

Kremer, J., de Bruijn, H.W.A. and Hindricks, F.R. (1980). Serum high density lipoprotein cholesterol levels in women using a contraceptive injection of depot-medroxyprogesterone acetate. *Contraception*, **22,** 359

Kurunmäki, H., Toivonen, J., Lähteenmäki, P. and Luukkainen, T. (1981). Intracervical release of levonorgestrel for contraception. *Contraception*, **23,** 473

Labrie, F., Auclair, C., Cusan, L., Kelly, P.A., Pelletier, G. and Ferland, F. (1978). Inhibitory effects of LHRH and its agonists on testicular gonadotropin receptors and spermatogenesis in the rat. *Int. J. Androl.* (Suppl.) **2,** 303

Landgren, B.M., Adedo, A.R., Hagenfeldt, F. and Diczfalusy, E. (1979). Clinical effects of orally administered extracts of *Montanoa zoapatle* in early human pregnancy. *Am. J. Obstet. Gynecol.*, **135,** 480

Lawley, P.D. and Brookes, P. (1963). Further studies on the alkylation of nucleic and their constituent nucleotides. *Biochem. J.*, **89,** 127

Lee, C.Y., Moon, Y.S., Duleba, A. and Chan, A.F. (1982). The instability of gossypol. In *Proceedings of the International Symposium of Reproductive Health Care: Contraceptive Delivery Systems*, Maui, Hawaii. Vol. 3, no. 3/4, Abstract no. 274

Lee, C.Y., Moon, Y.S. and Gomel, V. (1982). Inactivation of lactate dehydrogenase-X by gossypol. In *Proceedings of the International Symposium on Reproductive Health Care: Contraceptive Delivery Systems*, Maui, Hawaii. Vol. 3, no. 3/4, Abstract no. 275

Lee, D.L., Kollmann, P.A., Mash, F.J. and Wolff, M.E. (1975). Quantitative relationships between steroid structure and binding to putative progesterone receptors. *J. Med. Chem.*, **20,** 1139

Leonhard, J.M. and Paulsen, C.A. (1978). Contraceptive development studies for males: oral and parenteral steroid hormone administration, p. 1078. In Patanelli, D.J. (ed.) *Hormonal Control of Male Fertility*, DHEW Publ. (NIH)

Levi, A.J., Smethurst, P. and O'Morain, C.A. (1982). Sulphasalazine induced male fertility in man and rats. In *Proceedings of the International Symposium on Reproductive Health Care: Contraceptive Delivery Systems*, Maui, Hawaii. Vol. 3, no. 3/4. Abstract no. 289

Lewis, D.H., Tice, T.R., Meyers, W.E., Cowsar, D.R. and Beck, L.R. (1983). Biodegradable microcapsules for contraceptive steroids. In *Proceedings of the International Symposium on Reproductive Health Care: Contraceptive Delivery Systems*, Maui, Hawaii. Vol. 3, Abstract no. 55

Liu, Q.Z. (1980). Clinical trial of gossypol as a male antifertility agent. In Chang, C.F. (ed.) *Recent Advances in Fertility Regulation*. Proc. Symp. Beijing, September 1980

Lobl, T.J. (1979). 1-(2,4-Dichlorobenzyl)-1*H*-indazole-3-carboxylic acid (DICA), an exfoliative antispermatogenic agent in the rat. *Arch. Androl.*, **2**, 353

Lobl, T.J., Forbes, A.D., Kirton, K.T. and Wilks, J.W. (1979). Characterization of the exfoliative antispermatogenic agent 1-(2,4-dichlorobenzyl)-1*H*-indazole-3-carboxylic acid in the rhesus monkey. *Arch. Androl.*, **3**, 67

Lobl, T.J. and Porteus, S.E. (1978). Antifertility activities of 5-thio-D-glucose in mice and rats. *Contraception*, **17**, 123

Lucier, G.W., Lee, I.P. and Dixon, R.L. (1977). Effects of environmental agents on male reproduction. In Johnson, A.D. and Gomes, W.R. (eds.) *The Testis*. Vol. 4, pp. 578-604 (New York: Academic Press)

MacNatty, K.P., Henderson, K.M. and Sawers, R.S. (1975). Effect of prostaglandins F₂ and E₂ on the production of progesterone by human granulosa cells in tissue culture. *J. Endocrinol.*, **67**, 231

Mahmoud, K.Z., Abou Fadl, W.S., Abdou, M.S.S., Sharawi, M., Badawi, A.B.A., Safouri, L.S., Hemeida, N.A., Ragab, R.S. and Girgis, S.M. (1982). Contraceptive value of circumvasal copper-200 wire in male rats. In *Proceedings of the International Symposium on Reproductive Health Care: Contraceptive Delivery Systems*, Maui, Hawaii. Vol. 3, no. 3/4, Abstract no. 301

Mancini, R.E. (1974). Immunological approaches to fertility control. In Diczfalusy, E. and Borell, V. *Control of Human Fertility*, pp. 157-178. Nobel Symposium no. 15. (Stockholm: Almquist and Wiksell)

Manson, J.M. and Simons, R. (1979). Influence of environmental agents on male reproductive failure. In Hunt, V.R. (ed.) *Work and the Health of Women*, pp. 155-179. (Boca Raton, Florida: CRC Press)

Marek, J. and Horky, K. (1970). Aminogluthethimide administration in pregnancy. *Lancet*, **ii**, 1312

Mauss, J., Börsch, G., Bormacher, K., Richter, E., Leyendecker, G. and Nocke, W. (1975). Effect of longterm testosterone oenanthate administration on male reproductive function: clinical evaluation, serum FSH, LH, testosterone and seminal fluid analyses in normal men. *Acta Endocrinol. (Copenh.)*, **78**, 373

Mauss, J., Börsch, G., Richter, E. and Bormacher, K. (1974). Investigation on the use of testosterone oenanthate as a male contraceptive agent. *Contraception*, **10**, 281

Meyer, R.K. (1972). Chorionic gonadotropin, corpus luteum function and embryo implantation in the rhesus monkey. In Diczfalusy, E. and Standley, C.C. (eds.) *The Use of Nonhuman Primates in Research on Human Reproduction*, pp. 214-217 (Geneva: WHO)

Mishell, D.R. (1982). *Advances in Fertility Research*. Vol. 1. (New York: Raven Press)

Mora, G., Faundes, A. and Johansson, E.D.B. (1975). Lack of clinical contraceptive efficacy of large doses of R 2323 given before implantation of after a missed period. *Contraception*, **12**, 211

Mori, R., Hoshiai, H., Uehara, S., Imaitumi, H., Hirano, M. and Suzuki, M. (1983). 'Gossypol' as oral contraceptive for men. In Harrison, R. (ed.) *Eleventh World Congress on Fertility and Sterility*, Dublin. Abstract no. 369

Morton, D.M. and McAnulty, P.A. (1979). The effect on fertility of immunizing female sheep with ram sperm acrosin and hyaluronidase. *J. Reprod. Immunol.*, **1**, 61

Nassar, M.F. and Tierney, T.T. (1982). Contrasperm™: A contraceptive for men. In *Proceedings of the International Symposium on Reproductive Health Care: Contraceptive Delivery Systems*, Maui, Hawaii. Vol. 3, no. 3/4, Abstract no. 299

Neill, J.D., Johansson, E.D.B. and Knobil, E. (1969). Failure of hysterectomy to influence the normal pattern of cyclic progesterone secretion in the rhesus monkey. *Endocrinology*, **84**, 464

Neill, J.D. and Knobil, E. (1972). On the nature of gestation and chorionic gonadotropin levels in the monkey after ovariectomy in early pregnancy. *Endocrinology*, **78**, 1076

Neri, R.O. and Mylecraine, L. (1982). Effect of chronic administration of flutamide on the pituitary–gonadal axis in male rats. In *Proceedings of the International Symposium on Reproductive Health Care: Contraceptive Delivery Systems*, Maui, Hawaii. Vol. 3, no. 3/4, Abstract no. 304

Neumann, F. and Elger, W. (1971). Kritische Überlegungen zu den biologischen Grundlagen von Toxizitätsstudien mit Seroid-(Sexual-)hormonen. In Plotz, E.J. and Haller, J. (eds.) *Methodik der Steroidtoxikologie*, pp. 6–48. (Stuttgart: Georg Thieme)

Neumann, F., Schenck, B. and Steinbeck, H. (1977). Present state of male contraception and future possibilities. In Haspels, A.A. (ed.) *International Symposium on Hormonal Contraception, Utrecht*. (Amsterdam, Oxford: Excerpta Medica)

Neumann, F., Schleusener, A. and Hümpel, M. (1979). Antiandrogene. *Gynaekologie*, **12**, 228

Nieschlag, E., Hoogen, H., Bölk, M., Schuster, H. and Wickings, E.J. (1978). Clinical trial with testosterone undecanoate for male fertility control. *Contraception*, **18**, 607

Nilsson, C.G. (1982). Fertility after discontinuation of levonorgestrel-releasing intrauterine devices. *Contraception*, **25**, 273

Nilsson, C.G., Allonen, H., Diaz, J. and Luukkainen, T. (1983). Two years' experience with two levonorgestrel-releasing intrauterine devices and one copper-releasing intrauterine device: a randomized comparative performance study. *Fertil. Steril.*, **39**, 187

Nilsson, C.G., Luukkainen, T., Diaz, J. and Allonen, H. (1981). Clinical performance of a new levonorgestrel-releasing intrauterine device. A randomized comparison with a Nova-T-copper device. *Contraception*, **25**, 345

Niswender, G.D., Menon, K.M.J. and Jaffe, R.B. (1972). Regulation of the corpus luteum during the menstrual cycle and early pregnancy. *Fertil. Steril.*, **23**, 432

Oikawa, T. and Yanagimachi, R. (1975). Block of hamster fertilisation by anti-ovary antibody. *J. Reprod. Fertil.*, **45**, 487

O'Rand, M.G. (1980). Antigens of spermatozoa and their environment. In Dhinsda, D.S. and Schumacher, G.F.B. (eds.) *Immunological Aspects of Infertility and Fertility Regulation*, pp. 155–163. (New York: Elsevier-North Holland)

Oriol-Bosch, A. and Cortes, J. (1975). Effects of postovulatory estradiol benzoate administration on women's ovarian function. *Fertil. Steril.*, **26**, 405

Oriowo, M.A., Landgren, B.M., Stenström, B. and Diczfalusy, E. (1980). A comparison of the pharmacokinetic properties of three estradiol esters. *Contraception*, **21**, 415

Osterberg, R.E., Bierbower, G.W. and Hehir, R.M. (1977). Renal and testicular damage following dermal application of the flame retardant tris(2,3-dibromopropyl)phosphate. *J. Toxicol. Environ. Hlth.*, **3**, 979

Page, E. (1981). Experiences with a tampon-spermicide device. *Contraception*, **23**, 37

Pakrashi, A. and Chakrabarty, S. (1981). Biological profile of the steroid 5-Stigmastane-3β,5,6β-triol-monobenzoate. *Contraception*, **23**, 315

Pakrasi, P.L. and Pakrasi, A. (1980). Role of p-coumaric acid in experimentally induced delayed implantation in mice reproduction. *Obstet. Gynecol.*, **8**, 573

Parrish, R.F., Strauss, J.W., Paulsen, J.D., Polakoski, K.L., Tidwell, R.R., Geratz, J.D. and Stevens, F.M. (1978). Structure–activity relationships for the inhibition of acrosin by benzaminidine derivates. *J. Med. Chem.*, **21**, 1132

Paulsen, C.A., Leonard, J.M., Burgess, E.C. and Ospina, L.F. (1978). Male contraceptive development: reexamination of testosterone enanthate as an effective single entity agent. In Patanelli, D.J. (ed.) *Hormonal Control of Male Fertility*, p. 17. DHEW Publ No (NIH)

Petersen, P. (1977). Seelische Folgen nach legalem Schwangerschaftsabbruch. Ergebnisse einer Sammelstatistik der internationalen Literatur. *Dtsches Ärztl.*, **18**, 1205

Philibert, D., Dereadt, R. and Teutsch, G. (1981). RU 38486, a potent antiglucocorticoid *in vivo*. In *Eighth International Congress of Pharmacology*, Tokyo. Abstract no. 1463

Philibert, D. and Raynaud, J.P. (1974). Binding of progesterone and R 5020, a highly potent progestin, to human endometrium and myometrium. *Contraception*, **10**, 457

Pincus, G. (1965). *The Control of Fertility*, pp. 24–34. (New York: Academic Press)

Population Reports (1976). Sterilization. Tubal sterilization—Review of methods. Series C, No. 7, C-75, C-79, C-82, C-83, C-86, C-90. Department of Medical and Public Affairs, George Washington University Medical Center, Washington

Population Reports (1978). Special topic monographs. Voluntary sterilization: world's leading contraceptive method. No. 2, M-37. Department of Medical and Public Affairs, George Washington University Medical Center, Washington

Population Reports (1979). Intrauterine devices. IUDs—Update on safety, effectiveness and research. Series B, No. 3, Population Information Program. John Hopkins University, Baltimore

Population Reports (1983). *Migration, Population Growth and Development*. Vol. 7, September/October

Potashnik, G., Ben-Adere, N., Israeli, R., Yanai-Inbar, I. and Sober, I. (1978). Suppressive effect of 1,2-dibromo-3-chloropropane on human spermatogenesis. *Fertil. Steril.*, **30**, 444

Potashnik, G., Israeli, R. and Yanai-Inbar, I. (1982). Suppressive effect of dibromochloropropane on human testicular function. In *Proceedings of the International Symposium on Reproductive Health Care: Contraceptive Delivery Systems*, Maui, Hawaii. Vol. 3, no. 3/4, Abstract no. 296

Powers, M.B., Voelker, R.W., Page, N.P., Weisburger, E.K. and Kraybill, H.F. (1975). Carcinogenicity of ethylene dibromide (EDB) and 1,2-dibromo-3-chloropropane (DBCP) after oral administration in rats and mice. *Toxicol. Appl. Pharmacol.*, **33**, 171

Prakash, A. (1979). Protein concentration in the rat uterus under the influences of *Hibiscus rosa-sinensis* Linn. extracts. *Proc. Indian Acad. Sci.*, **4**, 327

Prakash, A.O. (1978). Antiestrogenic mode of action of leaf extracts *Artobotrys odoratissimus* Linn. *Indian J. Exp. Biol.*, **16**, 214

Prakash, A.O. (1979). Effect of *Embelia ribes* on uterine weight of normal and ovariectomized rats. *Planta Med.*, **35**, 370

Prakash, A.O. and Mathur, R. (1979). Studies on oestrus cycles of albino rats: Response to *Embelia ribes* extracts. *J. Med. Plant Res.*, **36**, 134

Prasad, M.R.N., Kalra, S.P. and Segal, S.J. (1965). Effect of clomiphene on blastocyts during delayed implantation in the rat. *Fertil. Steril.*, **16**, 101

Prema, K., Gayathiri, T.L., Ramalaskshimi, B.A., Madhavapeddi, R. and Philips, F.S. (1981). Low doses injectable contraceptive norethisterone enanthate 20 mg monthly. I. Clinical trials. *Contraception*, **23**, 11

Quai, S.Z. (1982). Participation of prostaglandin in the mechanism of action of gossypol. In *Proceedings of the International Symposium on Reproductive Health Care: Contraceptive Delivery Systems*, Maui, Hawaii. Vol. 3, no. 3/4, Abstract no. 276

Rabe, T., Kiesel, L., Kellermann, J., Weidenhammer, K., Runnebaum, B. and Potts, G. (1983). Inhibition of human placental progesterone synthesis and aromatase activity by synthetic steroidogenic inhibitors in vitro. *Fertil. Steril.*, **39**, 829

Rabe, T., Rabe, D. and Runnebaum, B. (1982). Aminogluthethimid-Pharmakologie und Klinik eines neuen Pharmakons. *Therapiewoche*, **32**, 1169

Rabe, T. and Runnebaum, M. (1982). *Kontrazeption*. (Heidelberg: Springer)

Randic, L. and Balogh, S. (1982). Effect of hydrogel on the reduction of bleeding associated with IUD use. In *XIth World Congress of Gynecology and Obstetrics*, San Francisco, USA. Abstract no. 1605

Rao, B.R., Wiest, W.G. and Allen, W.M. (1973). Progesterone 'receptor' in rabbit uterus. I. Characterization and estradiol-17β augmentation. *Endocrinology*, **92**, 1229

Rao, V.S.N., Dasaradhan, P. and Krishnaiah, K.S. (1979). Antifertility effect of some indigenous plants. *Indian J. Med. Res.*, **70**, 517

Rathinam, K., Shanthakumari, G. and Ramiah, H. (1976). Studies on the antifertility activity of Embelin. *J. Res. Indian Med. Yoga Homeopathy*, **11**, 84

Ratnam, S.S. and Prasad, R.N.V. (1980). Recent developments in steroidal contraception. *Singapore J. Obstet. Gynaecol.*, **3**, 7

Raynaud, J.P., Bonne, C., Bouton, M.M., Mogivelewsky, M., Philibert, D. and Azadian-Boulanger, G. (1975). Screening for anti-hormones by receptor studies. *J. Steroid Biochem.*, **6**, 615

Reddy, P.R.K. and Rao, J.M. (1972). Reversible antifertility action of testosterone propionate in human males. *Contraception*, **5**, 520

Reddy, P.R.K. and Rukmini, V. (1981). α-Difluoromethylornithine as a postcoitally effective antifertility agent in female rats. *Contraception*, **24**, 215

Reed, T. and Erb, R. (1982). Hysteroscopic sterilization with form-in-place silicone rubber plugs. In *XIth World Congress of Gynecology and Obstetrics*, San Francisco, USA. Abstract no. 1300

Reinius, S., Fritz, G.R. and Knobil, E. (1973). Ultrastructure and endocrinological correlation of an early implantation site in the rhesus monkey. *J. Reprod. Fertil.*, **32**, 171

Richart, R.M. (1981). Female sterilization using chemical agents. *Res. Front. Fertil. Reg.*, **1**, 12

Rimkus, V. and Semm, K. (1976). Hysteroscopic sterilization—a routine method? *Int. J. Fertil.*, **22**, 121

Rivier, J., Rivier, C., Perrin, M., Porter, M. and Vale, W. (1981). Gn-RH analogues: structure–activity relationships. In Zatuchni, G., Shelton, J. and Sciarra, J. *LH-RH Peptides as Female and Male Contraceptives*, pp. 13–23. Proceedings of an International Workshop, Chicago, 1981

Robertson, D.N., Alvarez, F., Sivin, I., Brache, V., Stern, J., Leon, P. and Faundes, A. (1981). Lipoprotein patterns in women in Santo Domingo using a levonorgestrel/estradiol contraceptive ring. *Contraception*, **24**, 469

Rosenfield, S.S. (1926). Semen injections with serologic studies. *Am. J. Obstet. Gynecol.*, **12**, 385

Roy, S., Wilkins, J. and Mishell, D. (1981). The effect of a contraceptive vaginal ring and oral contraceptives on the vaginal flora. *Contraception*, **24**, 481

Ruh, T.S. and Ruh, M.F. (1974). The effect of antiestrogens on the nuclear binding of the estrogen receptor. *Steroids*, **24**, 209

Runnebaum, B. and Rabe, T. (1979). Neue Aspekte zur hormonalen Kontrazeption. *Medizin. Forum*, **3**, 15

Sacco, A. and Shivers, C.A. (1973). Localisation of tissue-specific antigens in the rabbit ovary, oviduct and uterus by fluorescent antibody technique. *J. Reprod. Fertil.*, **32**, 415

Sakai, C.N., Engel, B. and Channing, C.P. (1977). Ability of extract of pig corpus luteum to inhibit binding of ^{125}I-labelled human chorionic gonadotropin to porcine granulosa cells. *Proc. Soc. Exp. Biol.*, **155**, 373

Sakiz, E. and Azadian-Boulanger, G. (1971). R 2323—a contraceptive compound. In James, V.H.T. and Martini, L. (eds.) *Proceedings of the Third International Congress on Hormonal Steroids*, pp. 865–871. (Amsterdam: Excerpta Medica)

Sakiz, E., Azadian-Boulanger, G., Laraque, F. and Raynaud, J.P. (1974). A new approach to estrogen-free contraception based on progesterone receptor blockage by mid-cycle administration of ethyl norgestrienone (R 2323). *Contraception*, **10**, 467

Sakiz, E., Azadian-Boulanger, G., Ojasoo, T. and Laraque, F. (1976). Contraceptive efficacy of one-weekly oral administration of 2.5 mg R 2323. *Contraception*, **14**, 275

Saluja, A.K. and Santani, D.D. (1981). Antifertility activity of *Hyptis suaveolens* Poir. *Indian Drugs*, **12**, 127

Sandow, J., Rechenberg, W.F. and Jerzabek, G. (1977). Endocrine effects of chronic treatment with LHRH analogue D-Ser (TBU)[6] ethylamide. *Acta Endocrinol. (Copenh.)*, **208**, Suppl., 208

Saxena, B.B., Hasan, S.H., Haour, F. and Schmidt-Gollwitzer, M. (1974). Radioreceptor assay of human chorionic gonadotropin: detection of early pregnancy. *Science, N.Y.*, **184**, 793

Schenkel-Hulliger, L., Krähenbühl, Ch., Talwalker, P.K. and Bischof, P. (1979). Experimental models in the search for antigestrogenic compounds with menses-inducing activity. *J. Steroid Biochem.*, **11**, 757

Schmidt-Gollwitzer, K. (1981a). Medikamentös induzierter Frühabort: Zyklus post abortum. In Hepp, H. and Schüßler, B. (eds.) *Prostaglandine in Geburtshilfe und Gynäkologie*, pp. 199–208. (Heidelberg: Springer)

Schmidt-Gollwitzer, M. and Schmidt-Gollwitzer, K. (1981). Abortinduktion mit Prostaglandinen. In Hepp, H. and Schüßler, B. (eds.) *Prostaglandine in Geburtshilfe und Gynäkologie*, pp. 182–191. (Heidelberg: Springer)

Schmidt-Gollwitzer, M., Schmidt-Gollwitzer, K., Schüßler, B., Koch, R. and Nevinny-Stickel, J. (1977). Erste Erfahrungen mit einem neuen Prostaglandin E2-Derivat. *Geburtshilfe Frauenheilk.*, **37**, 1030

Schmidt-Mathiessen, H. (1979). *Gynäkologie und Geburtshilfe*, p. 157. (Stuttgart, New York: Schatthauer)

Schneider, H. (1982). The microcomputer as an improved method for fertility awareness. In *Proceedings of the International Symposium on Reproductive Health Care: Contraceptive Delivery Systems*, Maui, Hawaii. Vol. 3, Abstract no. 52

Schreiner, W.E. (1976). Ovar. In Siegenthaler, W. (ed.) *Klinische Pathophysiologie*, p. 390. (Stuttgart: Thieme)

Seifert, R.M., Buttery, R.C. and Ling, L. (1968). Identification of some constituents of carrot seed oil. *J. Sci. Food Agric.*, **19**, 383

Semm, K. and Giese, K.P. (1981). Ernst Gräfenberg, das Leben und Werk des Kieler Facharztes. Zum 100. Geburtstag am 26. September 1981. *Geburtsh. Frauenheilk.*, **41**, 397

Seshardi, C., Suganthan, D. and Shanthakumari, G. (1978). Biochemical changes in the uterus and uterine fluid of mated rats treated with embelin—a non-steroidal oral contraceptive. *Indian J. Exp. Biol.*, **16**, 1187

Shamsuzzoha, R. and Ahmed, M. (1979). Antifertility activity of a medicinal plant of the genus *Andrographis* Wall. (family Acanthaceae). *Bangladesh Med. Res. Council Bull.*, **1**, 14

Sharma, M.M. and Jocob, D. (1976). Effect of a newly synthesized phenothiazine on gastric acid secretion and gastric ulcers in Shay rats. *Indian J. Exp. Biol.*, **14**, 340

Shaw, S.T., Macaulay, L.K., Aznar, R., Gonzalez-Angulo, A. and Roy, S. (1981). Effects of a progesterone-releasing intrauterine contraceptive device on endometrial blood vessels: A morphometric study. *Am. J. Obstet. Gynecol.*, **1**, 822

Shinada, T., Yokota, Y. and Igarashi, M. (1978). Inhibitory effect of various gestagens upon the pregnenolone 3β-ol-dehydrogenase-delta$^{5-4}$-isomerase system in human corpora lutea of menstrual cycles. *Fertil. Steril.*, **29**, 84

Shivers, C.A. (1975). Antigens of the ovum as a potential basis for the development of contraceptive vaccine. Presented at *Third Int. Symp. Imm. Reprod.*, Varna

Short, R.V. (1969). Implantation and the maternal recognition of pregnancy. In Wolstenholme, G.E.W. and O'Connor, M. (eds.) *Ciba Symposium on Foetal Autonomy*, pp. 2–31. (London: Churchill)

Short, R.V. (1976). The evolution of human reproduction. *Proc. R. Soc. London B*, **195**, 3

Silvesterini, B., Burberi, S., Catanese, B., Ciolo, V., Coulston, F., Lisciani, R. and Barcellona, P. (1975). Antispermatogenetic activity of I-*p*-chlorobenzyl-1*H*-indazole-3-carboxylic acid (AF 1312/TS) in rats. I. Trials of single short-term administration with the study of pharmacologic and toxicologic effects. *Exp. Molec. Pathol.*, **23**, 288

Sivin, I. and Stern, J. (1978). Long acting contraceptive implants. *Contraception*, **18**, 355

Sivin, I., Mishell, D.R., Victor, A., Diaz, S., Alvarez-Sanchez, F., Nielsen, N., Akinla, O., Pyrorala, T., Coutinho, E., Faundes, A., Roy, S., Brenner, P.F., Ahren, T., Pavez, M., Brache, V., Giwa-Osagie, O.F., Fasan, M.O., Zausner-Guelman, B., Darze, E., Gama da Silva, J.C., Diaz, J., Jackaicz, T.M., Stern, J. and Nash, H. (1981). A multicentre study of levonorgestrel-estradiol contraceptive vaginal rings. III. Menstrual patterns. *Contraception*, **24**, 377

Skoglund, R.D. and Paulsen, C.A. (1973). Danazol–testosterone combination; a potentially effective means for reversible male contraception. A preliminary report. *Contraception*, **7**, 357

Smith, K.D., Rodriguez-Rigau, L.J. and Steinberger, E. (1977). Relation between indices of semen analysis and pregnancy rates in infertile couples. *Fertil. Steril.*, **28**, 1314

Sod-Moriah, U.A., Shotland, I., Kaplanski, J., Potashnik, G., Hechtlinger, V. and Buchman, O. (1983). The effect of DBCP on reproduction of female rats. In Harrison, R.F. (ed.) *Eleventh World Congress on Fertility and Sterility* IFFS, Dublin. Abstract no. 374

Solo, A.J. and Gardner, J.O. (1968). Agents for alkylating steroid hormone receptors. I. Analogs derived from esters of 17-hydroxyprogesterone. *Steroids*, **11**, 37

Solo, A.J. and Gardner, J.O. (1971). Agents for alkylating steroid hormone receptors. III. ω-substituted esters of 17-hydroxyprogesterone. *J. Pharm. Sci.*, **60**, 1089

Steinberger, E. (1976). Recent advances in male fertility. In Moghissi, K. and Evans, T. (eds.) *Regulation of Human Fertility*, p. 274. (Detroit: Wayne State University Press)

Steinberger, E. and Smith, K.D. (1977). Effect of chronic administration of testosterone enanthate on sperm production and plasma testosterone, follicle-stimulating hormone and luteinizing hormone levels: a preliminary evaluation of a possible male contraceptive. *Fertil. Steril.*, **28**, 28

Steinberger, E., Smith, K.D. and Rodriguez-Gigau, L.J. (1978). Suppression and recovery of sperm production in men treated with testosterone enanthate for one year. A study of a possible reversible male contraceptive. *Int. J. Androl.*, **2** (Suppl.), 748

Stevens, V.C. (1975). Perspectives of development of a fertility control vaccine from hormonal antigens of the trophoblast. Presented at *Third Int. Symp. Imm. Reprod.*, Varna

Suganthan, D. and Santhakumari, G. (1979). Antifertility activity of an indigenous preparation Ayush-47. *Indian J. Med. Res.*, **70**, 504

Swerdloff, R.S., Peterson, M., Vera, A., Batt, R., Heber, D. and Bray, G.A. (1978). The hypothalamic pituitary axis in genetically obese (ob/ob) mice; response to luteinizing hormone releasing hormone. *Endocrinology*, **103**, 542

Tagaki, S., Sakata, H., Yoshida, T., Nakazawa, S., Fujii, K.T., Tominaga, Y., Ninawaga, T., Hiroshima, T., Tomida, Y., Ithoh, K. and Matuskawa, R. (1977). Termination of early pregnancy by ONO-802 (16,16-dimethyl-*trans*-2-PGE$_1$ methyl ester). *Prostaglandins*, **14**, 791

Talwar, G.P. and Sharma, N.C. (1976). Isoimmunization against human chorionic gonadotropin with conjugates of processed β-subunit of the hormone and tetanus toxoid. *Proc. Natl. Acad. Sci. USA*, **73**, 218

Taubert, H.D. and Kuhl, H. (1981). *Kontrazeption mit Hormonen.* (Stuttgart: Georg Thieme)

Teramoto, S.R., Saito, H., Aoyama, H. and Shirasu, Y. (1980). Dominant lethal mutation induced in male rats by 1,2-dibromo-3-chloropropane (DBCP). *Mutation Res.*, 77, 71

Thiery, M., Parewijck, W. and van der Pas, H. (1983). Immediate postpartum IUD insertion: Comparison of sutured and non-sutured devices. In *Proceedings of the International Symposium on Reproductive Health Care: Contraceptive Delivery Systems*, Maui, Hawaii. Vol. 3, Abstract no. 231

Timonen, H., Nylander, P., Kivijarvi, A., Hirvonen, E., Kajanoja, P., Kaivola, S., Koitilainen, A., Savia, E., Saure, A., Lonnblad, R., Terava, M., Venhola, M., Manniko, H., Kaar, K. and Vierola, H. (1983). Comparative performance of three copper IUD's (ML CU-375, Fincoid and Nova-T) after one year's follow-up in randomized multicenter trial. In *Proceedings of the International Symposium on Reproductive Health Care: Contraceptive Delivery Systems*, Maui, Hawaii. Vol. 3, Abstract no. 226

Toth, A. (1982). Reversible toxic effect of salicylazosulfpyridine (SASP) on male fertility. In *Proceedings of the International Symposium on Reproductive Health Care: Contraceptive Delivery Systems*, Maui, Hawaii. Vol. 3, no. 3/4, Abstract no. 387

Tsunoda, Y. and Chang, M.C. (1976a). The effect of passive immunization with hetero and isoimmune anti-ovary antiserum on the fertilization of mouse, rat and hamster eggs. *Biol. Reprod.*, 15, 361

Tsunoda, Y. and Chang, M.C. (1976b). Effect of anti-rat ovary antiserum on the fertilization of mouse, rat and hamster eggs in vivo and in vitro. *Biol. Reprod.*, 14, 354

Vickery, B.H. and McRae, G.I. (1980). Responses of the males of different laboratory species to continuous administration of an LHRH agonist. *J. Androl.*, 1, 37

Viinikka, L., Victor, A., Jänne, O. and Raynaud, J.P. (1975). The plasma concentration of a synthetic progestin R 2323, released from polysialastic vaginal rings. *Contraception*, 12, 309

Voisin, G.A. and Toullet, F. (1973). Auto-immune aspermatogenetic orchitis (AIAO) induced by different spermatozoa autoantigens and different immunopathological mechanisms. In *Immunology Reproduction.* (Sofia: Bulgarian Academy of Sciences Press)

Vorhauer, B.W. (1980). Excerpt from his presentation at the *MID-Atlantic Conference on Bio-fluid Mechanics. Times-Picayune*, New Orleans, May

Wang, S.S. and Shuy, S.D. (1970). Clinical analysis of 201 cases of midterm abortion induced with the Yuan-Hua terpin. *Chinese J. Obstet. Gynecol.*, 14, 290

Warren, L.A., McRae, G. and Vickery, B. (1979). Antifertility efficacy of twice daily oral administration of 6-chloro-6-deoxy-D-glucose (6CDG) in male rats. *Contraception*, 20, 275

Weinberger, M.A., Friedman, L., Farber, T.M., Moreland, F.M., Peters, E.L., Gilmor, G.I. and Khan, M.A. (1978). Testicular atrophy and impaired spermatogenesis in rats fed high levels of the methylxanthines, caffeine, theobromine, or theophylline. *J. Environ. Path. Toxicol.*, 1, 669

Weiner, E. and Johansson, E.D.B. (1975). Plasma levels of norethindrone after i.m. injection of 200 mg norethindrone enanthate. *Contraception*, 22, 359

Wheat, T.E. and Goldberg, E. (1981). Immunologically active peptide fragments of the sperm-specific lactate dehydrogenase C4 isoenzyme. In Rich, D.H., Gross, E. and Rockford, I.L. (eds.) *Peptides: Synthesis-Structure-Function*, pp. 557–560. (Pierce Chemical Company)

Wiechell, H. (1981). Intramurale Prostaglandinapplikation bei 328 Fällen von ambulantem Schwangerschaftsabbruch im 1. Trimenon. In Hepp. H. and Schüßler, B. (eds.) *Prostglandine in Gynäkologie und Geburtshilfe*, pp. 209–216. (Heidelberg: Springer)

World Health Organization (1978). Special Programme on Research, Development and Research Training in Human Reproduction, Geneva. *Seventh Annual Report.*

Yang, K.P., Samaan, N.A. and Ward, D.N. (1976a). Characterization of an inhibitor for luteinizing hormone receptor site binding. *Endocrinology*, 98, 233

Yang, K.P., Samaan, N.A. and Ward, D.N. (1976b). Lutropin receptors from male and female tissues: different responses to a lutropin receptor binding inhibitor. *Proc. Soc. Exp. Biol. Med.*, 152, 606

Yang, Y.C. (1979). Prematurity of the human endometrium after the oral administration of the progestin no. 1 compound tablet. *Acta Physiol. Sinica*, 31, 283

Ying, B.P. *et al.* (1976). Studies on the active principle of the root yuan-hua (*Daphne genkwa*). I. Isolation and structure of yanghuacine. *Acta Chim. Sinica (Shanghai)*, 35, 103

Yochim, J.M. and de Feo, V.J. (1962). Control of decidual growth in the rat by steroid hormones of the ovary. *Endocrinology*, 71, 134

Zatuchni, G.I., Labbok, M.H. and Sciarra, J.J. (eds.) (1980). *Research Frontiers in Fertility Regulation.* (Hagerstown, Md.: Harper and Row)

Zhang, S.Y. and Liu, X.G. (1982). Surface antigens of eggs: Immunological responses of zona pellucida material of heterologous species. In *Proceedings of the International Symposium on Reproductive Health Care: Contraceptive Delivery Systems*, Maui, Hawaii. Vol. 3, no. 3/4. Abstract no. 258

Zipper, J., Stachetti, A. and Medel, M. (1975). Transvaginal chemical sterilization: Clinical use of quinacrine plus potentiating adjuvants. *Contraception*, **12**, 11

Zysk, J.R., Bushway, A.A., Whistler, R.L. and Carlton, W.W. (1975). Temporary infertility produced in male mice by 5-thio-D-glucose. *J. Reprod. Fertil.*, **45**, 69

2
Steroidal contraception—
experimental background

F. NEUMANN

INTRODUCTION

Regression of germinal epithelium after administration of extracts from bull testes was shown in rats more than 50 years ago by Moore and Price[1]. Even as long ago as that, they assumed that the effect was accomplished via pituitary inhibition. In the following years the inhibitory effect of low and moderate androgen doses on the testes was described in numerous experiments[2-10].

Following the discovery of the negative feedback between testicular and hypophyseal function in 1932[11], it was assumed that the inhibitory effect of androgens and other steroid hormones on testes function and spermatogenesis is an indirect one and is accomplished by inhibition of gonadotrophin secretion. Because the inhibitory effect of steroid hormones on testes function has been known for so long, one wonders why preparations containing steroid hormones have not been developed before now for fertility control in men. The reasons for this will be discussed later, the different groups of steroid hormones being considered separately.

ANDROGENS AND ANABOLIC STEROIDS

The androgen requirement for the testis itself is higher than the androgen requirement for other androgen-dependent organs. The intratesticular androgen concentrations in the testes are consequently much higher than, for example, in the accessory sex glands or in serum. Table 1 gives one example.

Androgens or anabolic steroids inhibit LH secretion and consequently endogenous biosynthesis of androgens. In spite of the decreased androgen biosynthesis, exogenously administered androgens and anabolic steroids, while unable to support spermatogenesis, do maintain all other androgen-dependent functions, including libido. This is illustrated schematically in Figures 1 and 2.

As an example, Figure 3 shows the results of an experiment performed in adult male rats which were treated with increasing doses of testosterone

Table 1　Concentration of testosterone (nmol/ml) in serum and in testes cytosol of rats

Serum	Testes cytosol
11 ± 2	83 ± 14

propionate over a period of 6 weeks. Testosterone doses of approximately 0.1–0.3 mg/day decreased testicular weight drastically and inhibited spermatogenesis. Prostate weight is not impaired in lower doses: higher doses stimulate the prostate. Figure 4 shows the effect of several anabolic steroids on testes weight of juvenile rats.

Following administration of anabolic steroids, there is at first an androgen deficit in the testis itself, as can be seen from the drop in weight. With larger doses the deficit of endogenous androgens is increasingly compensated and the decrease in testicular weight is less extensive. This is shown by the descending part of the curve.

In this connection, danazol, an ethinyl testosterone derivative, should be mentioned, because several clinical studies have been performed with this steroid[12]. Danazol is characterized by its relatively strong antigonadotrophic effect, compared with its androgenic anabolic activity. Daily doses of 600 mg of danazol have to be administered in addition to an androgen

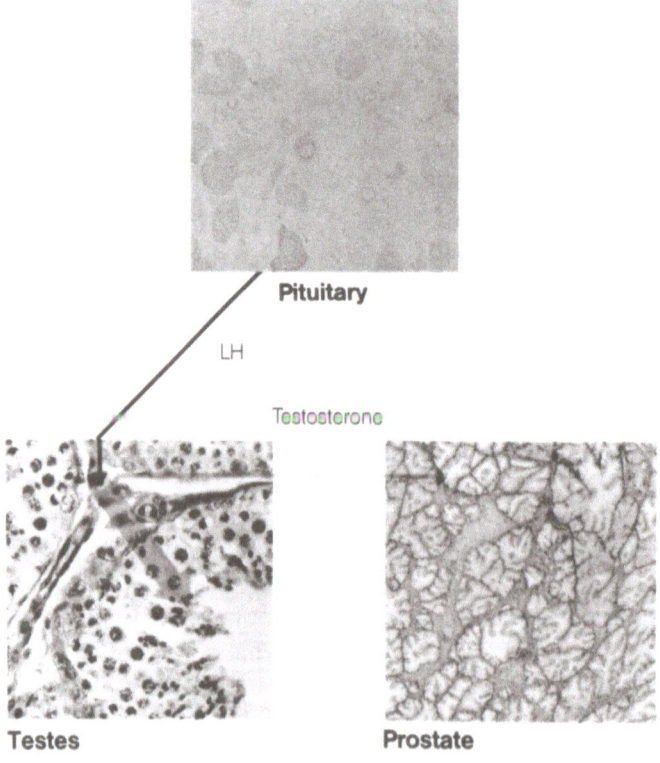

Pituitary

LH

Testosterone

Testes　　　　　　Prostate

Figure 1　Intratesticular and serum testosterone concentrations: normal situation

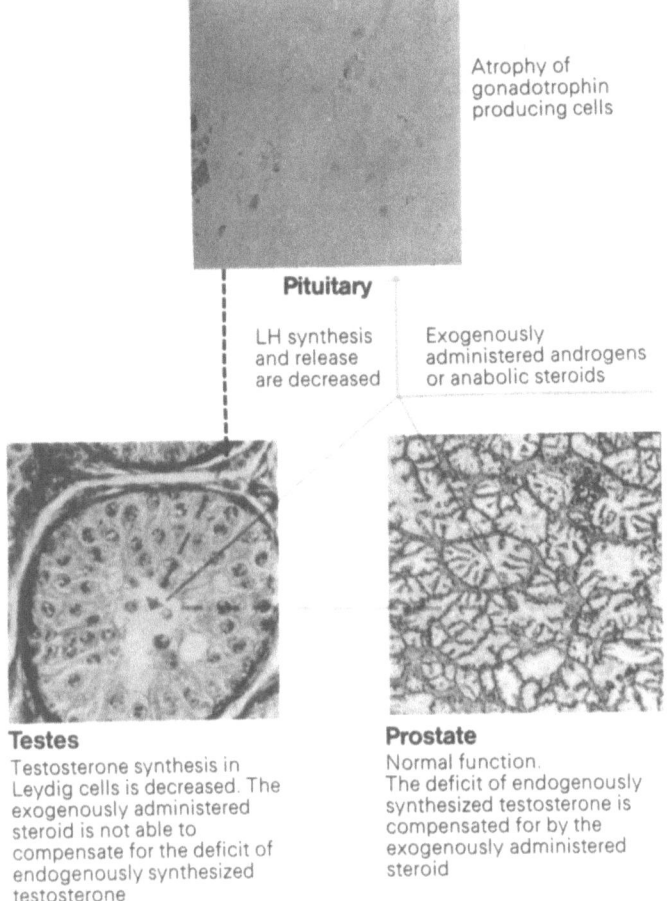

Pituitary

Atrophy of gonadotrophin producing cells

LH synthesis and release are decreased

Exogenously administered androgens or anabolic steroids

Testes
Testosterone synthesis in Leydig cells is decreased. The exogenously administered steroid is not able to compensate for the deficit of endogenously synthesized testosterone

Prostate
Normal function. The deficit of endogenously synthesized testosterone is compensated for by the exogenously administered steroid

Figure 2 Intratesticular and serum testosterone concentrations after treatment with androgens or anabolic steroids

in order to substitute for the peripheral androgen deficiency and to achieve azoospermia. Because this steroid is alkylated in position 17, toxic effects on liver function can not be excluded. Danazol offers no advantages as compared with other anabolic steroids; rather, disadvantages.

Numerous experiments of this type have been performed during the last 40 or 50 years. The outcome in each case was more or less identical: with a certain dose of an androgen or anabolic steroid it is possible to inhibit spermatogenesis without interfering with other androgen-dependent functions, including libido (potentia coeundi) and accessory sexual glands. On the basis of this pharmacological–endocrinological background, androgens and anabolic steroids can be used for male fertility control, and several clinical trials have been performed during the last 10–15 years. Some of these studies[12–23] are mentioned in Table 2.

The clinical data will not be discussed, because this aspect is covered elsewhere in this book.

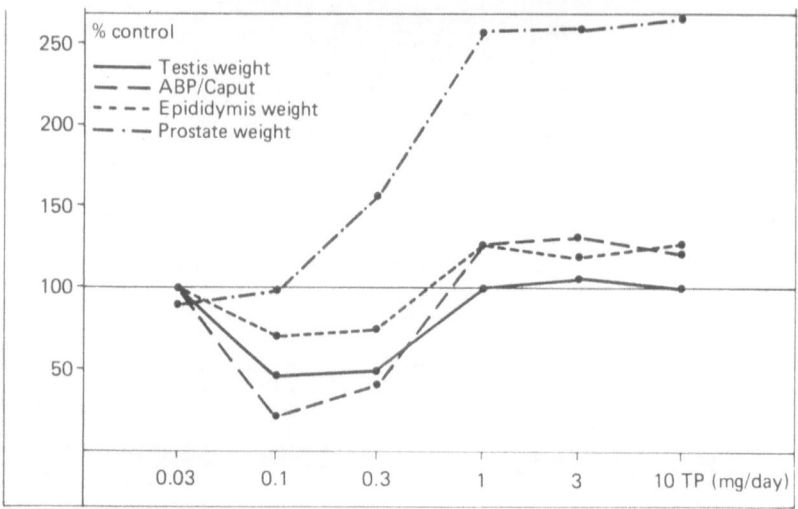

Figure 3 Effect of testosterone propionate (TP) on weight of prostate, epididymis and testes and androgen binding protein (ABP) content in the caput epididymidis. Rats with an initial body weight of about 200 g were treated for 6 weeks with increasing doses of TP (0.03–10 mg per animal per day s.c.). Note the biphasic effect of TP on testes, epididymis and ABP, which is due to the decrease of intratesticular testosterone concentrations while stimulation of the prostate occurs dose-dependently

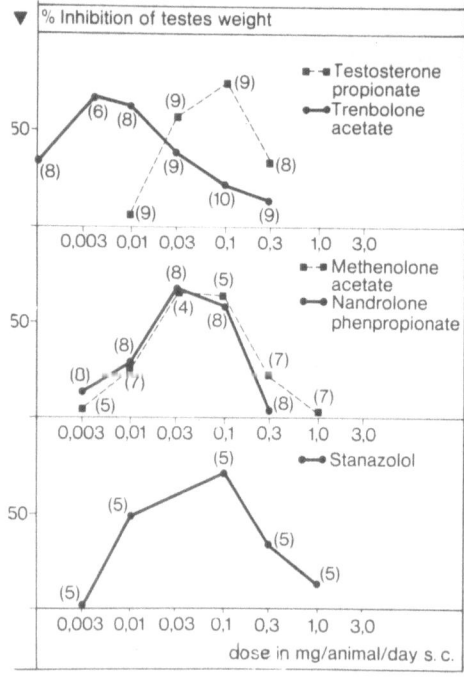

Figure 4 Effect of several anabolic steroids on weight of testes in juvenile rats treated for 14 days

Table 2 Effects of different steroids or steroid combinations on inhibition of spermatogenesis in men

Steroids	Dose	Effectiveness	Side-effects	References
Oestrogens				
Mestranol	450 µg/day p.o.	++	++	13
Progestogens				
Medroxyprogesterone acetate	125, 250 or 1000 mg i.m.	+	+	14
Chlormadinone acetate	200–500 mg i.m.	(+)	–	15
Gestonorone capronate	100 or 200 mg/week i.m.	(+)	–	16
Norethisterone enanthate	200 mg/3 weeks i.m.	++	+	16
Norethandrolone	30 mg/day p.o.	++	++	13
Norethisterone	30 mg/day p.o.	++	++	13
Noretynodrel	30 mg/day p.o.	++	++	13
Progesterone	50 mg/day p.o.	++	++	13
Androgens				
Testosterone propionate	25 or 50 mg/day i.m.	++	–	17, 18
Testosterone enanthate	200 or 250 mg/week i.m.	++	–	14
	200 mg in different intervals	++	–	19, 20
Combinations				
Danazol + testosterone enanthate	600 mg/day p.o., 200 mg/month i.m.	+	–	12
Danazol + testosterone propionate	600 mg/day p.o., 10 mg 3 × /week i.m.	+	–	12
Norethisterone + testosterone	25 mg/day p.o., Silastic implants	+	(+)	21
Megestrol acetate + testosterone	30 mg/day p.o., Silastic implants	++	(+)	22
Norgestrienone + testosterone	100 mg/week p.o., Silastic implants	++	(+)	23
Norethisterone + testosterone	100 mg/week p.o., Silastic implants	(+)	(+)	23
Megestrol acetate + testosterone	Silastic implants	(+)	(+)	22
Norethisterone + testosterone	Silastic implants	+	(+)	22

A commercial preparation for male fertility control containing an androgen or anabolic steroid does not exist, because there are several disadvantages.

(1) In position C-17 alkylated oral active androgens or anabolic steroids, when given in doses needed to inhibit spermatogenesis, are liver-toxic.

(2) Weekly injections or administration of depot preparations every 14 days or 4 weeks are not practicable.

(3) Azoospermia or oligozoospermia does not occur immediately, and examination of the ejaculate would be necessary to be sure whether and when azoospermia is achieved.

(4) Patients with oligozoospermia are not always infertile and it is known from clinical studies with cyproterone acetate[24] that this is even more the case in men where oligozoospermia had been induced by hormone treatment.

(5) After discontinuation of treatment, 3–6 months is needed before spermatogenesis is restored.

(6) It is known from animal experiments and from prostatic carcinoma patients that after long-term suppression of pituitary function by treatment with steroid hormones the hypothalamic–pituitary system becomes adapted to the high hormone levels and starts to secrete gonadotrophins again. Consequently, spermatogenesis is no longer fully inhibited. Regular control of the ejaculate would be necessary to be sure that azoospermia still persists.

Since we know that patients with pronounced oligozoospermia of less than 20 million spermatozoa/ml can be fertile, it seems highly improbable that, for example, the reliability of oral contraceptives for women, Pearl index much less than 1, can be achieved.

Taking all aspects together, it is very unlikely that androgens or anabolic steroids will be used for male fertility control in the near future. The situation might change during the next century (because of pressure of overpopulation).

SYNTHETIC PROGESTOGENS

Spermatogenesis is also inhibited by most of the synthetic progestogens. 19-Nortestosterone derivatives are more potent than hydroxyprogesterone derivatives. The mechanism of action is the same, as has been discussed for androgens and anabolic steroids, namely mainly inhibition of LH secretion and endogenous testosterone biosynthesis. However, in contrast to androgens and anabolic steroids, synthetic progestogens do not substitute peripheral androgen-dependent organs or functions. That means that with synthetic progestogens libido and potency (potentia coeundi) and secretory activity of accessory sexual glands is also impaired. This is illustrated schematically in Figure 5.

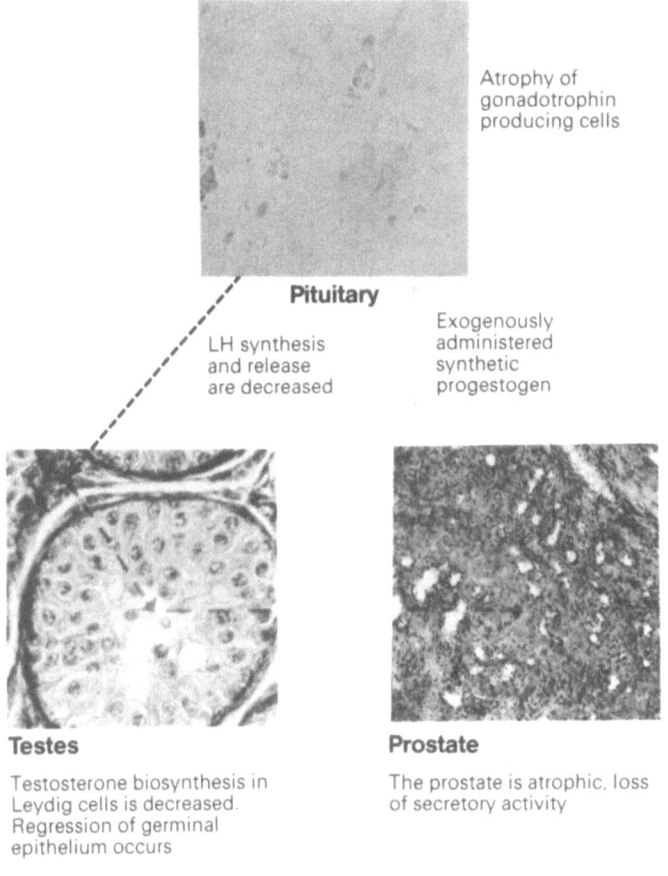

Atrophy of
gonadotrophin
producing cells

Pituitary

LH synthesis
and release
are decreased

Exogenously
administered
synthetic
progestogen

Testes

Testosterone biosynthesis in
Leydig cells is decreased.
Regression of germinal
epithelium occurs

Prostate

The prostate is atrophic, loss
of secretory activity

Figure 5 Intratesticular and serum testosterone concentrations after treatment with synthetic progestogen

One example is given in Figure 6, showing the effect of levonorgestrel on spermatogenesis and testes function in adult rats treated for 6 weeks. In contrast to androgens or anabolic steroids, there is also a pronounced decrease in prostate weight. This is a disadvantage, because male fertility control with progestogens demands additional substitution with androgens (see also Table 1).

As compared with the doses in oral contraceptives, the doses needed for inhibition of spermatogenesis are at least 10 times higher. The incidence of side-effects would be far inferior to all methods of contraception in the woman.

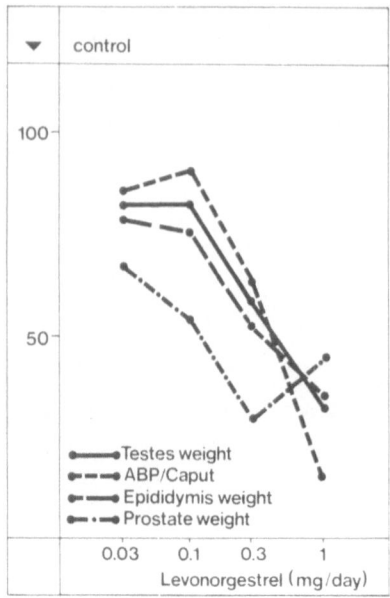

Figure 6 Effect of levonorgestrel on weight of prostate, epididymis and testes and ABP content in the caput epididymidis. Rats with an initial body weight of about 200 g were treated for 6 weeks with varying doses of levonorgestrel (0.03–30 mg per animal per day s.c.). Note the decrease between 0.03 and 1.0 mg/day, which is due to inhibition of gonadotrophin secretion

OESTROGENS

Oestrogens inhibit testicular function to a much higher degree than androgens, anabolic steroids or progestogens (see Figure 7 for an example). For several reasons, oestrogens are not suitable for fertility control in men.

(1) It is still unclear whether the testicular changes in men after long-term treatment with oestrogens are reversible or not.

(2) Oestrogens inhibit all androgen-dependent organs and functions, including libido.

(3) Oestrogens induce gynaecomastia and have cardiovascular side-effects when given in the higher doses needed for inhibition of spermatogenesis.

ANTIANDROGENS

Pure antiandrogens of the flutamide type inhibit spermatogenesis only partially. This has been discussed in detail elsewhere[25].

As early as 1966[26–28] we postulated that pure antiandrogens must also compete with androgens for receptor sites in those neural centres in which, under physiological conditions, androgens exert their negative feedback effect. Consequently, an androgen deficiency is simulated centrally, which

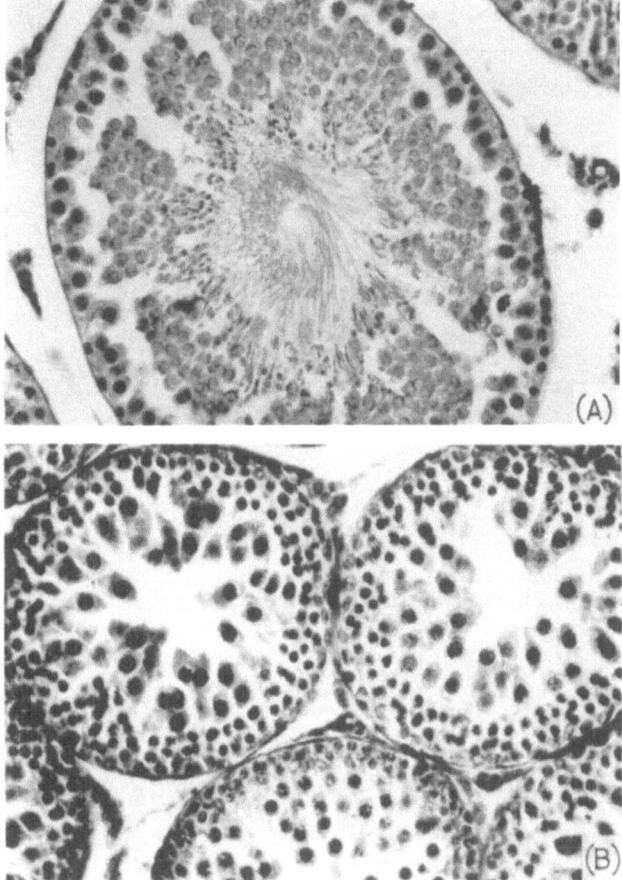

Figure 7 Histology of rat testes. (A) Untreated control. (B) Treated for 60 days with daily 1 mg/animal oestradiol s.c. Note the total atrophy of the tubules. Only Sertoli cells, spermatogonia and early spermatocytes are present. Staining, Azan; magnification, × 275

should result in an increased secretion of GnRH and gonadotrophins, i.e. the biosynthesis of androgens in the Leydig cells should be stimulated as a result of increased secretion of LH. This hypothesis is illustrated schematically in Figure 8, which shows the normal feedback and at that time the hypothetical effect of pure antiandrogens on the gonadal–hypothalamic-pituitary axis. The hypothesis put forward by us 16 years ago has since received substantial confirmation[29-35].

Two examples will show the influence of flutamide, a non-steroidal pure antiandrogen, and of cyproterone acetate on LH and testosterone plasma concentrations in adult male rats after one injection, 14 days or 6 weeks of treatment, respectively (Figures 9 and 10). There is a dramatic increase in both LH and testosterone concentrations under flutamide, whereas cyproterone acetate decreases LH and testosterone concentrations.

Intratesticular testosterone concentrations also are increased under

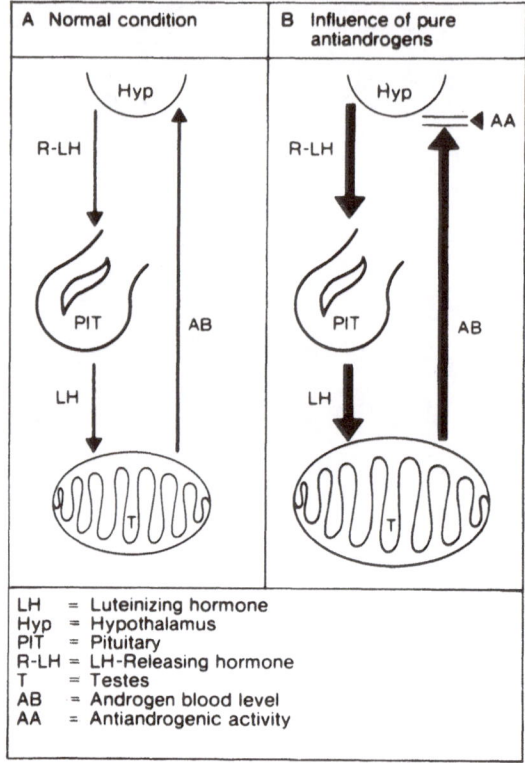

Figure 8   Normal feedback mechanism and feedback mechanism after treatment with a pure antiandrogen

flutamide. This is why pure antiandrogens lead at most to a transient disturbance of spermatogenesis and, thus, to only temporary infertility[36-39]. The intratesticular concentrations of androgens are, in fact, so high that the antiandrogen is no longer able to abolish the effect of androgens in the testis itself.

Antiandrogens of the cyproterone acetate type having additional progestogenic and antigonadotrophic activities inhibit spermatogenesis quite effectively (for review see Reference 39).

The extent of the inhibition of spermatogenesis is dose-dependent and naturally varies from species to species. A consistent finding, however, is that only spermatid maturation (spermiogenesis) is affected initially under medium doses. Meiosis fails to take place on administration of higher doses; secondary spermatocytes are the most advanced stages of spermatogenesis. Under extremely high doses, the convoluted tubules are completely depopulated and, apart from Sertoli cells, only spermatogonia and early spermatocyte forms are recognizable (Figure 11).

Whalen and Luttge[40] were the first to indicate that cyproterone acetate might be suitable for the control of fertility in men. They showed that daily treatment of rats with 10 mg cyproterone acetate subcutaneously leads to sterility but does not influence libido. This finding was confirmed by other

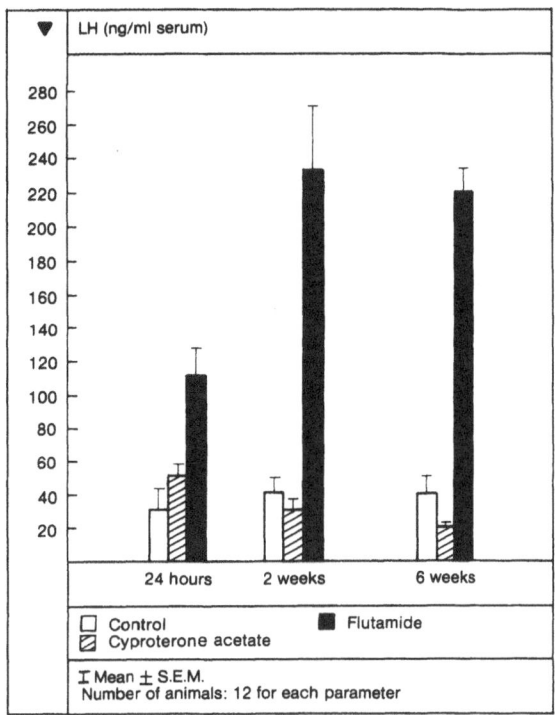

Figure 9 Effect of cyproterone acetate (20 mg per animal per day s.c.) and flutamide (10 mg per animal per day s.c.) on serum concentration of LH in adult male rats following treatment for 1 day and for 2 and 6 weeks

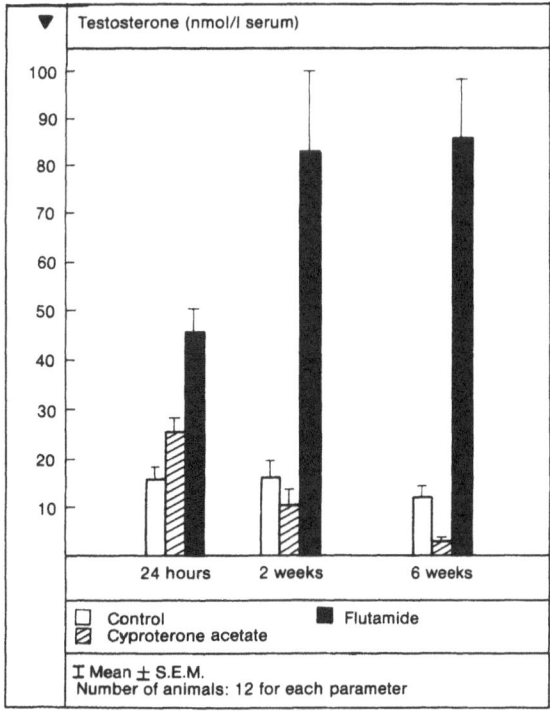

Figure 10 Effect of cyproterone acetate (20 mg per animal per day s.c.) and flutamide (10 mg per animal per day s.c.) on serum concentration of testosterone in adult rats following treatment for 1 day and for 2 and 6 weeks

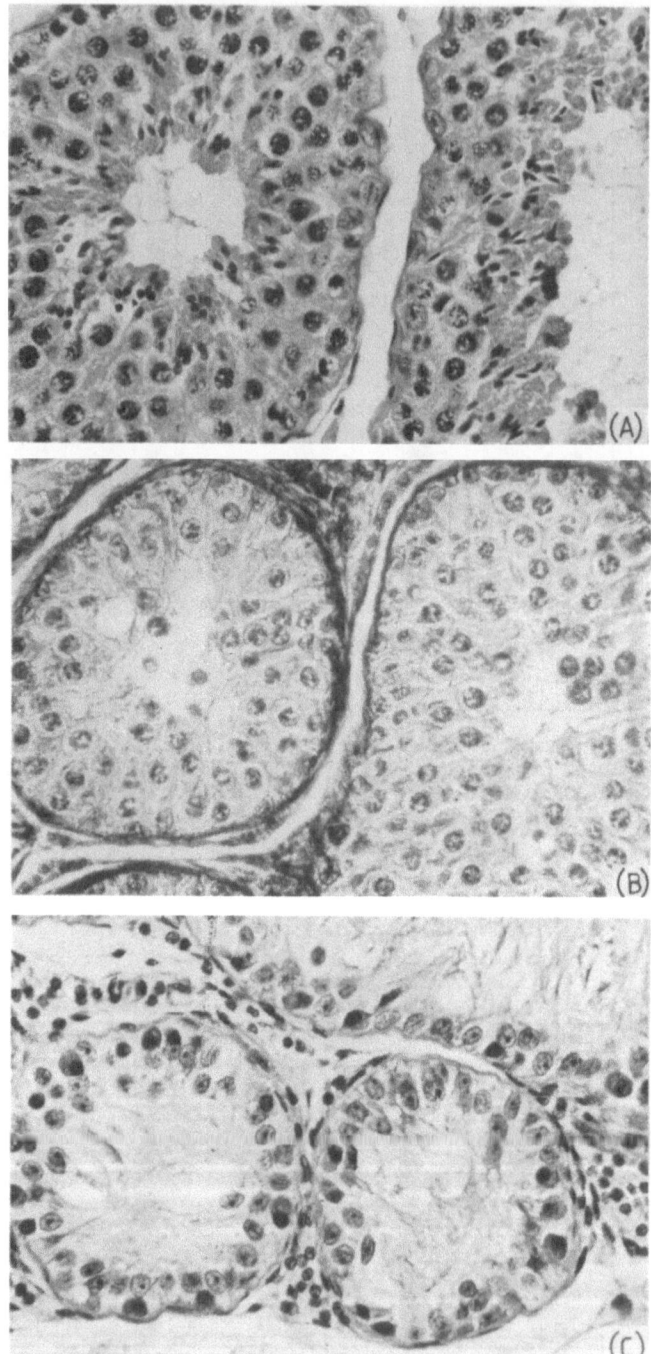

Figure 11 (A) Histology of dog testes. Control. (B) Histology of dog testes after 30 days of treatment with $10\,mg\,kg^{-1}\,day^{-1}$ cyproterone acetate i.m. Spermatogenesis is inhibited. (C) Histology of dog testes after 1 year of treatment with $100\,mg\,kg^{-1}\,day^{-1}$ cyproterone acetate p.o. Besides Sertoli cells, only spermatogonia and early spermatocytes are present. Staining, haematoxylin-eosin; magnification, (A) and (B) $\times$ 300, (C) $\times$ 240

researchers[41-44]. Because of the relatively rapid onset of action, Whalen and Luttge[40] suggested that, in addition to the inhibition of spermatogenesis, an effect on maturation processes in the epididymis must also be considered as a cause of the infertility.

The antifertility effect of cyproterone acetate has long been known. The idea of employing antiandrogens—and cyproterone acetate, in particular—for the control of fertility in men was not, however, taken up, because it was known that therapy with cyproterone acetate leads to a loss of libido in other species, e.g. dog[45], boar[46], rabbit[47] and, of course, man.

In 1970[48] an exciting experiment with rats was reported, which involved the implantation of cyproterone acetate containing silicone rubber capsules. The daily release rates were approximately 0.232 mg. Four months after the implantation, the animals were found to be infertile, although testicular function and the function of the accessory sex glands were not affected. Spermatozoa taken from the epididymis were found to be non-motile, the content of sialic acid in the epididymis was reduced, and degenerative changes were observed in the head and cauda of the epididymis. It has been concluded from these and other studies that the epididymis reacts more sensitively to antiandrogens than do other androgen–dependent organs, and that it therefore may be possible to influence selectively the processes of spermatozoal maturation in the epididymis by means of appropriate doses of antiandrogen (cyproterone acetate[48-52]). This would be an ideal method, i.e. via an influence on post-testicular mechanism, of achieving reversible sterility.

Following publication of these results, several workers attempted to reproduce this experiment, likewise using silicone rubber capsules containing cyproterone acetate[53-55]. The results were always negative. It was found that, although it is quite possible to induce partial inhibition of the function of the accessory sex glands (seminal vesicles, prostate), and the weight of the epididymes was also reduced, spermatogenesis and fertility remained unaffected[56]. Furthermore, it has been consistently shown in other studies in rats that infertility occurs only when spermatogenesis is inhibited, and that higher doses of cyproterone acetate are required for inhibition of spermatogenesis than for inhibition of the function of the accessory sex glands and for inhibition of epididymal function[54-57].

As could have been expected from all these data, in the human cyproterone acetate inhibits testosterone secretion even at low doses (5–10 mg/day) and consequently libido is also impaired[24, 58, 59]. But it will be impossible to find a dose for men which is reliably antifertile but which does not affect other androgen-dependent functions, including libido.

CONCLUSIONS

Inhibition of spermatogenesis is possible with many types of steroid hormones. Theoretically they could be used alone or in combination for male fertility control. For several reasons (side-effects, practicability, etc.) it is very unlikely that steroid hormones will be used for this purpose in the near future. In the 1983 annual report of WHO this approach is given a low priority. We agree with the statement made by Prasad and Diczfalusy[60]:

'A critical assessment of the promising leads which are pursued in attempts to develop an effective, safe and inexpensive male fertility regulating agent leads to the conclusion that, for the present, gossypol represents the only approach which has a reasonable chance to reach the stage of large scale clinical testing before the end of this decade.'

REFERENCES

1. Moore, C.R. and Price, D. (1932). Gonad hormone function, and the reciprocal influence between gonads and hypophysis with its bearing on the problem of sex hormone antagonism. *Am. J. Anat.*, **50**, 13

2. Dischreit, J. (1939). Wirkung des Testikelhormonpräparates Erugon auf den juvenilen Rattenhoden. *Klin. Wochenschr.*, **18**, 1493

3. Greene, R.R. and Burrill, M.W. (1940). The recovery of testes after androgen-induced inhibition. *Endocrinology*, **26**, 516

4. Gaarenstroom, J.H. (1939). Inhibition of the 'antimasculine effect' of oestrone by testosterone propionate. *Acta Brev. Neerl. Physiol.*, **9**, 134

5. Greep, R.O. and Chester Jones, I. (1950). Steroid control of pituitary function. *Recent Prog. Horm. Res.*, **5**, 197

6. Ludwig, D.J. (1950). The effect of androgen on spermatogenesis. *Endocrinology*, **46**, 453

7. Rössle, R. and Zahler, H. (1938). Experimentelle Untersuchungen über Hoden- und Prostataveränderungen durch Zufuhr von Hodenwirkstoffen. *Virchows Arch. Pathol. Anat.*, **302**, 251

8. Rubinstein, H.S. and Kurland, A.A. (1941). The effect of small doses of testosterone propionate on the testis and accessory sex organs. *J. Urol.*, **45**, 780

9. Zahler, H. (1947). Über die Wirkung verschiedener Gaben von Testosteronpropionat auf infantile Rattenhoden. *Virchows Arch. Pathol. Anat.*, **314**, 23

10. Zahler, H. (1947). Über das Verhalten der Hoden und Hypophysen A-vitaminotischer Ratten und ihre Beeinflußbarkeit durch androgenen Wirkstoff. *Virchows Arch. Pathol. Anat.*, **314**, 45

11. Hohlweg, W. and Junkmann, K. (1932). Die hormonal-nervöse Regulierung der Funktion des Hypophysenvorderlappens. *Klin. Wochenschr.*, **11**, 321

12. Skoglund, R.D. and Paulsen, C.A. (1973). Danazol-testosterone combination. A potential effective means for reversible male contraception. A preliminary report. *Contraception*, **7**, 357

13. Heller, C.G., Moore, D.J., Paulsen, C.A., Nelson, W.O. and Laidlaw, W.M. (1959). Effects of progesterone and synthetic progestins on the reproductive physiology of normal men. *Fed. Proc.*, **18**, 1057

14. McLeod, J. (1965). Human seminal cytology following the administration of certain antispermatogenic compounds. In Austin, C.R. and Perry, J.S. (eds.) *Agents Affecting Fertility*, pp. 93–123. (London: Churchill)

15. Jarpa, A. and Donoso, J. (1969). Untersuchungen über die Hemmung der Spermiogenese durch Depot-Gestagene. *Andrologie*, **1**, 107

16. Petry, R., Mauss, J., Senge, Th. and Rausch-Stroomann, J.-G. (1970). Über den Einfluß von Cyproteronacetat, Norethisteronönanthat und Gestonoroncapronat auf die Hypophysen-Gonadenachse beim Mann. In *Symposium der Deutschen Gesellschaft für Endokrinologie*, pp. 428–430. (Berlin, Heidelberg, New York: Springer Verlag)

17. Heller, C.G., Nelson, W.O., Hill, I.C., Henderson, E., Maddock, W.O., Jungck, E.C., Paulsen, C.A. and Mortimore, G.E. (1950). Improvement in spermatogenesis following depression of human testes with testosterone. *Fertil. Steril.*, **1**, 415

18. Heller, C.G., Nelson, W.O., Hill, I.C., Henderson, E., Maddock, W.O. and Jungck, E.C. (1950). The effect of testosterone administration upon the human testis. *J. Clin. Endocrinol. Metab.*, **10**, 816

19. Mauss, J., Richter, E. and Bormacher, K. (1974). Investigations on the use of testosterone oenanthate as a male contraceptive agent. *Contraception*, **10**, 281

20. Steinberger, E., Cervantes, A. and Smith, K.D. (1976). A preliminary report on the investigation of testosterone enanthate (TE) as a potential male contraceptive [Abstract]. *Fertil. Steril.*, **27**, 216

21. Johansson, E.D.B. and Nygren, K.-G. (1973). Depression of plasma testosterone levels in men with norethindrone. *Contraception*, **8**, 141
22. Frick, J. (1973). Control of spermatogenesis in men by combined administration of progestin and androgen. *Contraception*, **8**, 191
23. Coutinho, E.M. and Melo, J.F. (1973). Successful inhibition of spermatogenesis in man without loss of libido: A potential new approach to male contraception. *Contraception*, **8**, 119
24. Roy, S., Chatterjee, S., Prasad, M.R.N., Poddar, A.K. and Pandey, D.C. (1976). Effects of cyproterone acetate on reproductive functions in human males. *Contraception*, **14**, 403
25. Neumann, F., Habenicht, U.-F. and Schacher, A. (1984). Antiandrogens and target cell response—different in vivo effects of cyproterone acetate, flutamide and cyproterone. In McKerns, K.W., Aakvaag, A. and Hansson, V. (eds.) *Regulation of Target Cell Responsiveness*, pp. 489–527. (New York: Plenum)
26. Neumann, F. (1966). Antagonismus von Testosteron und 1.2-Methylen-6-chlor-pregna-4.6-dien-17-ol-3.20-dion (Cyproteron) an den die Gonadotropinsekretion regulierenden Zentren bei männlichen Ratten. *Acta Endocrinol. (Copenh.)*, **53**, 382
27. Neumann, F., Elger, W. and von Berswordt-Wallrabe, R. (1966). Effects of an anti-androgen on the hypothalamic pituitary system in male and female rats [Abstract 276]. *Excerpta Medica Int. Congr. Ser.*, **111**
28. Neumann, F., Elger, W., von Berswordt-Wallrabe, R. and Kramer, M. (1966). Beeinflussung der Regelmechanismen des Hypophysenzwischenhirnsystems von Ratten durch einen Testosteron-Antagonisten (1.2α-Methylene-6-chlor-Δ4.6-pregnadien-17α-ol-3.20-dion). *Naunyn Schmeidebergs Arch. Pharmak. Exp. Pathol.*, **255**, 221
29. Mietkiewski, K. and Lukaszyk, A. (1969). The response of the rat testis to prolonged administration of an androgen antagonist (cyproterone). *Acta Endocrinol. (Copenh.)*, **60**, 561
30. Neri, R.O. and Monahan, M. (1972). Effects of a novel non-steroidal anti-androgen on canine prostatic hyperplasia. *Invest. Urol.*, **10**, 123
31. Neri, R., Florance, K., Koziol, P. and van Cleave, S. (1972). A biological profile of a non-steroidal anti-androgen SCH 13521 (4′-nitro-3′-trifluoromethylisobutyranilide). *Endocrinology*, **91**, 427
32. Kliman, B., MacLaughilin, R., Irwin, R.J. and Prout, G.R. (1974). Anti-androgen stimulation of plasma luteinizing hormone (LH) and testosterone (T). *Clin. Res.*, **22**, 342a
33. Sizonenko, P.C., Paunier, L. and Cuendet, A. (1974). Evaluation of the hypothalamic-pituitary-gonadal axis by a new antiandrogen (SCH 13521) in boys [Abstract]. *Acta Paediat. Scand.*, **63**, 328
34. Södersten, P., Gray, G., Damassa, A.D., Smith, E.R. and Davidson, J.M. (1975). Effects of a non-steroidal anti-androgen on sexual behavior and pituitary gonadal function in the male rat. *Endocrinology*, **97**, 1468
35. Reznikov, A.G., Demchenko, V.N., Varga, S.V. and Bozhok, Y.M. (1978). Hypothalamo-hypophyseal-gonadal system in male rats and guinea pigs treated with the anti-androgen 4-nitro-3-trifluormethylisobutyranilide. *Endocrinology*, **72**, 276
36. Dhar, J.E. and Setty, B.S. (1976). Studies on the physiology and biochemistry of mammalian epididymis: Effect of flutamide, a non-steroidal anti-androgen, on the epididymis of the rat. *Fertil. Steril.*, **27**, 566
37. Setty, B.S. (1976). Remark during general discussion. *IPPF Congress on Agents Affecting Control of Fertility in the Male*, New Delhi, 1974. *J. Reprod. Fertil. (Suppl.)*, **24**, 175
38. Vojtisková, M., Poláčková, M., Viklický, V. and Khoda, M.E. (1978). Reversible inhibitory effect on the non-steroidal anti-androgen flutamide (SCH 13521) on spermatogenesis in mice. *Endocrinology*, **71**, 135
39. Neumann, F. and Schenck, B. (1980). Anti-androgens: Basic concepts and clinical trials. In Cunningham, G.R., Schill, W.-B. and Hafez, E.S.E. (eds.) *Regulation of Male Fertility*, pp. 93–104. (The Hague, Boston, London: Martinus Nijhoff)
40. Whalen, R.E. and Luttge, W.G. (1969). Contraceptive properties of the antiandrogen cyproterone acetate. *Nature (London)*, **223**, 633
41. Beach, F. and Westbrook, W. (1968). Morphological and behavioral effects of an anti-androgen in male rats. *J. Endocrinol.*, **42**, 379
42. Whalen, R.E. and Edwards, D.A. (1969). Effects of the anti-androgen cyproterone acetate on mating behavior and seminal vesicle tissue in male rats. *Endocrinology*, **84**, 155
43. Zucker, I. (1966). Effects of an anti-androgen on the mating behaviour of male guinea-pigs and rats. *J. Endocrinol.*, **35**, 209

44. Bloch, G.J. and Davidson, J.M. (1971). Behavioral and somatic responses to the anti-androgen cyproterone (1.2α-methylene-6-chloro-Δ6-17α-hydroxyprogesterone). *Horm. Behav.*, **2,** 11
45. Schmidtke, D. and Schmidtke, H.O. (1968). Ein neues Anti-androgen beim Hund. *Kleintier-Prax.*, **13,** 146
46. Horst, P. and Bader, J. (1969). Untersuchungen zur Bedeutung der Jungebermast. 2. Mitteilung: Versuche zur Unterdrückung des Sexualgeruches. *Züchtungskunde*, **41,** 248
47. Neumann, F. (1979). Antiandrogens. In Jacobs, H.S. (ed.) *Advances in Gynaecological Endocrinology*, pp. 335-336. Proceedings of the Sixth Study Group of the Royal College of Obstetricians and Gynaecologists, London, 1978
48. Prasad, M.R.N., Singh, S.P. and Rajalakshmi, M. (1970). Fertility control in male rats by continuous release of microquantities of cyproterone acetate from subcutaneous silastic capsules. *Contraception*, **2,** 165
49. Prasad, M.R.N., Rajalakshmi, M. and Reddy, P.R.K. (1971/1972). Action of cyproterone acetate on male reproductive functions. *Gynecol. Invest.*, **2,** 202
50. Rajalakshmi, M., Singh, S.P. and Prasad, M.R.N. (1971). Effects of microquantities of cyproterone acetate released through silastic capsules on the histology of the epididymis of the rat. *Contraception*, **3,** 335
51. Prasad, M.R.N. (1973). Limiting male fertility by selectively depriving the epididymis of androgen. *Res. Reprod.*, **5,** 3
52. Rajalakshmi, M. and Prasad, M.R.N. (1975). Action of cyproterone acetate on the accessory organs of reproduction in prepubertal and sexually mature rats. *Fertil. Steril.*, **26,** 137
53. Elger, W. and von Berswordt-Wallrabe, R. (1973). Failure to induce sterility in male rats with continuously released micro-quantities of cyproterone acetate and norgestrel [Abstract 120]. *Acta Endocrinol. (Copenh.), Suppl.*, **173,** 120
54. Chatterjee, A., Ray, P., Gupta M., Pal, A.K. and Kolay, A.R. (1977). Cyproterone acetate. I. Microquantity releasing device of cyproterone acetate and its failure in inducing functional sterility in male rats. *Andrologia*, **9,** 70
55. Schenck, B., Elger, W., Schöpflin, G. and Neumann, F. (1975). Failure to induce sterility in male rats with microdoses of cyproterone acetate (CPA). *Contraception*, **12,** 517
56. Neumann, F. and Schenck, B. (1976). New antiandrogens and their mode of action. Presented at *IPPF Congress on Agents Affecting Control of Fertility in the Male*, New Delhi, 1974. *J. Reprod. Fertil.*, **24,** 129
57. Steinbeck, H., Mehring, M. and Neumann, F. (1971). Comparison of the effects of cyproterone, cyproterone acetate and estradiol on testicular function, accessory sexual glands and fertility in a long-term study on rats. *J. Reprod. Fertil.*, **26,** 65
58. Koch, U.J., Lorenz, F., Danehl, K., Ericsson, R., Hasan, S.H., von Keyserlingk, D., Lübke, K., Mehring, M., Römmler, A., Schwartz, U. and Hammerstein, J. (1976). Continuous oral low-dosage cyproterone acetate for fertility regulation in the male? A trend analysis in 15 volunteers. *Contraception*, **14,** 117
59. Moltz, L., Neumann, F. and Hammerstein, J. (1980). Beeinflussung der Fertilität des Mannes durch Antiandrogene. *Gynäkologe*, **13,** 18
60. Prasad, M.R.N. and Diczfalusy, E. (1982). Gossypol. Presented at *Second International Congress of Andrology*, Tel Aviv, 1981. *Int. J. Androl., Suppl.* 5, 53

3
Male contraception in the preclinical evaluation

K.-W. VON EICKSTEDT

In women the inhibition of ovulation is a successful way of excluding germ cells from fertilization. In men the function of the germ cells cannot be inhibited as easily. The close association, both morphological and functional, of spermatogenesis and androgen synthesis presents problems which have not yet been solved. The consideration of sperms as a single compartment is wrong, since libido and sperm function are closely linked together. All methods which have been developed to directly inhibit the spermatogenesis or the spermiogenesis did not produce satisfactory results. Acylating or heterocyclic substances which were effective inhibitors were too toxic in animal experiments. One such substance which affects spermatogenesis is gossypol (Figure 1). This binaphthalene isolated from cotton seeds inhibits sperm maturation.

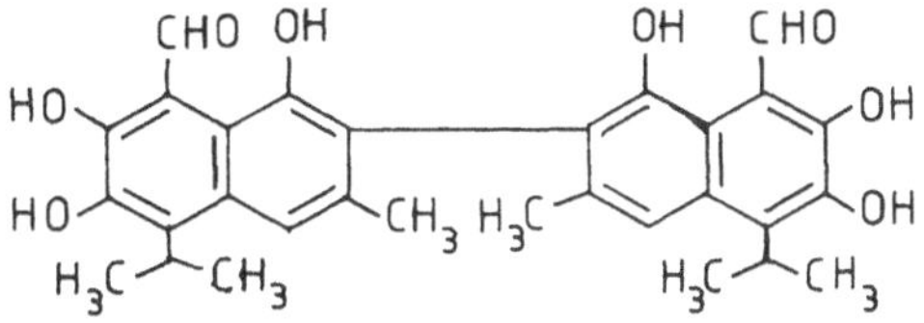

Figure 1   Structure of gossypol

Interference of gossypol with spermatogenesis has been found in hamsters, rats, dogs and monkeys. For safety evaluations long-term studies have been performed in rats, dogs and monkeys. Toxic effects were found mainly in dogs, with doses near to therapeutic. In rats and monkeys no such toxic effects were seen. If one compares the chemical structure of gossypol with that of antimalarial or antiamoebal drugs, the explanation can be found for the difference in toxicity in the various animal species. Dogs are more sensitive to such drugs, since they cannot metabolize such substances as easily as rats, monkeys and humans. Their paths of elimination are different. Therefore, species differences have to be detected before long-term toxicological studies can be started with such substances.

One adverse effect of gossypol has uniformly been found in all species, including humans: a decline of the potassium plasma levels during long-term treatment[1]. The evaluation of this untoward effect is the task of the clinicians who perform the clinical trials.

Systemic immunization is another possible means of affecting sperm activity directly. Studies on this are still in the stage of animal experimentation. Direct effects on the post-testicular activity of sperms primarily concern women. For instance, drugs which damage sperms have to be applied intravaginally. This method of contraception, therefore, will not be discussed in this chapter.

The most promising method now under investigation is the inhibition of spermatogenesis via hormonal regulation. The inhibition of androgen production in the Leydig cells is one of the methods which have been developed in order to attain azoospermia[2]. Hormonal regulation of spermatogenesis has been studied mainly in rodents and less extensively in monkeys. In the human the feasibility of such experiments is limited, in spite of the fact that the antifertility effects of gossypol and ketoconazole were first accidentally found in humans and then proven in animals.

In non-human primates Nieschlag and Marshall[3] found that the onset of spermatogenesis can occur with testosterone alone, but the complete normal process requires further hormonal stimulation. Nieschlag and Marshall's interpretation is that FSH and LH are involved. Barr and Pomerantz[4] studied the physiological role of oestradiol in controlling testosterone production via intratesticular mechanisms in rats. They found that oestradiol treatment can increase the FSH–LH stimulus on the Leydig cell function in hypophysectomized animals. This would mean, if the results of experiments in rats can be transferred to the human, we are dealing not only with gonadotrophins, but also with steroids which maintain testosterone production.

To suppress the synthesis of testosterone in the Leydig cells by suppressing the gonadotrophin release, different steroids have already been used in the human; for instance, testosterone enanthate and ethinylnortestosterone. Both of these had to be applied in a high dosage and therefore produced unwanted effects, such as changes in metabolism and loss of libido. Changes in libido cannot sufficiently be proven in male animals, because of seasonal changes in fertility. The antiandrogen cyproterone acetate and other progestogens, as well as combinations of progestogens and androgens, are also able to suppress spermiogenesis when used in a high dosage.

The high dosage of sex steroids needed to achieve azoospermia in men results in adverse effects which prevent the introduction of this kind of contraception, which seemed promising in animal experiments.

The mechanism by which azoospermia is achieved is understood to be a complete blocking of the FSH and LH output from the pituitary. Such a suppression of gonadotrophin secretion can be more easily obtained with a non-physiological high dosage of LHRH or its analogues.

In contrast to the steroid overdosage, overdosage of LHRH and some of its analogues induces side-effects, which can be tolerated, with the exception of loss of libido and sexual activity. However, loss of libido is a special aspect of male contraception in humans, with which the clinician has to deal.

The suppression of testosterone synthesis in the Leydig cells by LHRH agonists seems to be insufficient to produce complete azoospermia. This

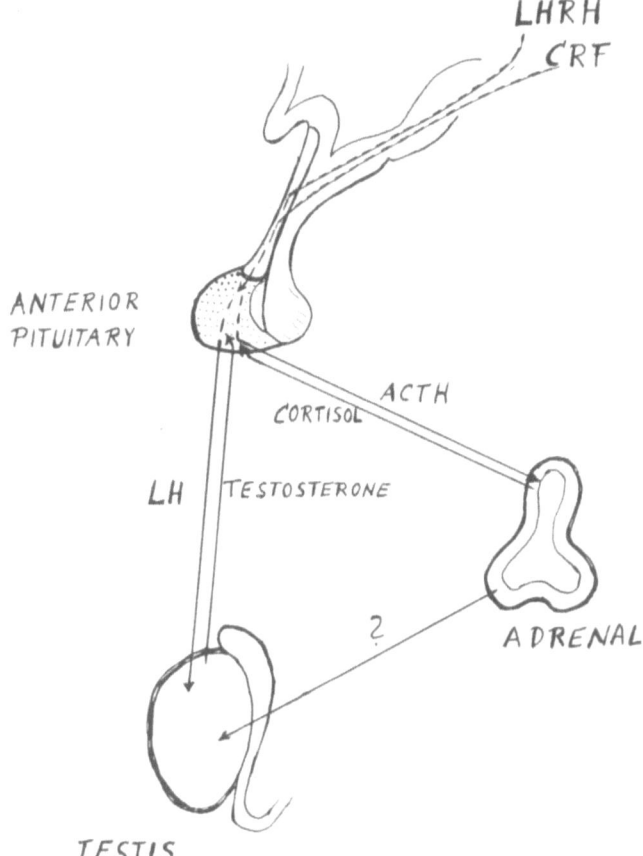

Figure 2   Hormonal control of the testis

raises the question: which hormonal regulations are involved in testicular androgen production and spermatogenesis?

Both androgen and oestrogen production by the adrenal gland have to be taken into account if the down-regulation of testicular functions is to be achieved.

In the normal male the Leydig cells are the main source of androgens. Their testosterone production is induced by LH from the pituitary. But which role do the androgens and perhaps even the oestrogens which are produced by the adrenal cortex play when testicular hormone production falls? Labrie[5] postulated that adrenal androgens are stimulated by ACTH, which is independent of LHRH. However, whether these androgens and their precursors can support androgen functions in the case where gonadal testosterone synthesis is down-regulated by overdosage of an LHRH analogue is still an open question (Figure 2).

It is well known that the adrenal secretes considerable amounts of Δ_4-androstenedione. In addition, dehydroepiandrosterone sulphate and 11β-hydroxyandrostenedione are produced by the adrenal. 11β-Hydroxyandros-

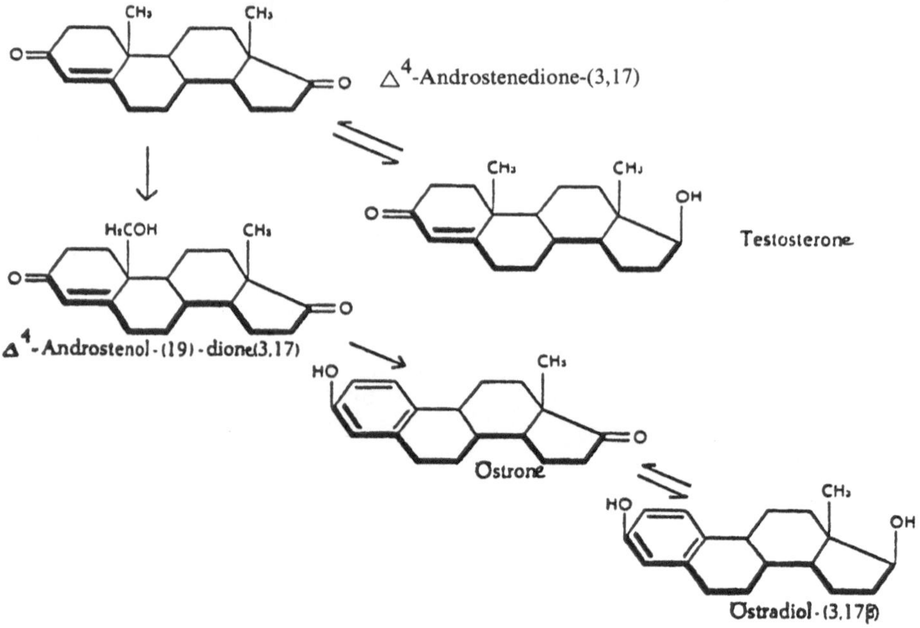

Figure 3 Androstenedione metabolites

tenedione can be regarded as a metabolite of Δ_4-androstenedione. Whether dehydroepiandrosterone sulphate exerts relevant hormonal effects is uncertain. The amounts of testosterone itself which are synthesized by the adrenal gland are too small to serve as a substitute for the normal physiological amounts of this androgen in the case of castration. Our knowledge of the physiological role of the adrenal Δ_4-androstenedione is still small. Whether it may serve as a precursor of the testicular testosterone in abnormal states has not yet been studied sufficiently. It is converted not only into testosterone, but also into oestrone. Its metabolite oestradiol supports the gonadotrophin stimulus on the Leydig cells, as Barr and Pomerantz found in rodents. The question is whether the oestrogens play a role when spermatogenesis is suppressed by hormonal down-regulation. This question has partly been investigated in animals. At the moment our understanding is that only testosterone production has to be suppressed completely in order to achieve azoospermia.

The new LHRH analogues seem to be the hormones by which a complete down-regulation of testosterone in the testis can successfully be performed (Figure 4). Nieschlag and his co-workers[6] reported that an LHRH agonist such as buserelin could not achieve complete azoospermia. He reported that the results which he got with an LHRH antagonist in *Cynomolgus* monkeys were more promising[7]. One explanation for this success is the immediate suppression of the pituitary by the LHRH antagonist. In contrast to the LHRH antagonists, the LHRH agonists initially stimulate the pituitary and the testis and thereby induce testosterone production, which then stimulates spermatogenesis.

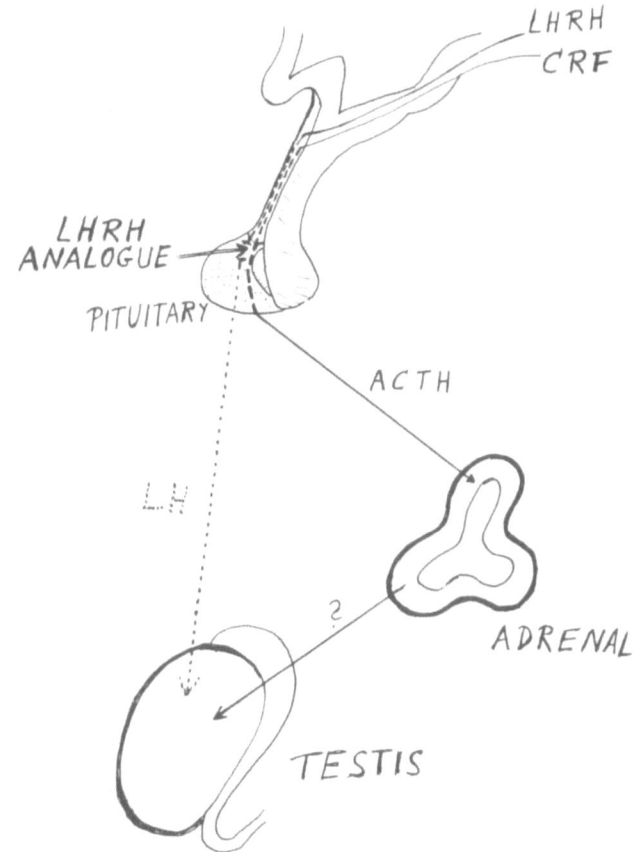

Figure 4 Down-regulation of testicular functions

In addition to this hormonal feed-back regulation, which includes the releasing hormone from the hypothalamus, the LH from the pituitary and the testosterone from the testis, still other hormones are of interest (Figure 4). The oestrogens have already been mentioned. Whether they can have a significant influence during the down-regulation of testosterone synthesis is at the moment uncertain. The androgens and their precursors from the adrenal cortex are also of interest. They should be taken into account with respect to hypothalamic regulations. The feed-back control of the ACTH results from the plasma levels of the corticoids. Whether adrenal androgens can become involved in such circuits at the hypothalamic level is not known. In the steroid feed-back control of the testicular function, not only is testosterone itself involved, but also various metabolites. We have to distinguish between those metabolites which are formed in the midbrain tissues and the anterior pituitary and those which are formed in peripheral tissues. In normal males testosterone is the main steroid hormone which controls the output of LHRH and gonadotrophins. In male mammals it is metabolized not only in peripheral tissues such as the liver, but also in the anterior pituitary and several brain regions such as the hypothalamus, mid-brain and amygdala. Figure 5 shows the metabolic pathways of testosterone and the converting enzymes in several central nervous structures, as they have been described by Motta et al.[8].

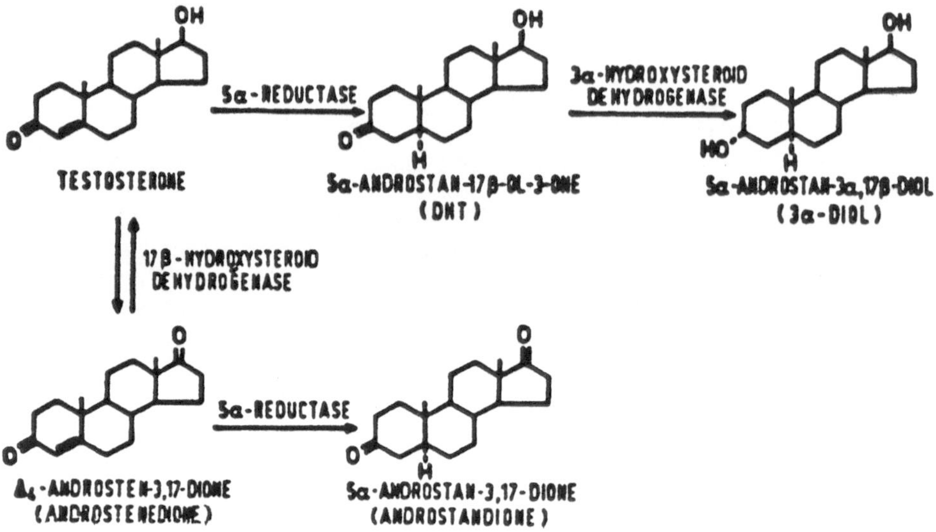

Figure 5   Hypothalamic steroids

Motta, Martini and their co-workers performed experiments in rats and found that castration has an influence on the metabolism of testosterone in the anterior pituitary and hypothalamus. There is an increase in the activity of the 5α-reductase after castration. This means that the metabolism of testosterone and also Δ_4-androstenedione in the hypothalamus and anterior pituitary is enhanced after castration. The testosterone metabolites 5α-di-hydrotestosterone (DHT) and 3α-diol have already been studied with respect to their pituitary and hypothalamic functions. The increase in these metabolites after castration results in a negative feed-back on LH secretion at the hypothalamic level. In the anterior pituitary the 3α-diol increases LH secretion. This has been observed in rats.

In humans we have two different kinds of castration: surgical castration and so-called 'chemical castration'. The latter is achieved by down-regulation of testosterone synthesis by overdosage of an LHRH analogue. We have to expect that the two treatments result in different effects on the pituitary. This first has to be studied in animals and then compared with measurable steroid levels in humans.

The central areas in which the feed-back control takes place are of interest, not only with respect to steroid hormone metabolism. The influence of these hormones on midbrain and hypothalamic receptors such as the dopaminergic, the serotoninergic and the adrenergic receptors is also of interest, since some side-effects will have their origin there. In addition, we assume that the libido is regulated in these central regions. Oestradiol may be involved in this regulation.

We already know many pathways of steroid metabolism in peripheral tissues which can be compared in animals and humans. Therefore, many predictions from animal experiments are possible in this field. The metabolic pathways of the steroids in the central nervous tissues should also be studied with respect to their effects on the feed-back control of releasing hormones, even if a direct comparison with the human seems impossible.

The side-effects differ greatly among the various types of male contraception. For instance, the down-regulation of testosterone by a substance such as ketoconazole differs from down-regulation by LHRH analogues such as buserelin or leuprolide. Ketoconazole acts directly on enzymes in the Leydig cells. However, it also inhibits adrenal enzymes which are involved in the synthesis of glucocorticoids. This latter effect is undesirable. The suppression of adrenal androgens may perhaps be a desired effect. The benefit–risk calculation has to take both the wanted suppression of androgen production and the unwanted inhibition of corticoid synthesis into account. Such various effects should be studied preclinically to evaluate the dose-dependent differences in the enzyme systems concerned. Dose-dependent studies must include testing up to toxic doses, and therefore the use of humans for such studies must be excluded. In the human, the benefit–risk ratio can be studied at steroid plasma levels.

Animal models are needed for preclinical investigations of new drugs. Usually one or two rodent species are used and one or two non-rodent species. As already mentioned, species differences have to be detected before long-term toxicity studies can be started with a new substance. Monkeys usually provide the best subspecies for such preclinical testing. In preclinical studies of male contraceptives in monkeys, we do not deal with cycle length, bleeding pattern or rutting season, as in studies of female contraceptives.

In discussing future aspects of male contraception, one has to consider slow-release systems for hormones. The combination of steroid hormones with LHRH analogues in biodegradable slow-release systems can solve problems of contraception in men as well as in women. The long-term application of LHRH agonists themselves already carries problems[10]. They can be applied intranasally, but then the application of a steroid hormone is also needed. The loss of libido in men caused by LHRH analogues requires the concomitant application of an adequate dose of an androgen. The best way to administer such a combination is by a biodegradable slow-release system. Biodegradable implant delivery systems have been tested in animals and some early clinical trials have also been performed. Such implants are made from polycaprolactone, an aliphatic polyester, or from synthetic polypeptides, or from copolymers of glutamic acid and ethylglutamate[11]. The latter can form biodegradable microcapsules, which are injected subcutaneously. The kinetics of hormone release from these systems usually differ among animal species. Again monkeys seem to be a species relevant to the human. The reactions of the subcutaneous tissue also have to be investigated. Experience with subcutaneous tissue reactions is already available, but the kinetics of the various hormones still have to be adapted to the long-term intervals needed. There are great differences in solubility between steroids and peptides. Therefore, one can imagine that further work will be needed to produce a suitable biodegradable slow-release system which delivers an LHRH analogue together with an androgen in such a way that constant blood levels are sustained for weeks. Therefore, it will be some time before a satisfactory male contraceptive is produced.

REFERENCES

1. Quian Shao-zhen (1981). Effect of gossypol on potassium and prostaglandin metabolism and mechanism of action of gossypol. In Chang Chai Fen, Griffin, D. and Woolman, A. (eds.) *Recent Advances in Fertility Regulation*, pp. 152–159. (Geneva: ATAR)
2. De Kretser, D.M. (1981) Fertility regulation in the male: recent developments. In Chang Chai Fen, Griffin, D. and Woolman, A. (eds.) *Recent Advances in Fertility Regulation*, pp. 112–121. (Geneva: ATAR)
3. Nieschlag, E. and Marshall, G.R. (1984). Hormonal regulation of spermatogenesis in primates. In *Seventh International Congress of Endocrinology*, 1–7 July, Quebec. (Amsterdam: Excerpta Medica). (In press)
4. Barr, D.B. and Pomerantz, D.K. (1984). Mode of maintenance with gonadotropin influences the response of the Leydig cell to estradiol in the hypophysectomized rat. In *Seventh International Congress of Endocrinology*, 1–7 July, Quebec. (Amsterdam: Excerpta Medica). (In press)
5. Labrie, F. (1984). Dramatic response to a new antihormonal treatment for prostate cancer. In *Seventh International Congress of Endocrinology*, 1–7 July, Quebec. (Amsterdam: Excerpta Medica). (In press)
6. Nieschlag, E., Akhtar, F.B., Weinbauer, G.F., Schürmeier, T. and Michel, E. (1984). LHRH analogues for male fertility control: Experiments in monkeys and men. In *International Symposium on LHRH and its Analogues*, 28–30 June, Quebec
7. Akhtar, F.B., Weinbauer, G.F. and Nieschlag, E. (1984). GNRH antagonist-mediated suppression of testicular function in monkeys. In *Seventh International Congress of Endocrinology*, 1–7 July, Quebec. (Amsterdam: Excerpta Medica). (In press)
8. Motta, M., Massa, R., Zanisi, M. and Martini, L. (1980). Mode of action of androgens and progestogens in neuroendocrine tissues. In Genazzani, E., *et al.* (eds.) *Pharmacological Modulation of Steroid Action*. (New York: Raven Press)
9. Zanisi, M., Motta, M. and Martini, L. (1975). Inhibitory effect of 5-α-reduced metabolites of testosterone on gonadotropin secretion. *J. Endocrinol.*, **56**, 315
10. Swerdloff, R.S. and Basin, S. (1984). Suppression of gonadal function by constant infusion of GNRH agonist in the human male. In *International Symposium on LHRH and its Analogues*, 28–30 June, Quebec
11. Langer, R.S. (1984). Polymers and drug delivery systems. In Zatuchni, G.A., *et al.* (eds.) *Long-acting Contraceptive Delivery Systems*. (Philadelphia: Harper and Row)

4
Long-acting steroids for male contraception

H. KUHL, H.-J. BORN, M. SCHNEIDER, J. SANDOW, W. SINGER and
H.-D. TAUBERT

INTRODUCTION

Inhibition of spermatogenesis by suppression of gonadotrophin release by steroid hormones is one of the most promising approaches for male contraception.

While progestogens and androgens given alone are effective in achieving azoospermia only at very high doses, the combination of both hormones allows of a marked reduction of the doses, since androgens and progestogens inhibit synergistically gonadotrophin secretion. These regimens may reduce the risk of adverse side-effects and maintain sufficient androgen levels, but as yet they have the disadvantage of requiring rather frequent injections to achieve a pronounced suppression of the sperm count[1].

Previous investigations have revealed that various dimeric steroid esters synthesized in our laboratory[2-4] show a very protracted hormone effect after a single injection of an oily solution into rats[5-7]. One of these compounds, the dimeric testosterone-ethynodiol succinate (Figure 1), which had previously been shown to exert both androgenic and progestogenic depot effects[7], was investigated with respect to its suitability as a contraceptive depot preparation in the male rat and rhesus monkey.

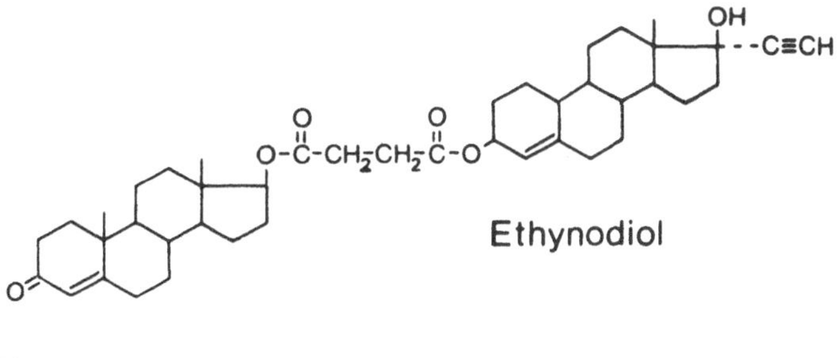

Figure 1 Structural formula of the dimeric testosterone-ethynodiol ester

MATERIAL AND METHODS

The dimeric testosterone-ethynodiol ester (3-oxo-4-androsten-17β-y1)-(17β-hydroxy-17α-ethynyl-4-estren-3β-yl)-succinate was synthesized as described previously[4].

Rats

Adult intact male SIV rats weighing 180–230 g were injected i.m. once with 10, 20 or 40 mg of the dimer dissolved in 0.5 ml arachis oil/benzyl benzoate (6:4). Groups of 6 or 7 animals were sacrificed under ether anaesthesia by decapitation 1, 2, 4, 6, 8, 12 and 16 weeks following the single injection. Various tissues were dissected, fixed in Bouin's solution for 24 h and weighed. One testis of every rat was prepared for histological and morphometrical evaluation of spermatogenesis. After fixation in Bouin's solution, the testes were embedded in paraffin and sections of 3 μm thickness were stained with haematoxylin-eosin. The diameter of the tubuli seminiferi and the height of the germinal epithelium were determined morphometrically with the MOP I (Kontron, Starnberg, FRG). The testis of each animal was divided into four parts. Sections were prepared from each, and 100 transversally cut tubuli each were measured. The histological examination of spermatogenesis was carried out microscopically (range of magnification × 160 to × 400).

Serum LH was measured by a double-antibody solid-phase method, as described previously[8]. The reagents (purified NIAMDD Rat LH-I-4, NIAMDD-Anti-Rat LH-S-4, NIAMDD Rat LH-RP-1) were kindly supplied by Dr A.F. Parlow (NIAMDD Rat Pituitary Hormone Distribution Program). Serum testosterone was measured after ether extraction by means of a commercial radio-immunoassay test kit.

Monkeys

Four mature male rhesus monkeys (*Macaca mulatta*) weighing 4.2, 4.7, 5.7 and 6.2 kg were used. They received a single i.m. injection of 50 mg/kg body weight of the dimeric steroid ester dissolved in arachis oil/benzyl benzoate (6:4) (concentration 100 mg/ml) on 9 November. Immediately before and 4, 6, 10, 14, 18 and 22 weeks after the injection testicular biopsies were taken under ketamine anaesthesia. After fixation in Bouin's solution, the specimen was embedded in paraffin, and step-sections of 3 μm thickness were stained with haematoxylin-eosin. The diameter of the tubuli seminiferi was determined morphometrically with the MOP I (Kontron, Starnberg, FRG). The histological examination of spermatogenesis was carried out microscopically (magnification × 120).

Serum LH was determined radio-immunologically according to a modification of the method of Monroe *et al.*[9]. The reagents (purified cynomolgus pituitary LH for radio-iodination, rabbit antiserum to hCG (R 13, pool D), and rhesus pituitary LH reference preparation (WP-XV-20)) were kindly supplied by Dr S. Raiti (NIADDK National Hormone and Pituitary Program). Serum testosterone was measured by means of a commercial radio-immunoassay test kit.

RESULTS

Rats

The histological evaluation of sections taken from the rat testes revealed a total suppression of spermatogenesis and a pronounced narrowing of the tubuli seminiferi depending upon the dose of the dimer and upon the time interval after the injection (Figures 2, 3). There was a complete arrest of spermatogenic activity within 4 weeks after the administration of 10 and 20 mg. The height of the germinal epithelium was considerably reduced and there were no mature spermatozoa. The morphological criteria of the germinal epithelium, however, had not changed and no necrobiotical alterations were discernible. As the inhibition of spermatogenesis occurred apparently before the second maturation division, the earlier stages appeared relatively unaffected. No direct toxic effect was observed at any time after the injection. The examination of the interstitium revealed no alteration of the basal membrane and only a slight hypoplasia or hypotrophy of the Leydig cells. The reversibility of the arrest of spermatogenesis was demonstrated by the restoration of spermatogenesis 12 weeks after the injection of 10 mg and 16 weeks after 20 mg of the dimeric steroid ester (Figure 2). When 40 mg had been injected, there was a significant decrease in the height of the germinal epithelium, but not before a time interval of 6 weeks. The suppression, however, lasted for at least 16 weeks after the single injection (Figure 2). For comparison, the single injection of 24 mg norethisterone enanthate, a depot progestogen, had only a slight inhibitory effect upon spermatogenesis (Figure 2).

The results of the morphometrical evaluation of the tubuli seminiferi corresponded to the histological findings. Four weeks after the administration of 10 mg, a marked reduction in the diameter of the tubules could be demonstrated, which lasted for 2–4 weeks (Figure 3). A similar effect could be observed after the injection of 20 mg, while the dose of 40 mg did not become effective before 6 weeks, but the reduction in the diameter of the tubules lasted at least 16 weeks after the injection (Figure 3).

The reversible suppression of rat spermatogenesis by the dimeric testosterone-ethynodiol ester is exemplified by Figures 4–9. As early as 1 week after the injection of 10 mg, there was a reduction in the diameter of the tubuli seminiferi as compared with untreated controls, while spermatogenesis still appeared to be unaffected. After 2 weeks the height of the germinal epithelium continued to decrease, and 4 weeks after the administration of 10 mg no mature spermatozoa could be observed. Eight weeks after the injection the germinal epithelium had fairly regenerated, but the diameter of tubuli was still reduced.

Serum LH was rapidly suppressed after the injection of each dose to values 70–50% below those of the control groups (Figure 10). When 20 or 40 mg had been injected, the suppression of gonadotrophin secretion lasted for at least 16 weeks.

In contrast, there was a steep initial rise in the testosterone levels during the first 2 weeks after the injection of 40 mg, probably due to an initial hydrolysis of the circulating dimeric ester. Thereafter, serum testosterone was significantly suppressed until at least 16 weeks after the injection.

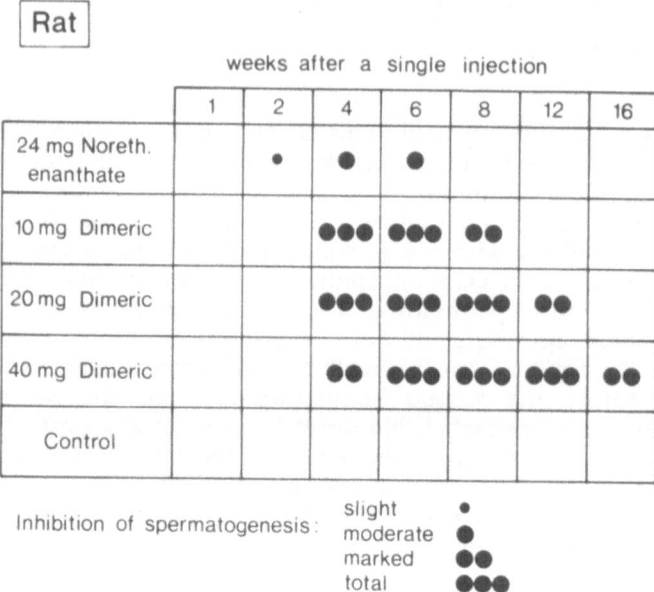

Figure 2 Inhibition of spermatogenesis in the rat in dependency upon the time interval after a single injection of 12 mg norethisterone enanthate or 10, 20 or 40 mg of the dimeric testosterone-ethynodiol

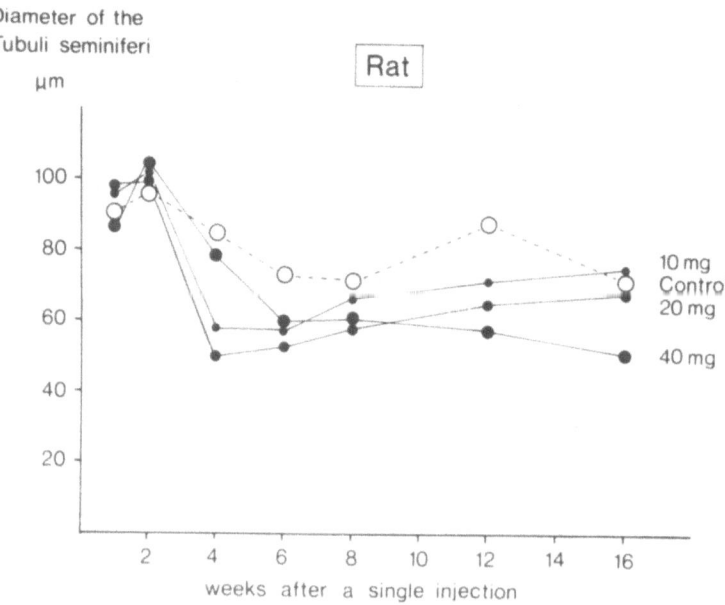

Figure 3 Effect of a single injection of various doses of the dimeric testosterone-ethynodiol upon the diameter of the seminiferous tubules of the rat (mean values of 6–7 rats)

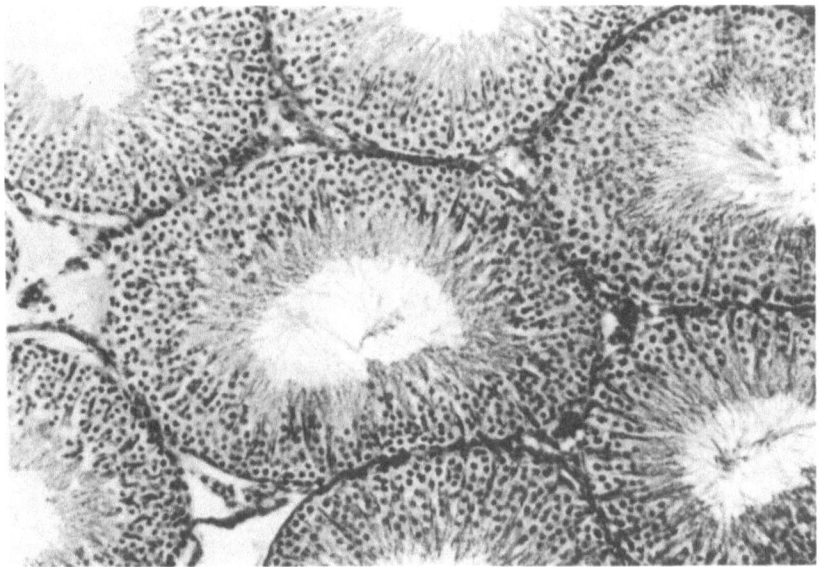

Figure 4 Photomicrograph of testicular tissue of an untreated rat. Staining H.-E.; magnification × 160

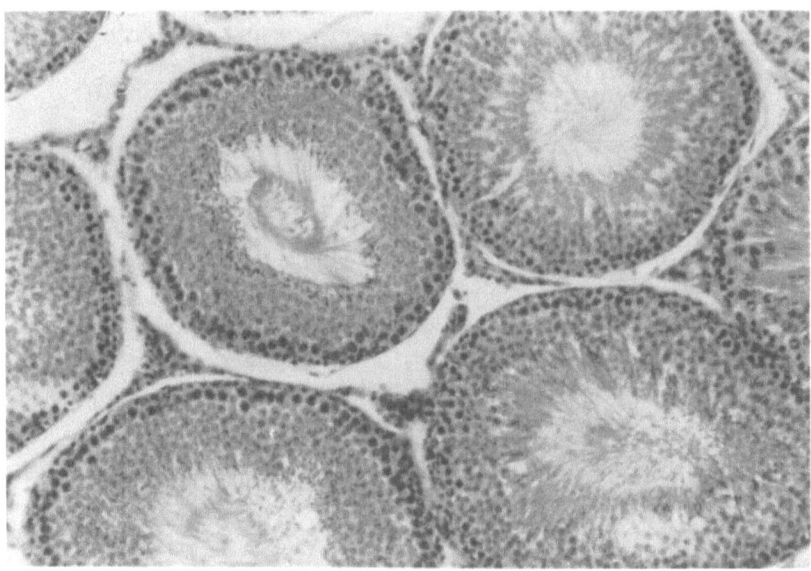

Figure 5 Histological section of rat testis 1 week after the injection of 10 mg of the dimeric testosterone-ethynodiol. Staining H.-E.; magnification × 160

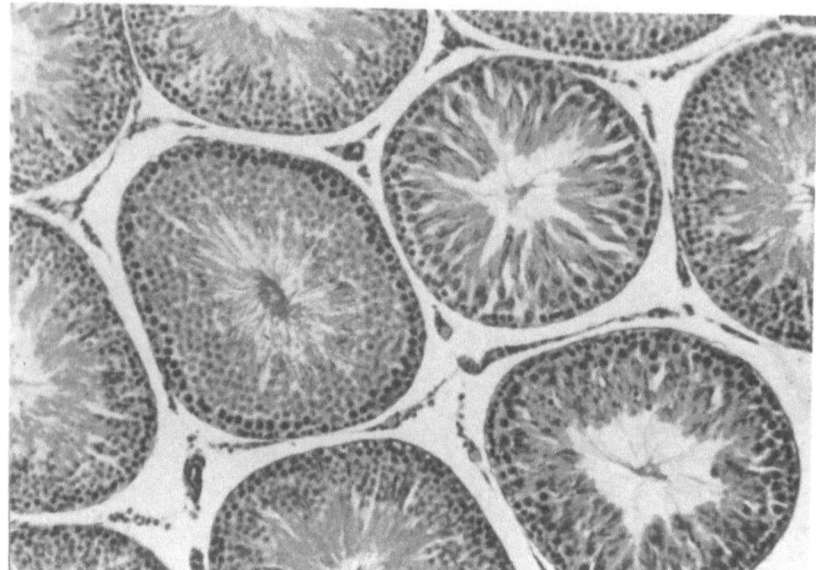

Figure 6 Histological section of rat testis 2 weeks after the injection of 10 mg of the dimeric testosterone-ethynodiol. Staining H.-E.; magnification × 160

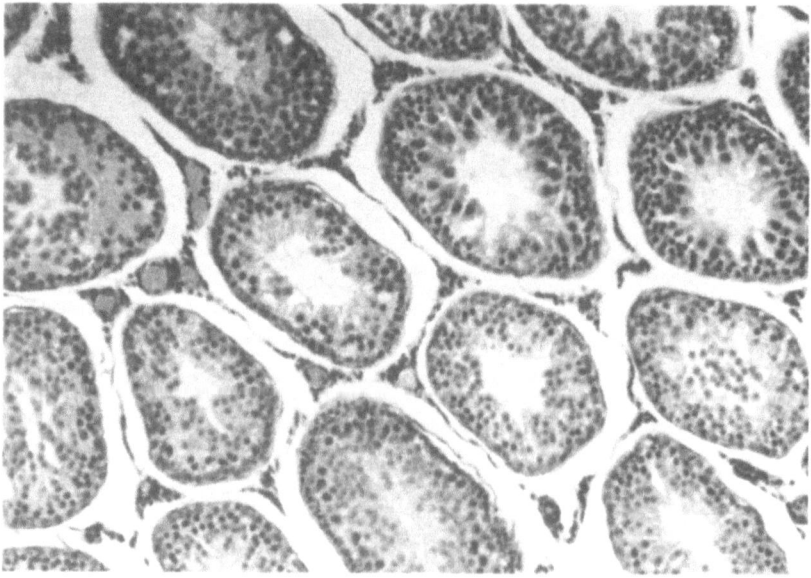

Figure 7 Histological section of rat testis 4 weeks after the injection of 10 mg of the dimeric testosterone-ethynodiol. Staining H.-E.; magnification × 160

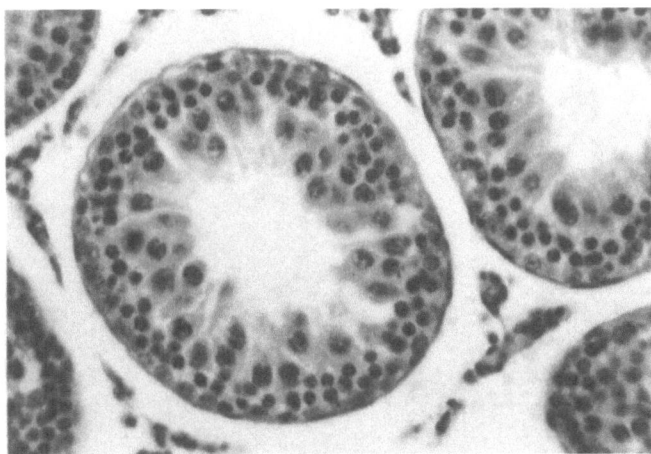

Figure 8 Photomicrograph of testicular tissue of a rat 4 weeks after the injection of 10 mg of the dimeric testosterone-ethynodiol. Staining H.-E.; magnification × 400

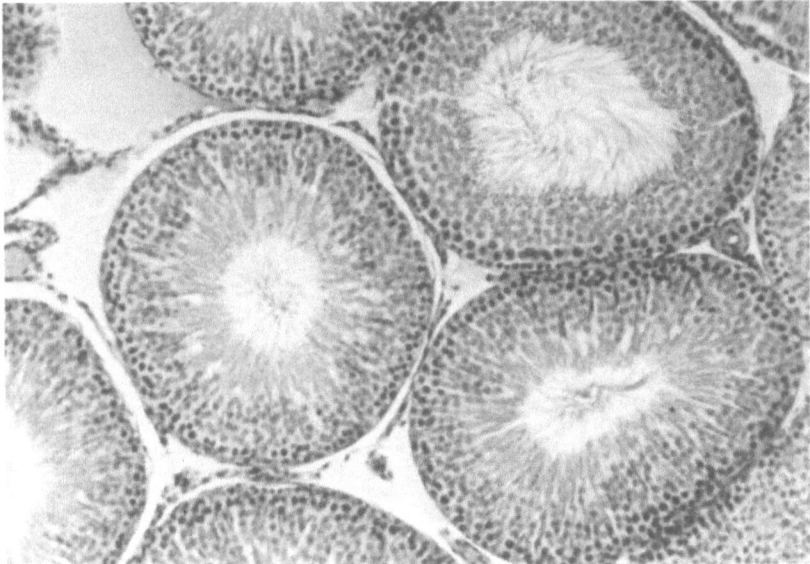

Figure 9 Histological section of rat testis 8 weeks after the injection of 10 mg of the dimeric testosterone-ethynodiol. Staining H.-E.; magnification × 160

The sexual activity of all rats treated with 10, 20 or 40 mg of the dimeric ester did not differ from that of untreated control rats when being coupled with pro-oestrous rats during the night.

Monkeys

The single injection of 50 mg/kg body weight of the dimeric ester resulted in a continuous decrease in the diameter of the tubuli seminiferi to a mini-

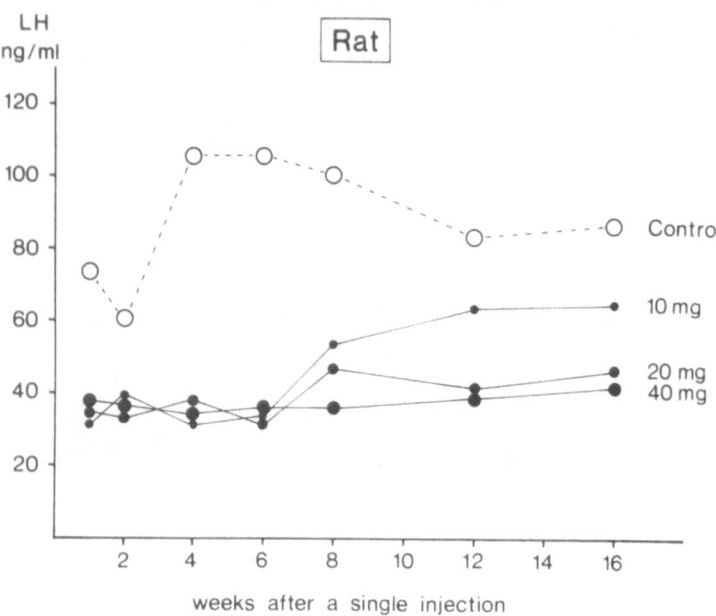

Figure 10   Effect of a single injection of various doses of the dimeric testosterone-ethynodiol ester upon serum LH of the rat (mean values of 6–7 rats)

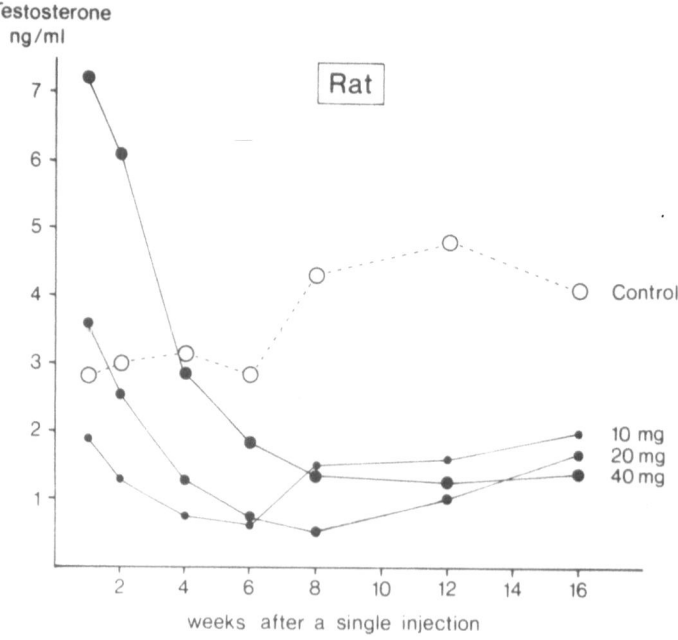

Figure 11   Effect of a single injection of various doses of the dimeric testosterone-ethynodiol ester upon serum testosterone of the rat (mean values of 6–7 rats)

mum after 10 weeks. Thereafter, a gradual reversion could be observed, and 22 weeks after the injection the tubuli showed a normal shape (Figure 12). Spermatogenesis was markedly inhibited 6 weeks after the injection and was totally abolished 4 weeks later. The suppression of spermatogenic activity lasted for at least 14 weeks, and 18 weeks after the injection there were only some mature spermatozoa. After 22 weeks the inhibition of spermatogenesis was shown to be completely reversible (Figure 12).

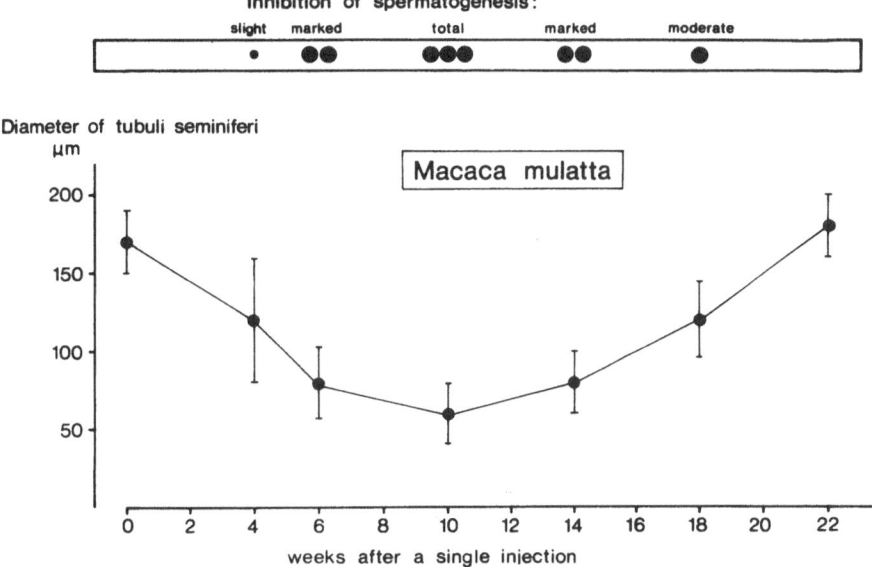

Figure 12 Inhibition of spermatogenesis and effect upon the diameter of the tubuli seminiferi of four rhesus monkeys after a single injection of 50 mg/kg of the dimeric testosterone-ethynodiol in dependency on time

The histological evaluation of testicular sections revealed a marked reduction in the diameter of the tubuli seminiferi and in the height of the germinal epithelium 6 weeks after the injection, as compared with those before treatment (Figures 13, 14). After 10 weeks the germinal epithelium had severely decreased, the tubuli were reduced to a minimum and no spermatozoa could be observed. Sperm development was arrested at the stage of spermatogonia; only some primary spermatocytes could be seen (Figure 15). The basal membranes and the Sertoli cells appeared to be unchanged, and the Leydig cells were hypotrophic.

Eighteen weeks after the administration of the dimeric steroid ester, the height of the germinal epithelium had markedly increased and the reduction in the diameter of the seminiferous tubules was fairly reversed (Figure 16). After 22 weeks there was a complete restoration of spermatogenesis. By morphological and morphometrical criteria the germinal epithelium did not differ from the stage before treatment (Figure 17).

There was no significant suppression of LH serum levels after the injection of the monkeys with 50 mg/kg of the dimeric compound, although in three of the four animals LH secretion seemed to be decreased at certain

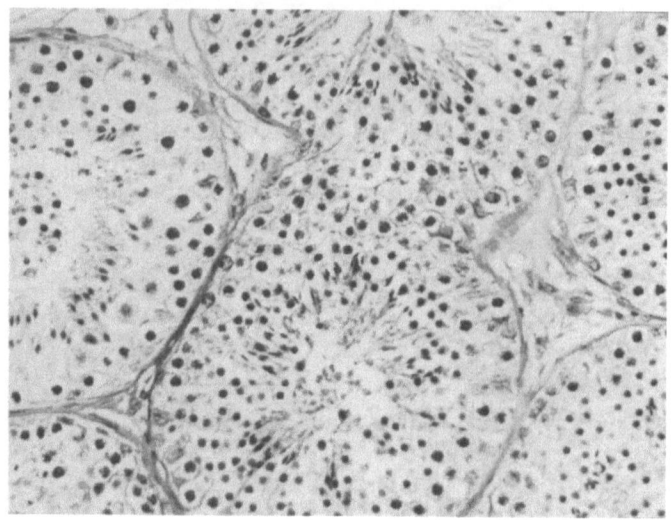

Figure 13 Photomicrograph of testicular tissue of an untreated rhesus monkey. Staining H.-E.; magnification × 120

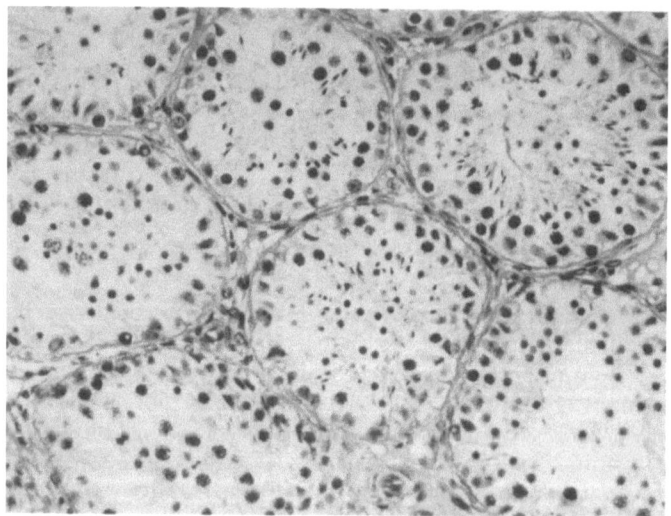

Figure 14 Histological section of the testis of a monkey 6 weeks after the injection of 50 mg/ kg of the dimeric testosterone-ethynodiol. Staining H.-E.; magnification × 120

time intervals (Figure 18). The testosterone levels, however, decreased continuously after the injection, but remained at all times above the level of 2 ng/ml (Figure 19).

The sexual activity of the dominant animal was not impaired during the whole experiment. Apart from a slight reduction in body weight and the decrease in testicular size, no adverse side-effects could be observed.

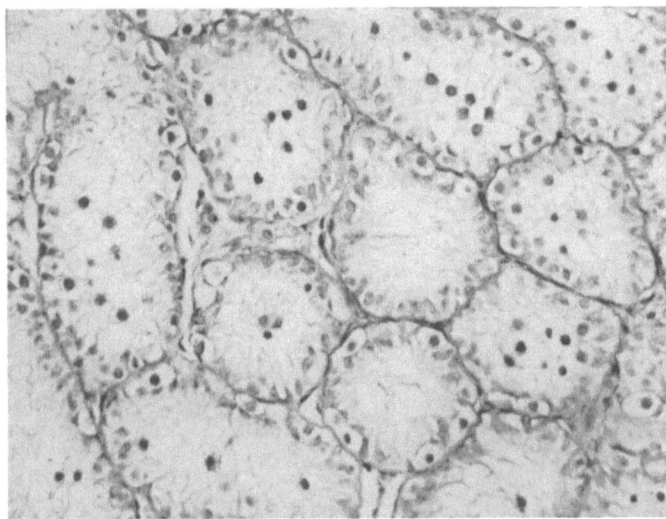

Figure 15   Histological section of the testis of a monkey 10 weeks after the injection of 50 mg/ kg of the dimeric testosterone-ethynodiol. Staining H.-E.; magnification × 120

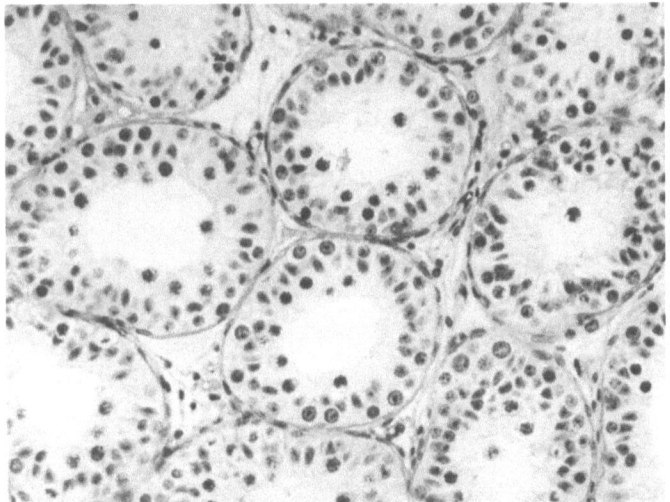

Figure 16   Histological section of the testis of a monkey 18 weeks after the injection of 50 mg/ kg of the dimeric testosterone-ethynodiol. Staining H.-E.; magnification × 120

DISCUSSION

The results demonstrate that a single injection of the dimeric testosterone-ethynodiol ester is capable of inhibiting reversibly spermatogenesis in both the rat and the rhesus monkey for a prolonged period of time. In the rat the suppression of fertility became evident 4 weeks after the injection, and outlasted the experimental period of 16 weeks when the dose was 40 mg. This contraceptive effect seemed to be mediated mainly by the pronounced

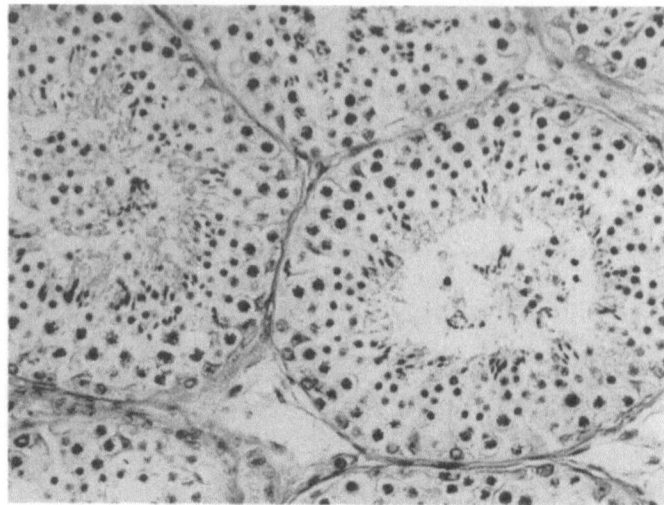

Figure 17   Histological section of the testis of a monkey 22 weeks after the injection of 50 mg/kg of the dimeric testosterone-ethynodiol. Staining H.-E.; magnification × 120

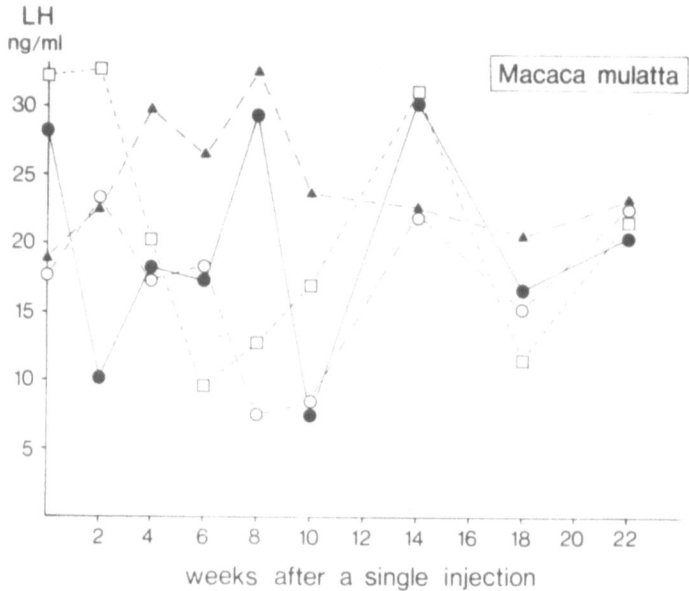

Figure 18   Effect of a single injection of 50 mg/kg of the dimeric testosterone-ethynodiol upon serum LH of four rhesus monkeys

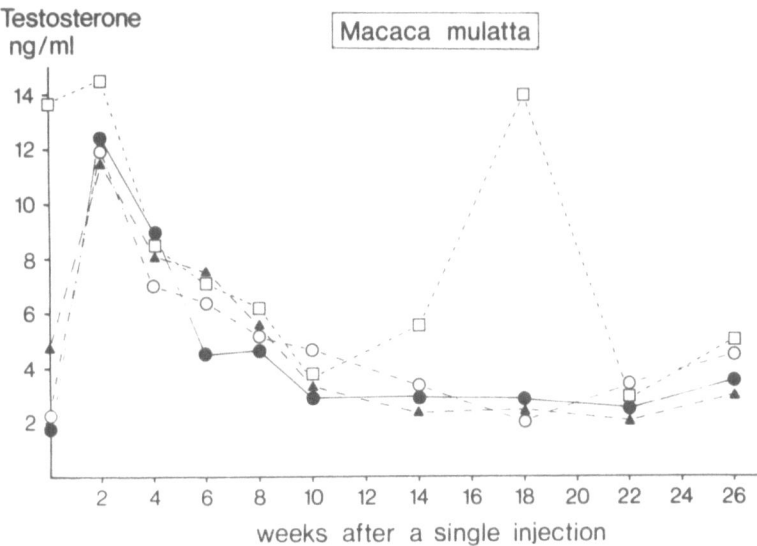

Figure 19   Effect of a single injection of 50 mg/kg of the dimeric testosterone-ethynodiol upon serum testosterone of four rhesus monkeys

suppression of gonadotrophin release. This may, in all probability, be due to a direct action of the intact dimeric compound upon the pituitary, as the relatively low serum levels of testosterone do not seem to be capable of inhibiting gonadotrophin secretion. A comparison of the suppressive effect of the dimeric ester upon serum LH and on spermatogenesis with that of an equivalent dose of norethisterone enanthate indicates that the dimer must have a direct inhibitory effect upon testicular germinal epithelium[7]. Although the level of LH was reduced to the same extent during the first 4 weeks after the injection of 24 mg of norethisterone enanthate, as compared with that after treatment with the dimer, the depot progestogen exerted only a moderate inhibition of spermatogenesis, while the testosterone-ethynodiol ester suppressed spermatogenesis completely for a long period of time[7].

In the monkey a single injection of 50 mg/kg resulted in a marked inhibition of spermatogenesis after 6 weeks, which had become complete after 10 weeks. Even 18 weeks after the injection, only few mature spermatozoa could be observed, even though the germinal epithelium showed a pronounced reversion of the suppression. Since serum LH was not consistently suppressed during the experiment, the inhibition of spermatogenesis seems to be due to a direct effect of the intact dimeric compound upon the testis.

It is known that spermatogenesis requires a high intratesticular testosterone concentration[10]. The androgen accumulation in the environment of the seminiferous tubules and in the epididymis is maintained by the androgen binding protein (ABP) produced by Sertoli cells[11]. The interaction between testosterone and ABP could possibly be impaired by the presence of the dimeric testosterone-ethynodiol, resulting in an inhibition of spermatogenesis.

The maintenance of libido during treatment, which in the monkey may be based on testosterone levels not below 2 ng/ml and supported by the androgenic partial effect of the intact dimer, as well as the lack of discernible adverse effects, lead to the conclusion that the dimeric testosterone-ethynodiol ester might be a promising approach for the development of a depot contraceptive in the male.

REFERENCES

1. Schearer, S.B., Alvarez-Sanchez, F., Anselmo, J., Brenner, P., Coutinho, E., Latham-Faundes, A., Frick, J., Heinild, B. and Johansson, E.D.B. (1978). Hormonal contraception for men. *Int. J. Androl., Suppl.* **2,** 680
2. Kuhl, H. and Taubert, H.-D. (1973). A new class of long-acting hormonal steroid preparation: synthesis of oligomeric estradiol derivatives. *Steroids,* **22,** 73
3. Kuhl, H. and Taubert, H.-D. (1974). A new class of long-acting hormonal steroid preparation: synthesis of dimeric ethynodiol and nortestosterone, of dimeric and trimeric androgens and of some dimeric combinations of steroids. *Steroids,* **24,** 613
4. Kuhl, H. and Taubert, H.-D. (1976). A new class of long-acting hormonal steroid preparation: synthesis of dimeric androgens coupled at C_3-C_3 and C_{17}-C_3 and of an androgen-progestogen combination. *Steroids,* **28,** 89
5. Kuhl, H., Auerhammer, W. and Taubert, H.-D. (1976). Oligomeric oestradiol esters: A new class of long-acting oestrogens. *Acta Endocrinol. (Copenh.),* **83,** 439
6. Kuhl, H., Braun, J., Dericks-Tan, J.S.E. and Taubert, H.-D. (1979). The biological activity of dimeric testosterone, a new long-acting androgen, and of testosterone enanthate in the castrated male rat. *Horm. Res.,* **10,** 252
7. Kuhl, H., Franz, I., Born, H.-J., Schneider, M. and Taubert, H.-D. (1981). Reversible inhibition of spermatogenesis by a long-acting dimeric ethynodiol-testosterone ester. *Contraception,* **24,** 61
8. Dericks-Tan, J.S.E. and Taubert, H.-D. (1975). Measurement of rat LH with a double-antibody solid-phase radioimmunoassay: effect of LH-RH and of testosterone oenanthate in castrated animals. *Acta Endocrinol. (Copenh.),* **78,** 451
9. Monroe, S.E., Peckham, W.D., Neill, J.D. and Knobil, E. (1970). A radioimmunoassay for rhesus monkey luteinizing hormone (RhLH). *Endocrinology,* **86,** 1012
10. Hunt, D.M., Lau, I.-F., Saksena, S.K. and Chang, M.-C. (1978). Endocrinological and physiological features after steroid treatment of male rats. *Arch. Androl.,* **1,** 311
11. Hutson, J.C. and Stocco, D.M. (1981). Peritubular cell influence on the efficiency of androgen-binding protein secretion by Sertoli cells in culture. *Endocrinology,* **108,** 1362

5
Relationship between ligand structure and affinity for androgen binding protein

T.J. LOBL, G.R. CUNNINGHAM, J.A. CAMPBELL and D.J. TINDALL

INTRODUCTION

Androgen binding protein (ABP) is an FSH stimulated secretory product of the Sertoli cell of the testis[1]. Under the dual control of FSH and androgen, ABP is secreted into the blood and seminiferous tubules. Once in the seminiferous tubule, ABP travels through the rete testis to the caput epididymis. It is in the initial segment and the caput epididymis that ABP is largely reabsorbed out of the luminal fluid. In the rat ABP binds testosterone and dihydrotestosterone (DHT), and is presumed to help maintain the high intraluminal concentration of these androgens in the seminiferous tubules and to transport them to the initial segment of the epididymis. This sequelae of events suggested that ABP may play a role in the androgen-dependent maturation of epididymal spermatozoa and male fertility in general. ABP is also found in much lower concentration in the serum of the rat, rabbit and other species. The study of serum ABP is confounded by a similar but not identical liver protein, testosterone-oestrogen binding globulin (TeBG), in many species but not the rat[2]. Serum hABP can be distinguished from serum hTeBG by concanavalin A chromatography[3]. Rat ABP has a molecular weight of about 90 000, an isoelectric point of 4.6–4.7 pH and an R_f of approximately 0.54 by polyacrylamide gel electrophoresis (PAGE)[2]. It is composed of protomers of 47 000 and 41 000 daltons. Although the physical-chemical properties of ABP have been well defined, the biological function remains to be elucidated.

Initially ABP was characterized by its binding of [³H]-testosterone and [³H]-DHT by the steady state PAGE method[4], which allowed of the quantification of ABP binding activity. A radio-immunoassay is now available for rat ABP which quantifies total ABP protein present rather than binding activity[5]. Binding studies to natural compounds showed that, unlike TeBG from many species, rat ABP had low affinity for oestradiol[6]. It also poorly bound non-androgens such as progesterone, cortisol and androstenedione[6]. The binding studies of natural steroids enabled scientists to distinguish rat ABP from TeBG (Table 1). The testicular origin of ABP and its preference for androgens suggested that ABP may have an

Table 1 Affinity (equilibrium dissociation constant, nM) of selected steroids to ABP and androgen receptor AR[21]. Extensive lists of affinities to ABP, AR and TeBG can be found in References 6, 7, 21 and 22

Steroid	ABP	AR
DHT	2.3	1.5
Testosterone	12	2.3
4-Androsten-3,17-dione	1180	520
Progesterone	120	90
17α-Hydroxyprogesterone	645	1590
Cyproterone acetate	1060	37
Cortisol	3830	⩾10 000

important function in the male reproductive system. In order to study this possibility, competitive affinity antagonists to ABP are needed to block the binding of the natural androgen. There were several reasons for studying the steroid structure–activity relationships (SAR)* to ABP. First, the studies provide clues to the protein's function. Second, they provide information about the tolerance of active sites for different structures and about the mechanism of binding. Third, they identify compounds which may interfere with the binding of natural androgens by competitive inhibition and compounds which may have binding properties superior to those of natural ligands. This chapter gives a selective review of the SAR for ABP and a summary of the potential for these compounds to be used as antifertility agents.

STRUCTURE–ACTIVITY RELATIONSHIPS OF SYNTHETIC STEROIDS

The structure–activity studies were designed to evaluate several components of typical SAR analysis. The first component considered the effects of functional group size and position. The second considered the polar effects and the ability to form hydrogen bonds at the key extremes (the 3 and 17 steroidal loci). Finally, the influence of functional groups on the hydrophilic and hydrophobic character of the steroid was examined. The following subsections will summarize our relevant observations on the SAR of ABP.

The A ring

The A ring provided insight into ABP binding[7] (Table 2). Substitution of alkyl groups such as methyl, ethyl or a bulky spirocyclopropyl group on to DHT at C-2 maintained good ABP affinity. In many cases these compounds enjoyed affinity enhancements by factors of 2–4 when complete displace-

---

* The structure–activity relationship describes how the binding affinity (activity, K_d, etc.) of synthetic ligands, which can be related simply to the natural ligands, changes with structural (functional group) changes. SAR studies allow of the empirical mapping of binding sites by successive modification of parent ligands. The method is particularly popular in drug development.

Table 2 Affinities of selected steroids with A-ring, D-ring substitutions on ABP and AR affinity[7]*

Steroid	% [³H]-DHT displaced	
	ABP	AR
17β-Hydroxy-5α-androstan-3-one (DHT)	100	100
17β-Hydroxy-2α-methyl-5α-androstan-3-one	100	72
2α-Fluoro-17β-hydroxy-5α-androstan-3-one	51	80
17β-Methoxy-5α-androstan-3-one	69	1
17β-Methoxy-2α-methyl-5α-androstan-3-one	100	11
17β-Methoxy-spiro(5α-androstan-2,1′-cyclopropan)-3-one	100	6
2α-Ethyl-17β-methoxy-5α-androstan-3-one	100	0
2α-Bromo-17β-methoxy-5α-androstan-3-one	34	3
17β-Benzyloxy-2α-methyl-5α-androstan-3-one	100	4
17β-Hydroxy-7α-methyl-5α-androstan-3-one	97	92
17β-Hydroxy-17α-methyl-5α-androstan-3-one	100	122
17α-Ethinyl-17-hydroxyl-5α-androstan-3-one	100	15
5α-Androstane-11β,17β-diol	33	10
11β,17β-Dihydroxy-5α-androstan-3-one	32	78
17β-Hydroxy-7α-methylestra-4,14-diene-3-one	100	110
5α-Androst-16-en-3-one	19	23
17α-Hydroxy-4-androsten-3-one (epitestosterone)	13	17

* Based upon displacement of [³H]-DHT by 10 nM of test compound

ment curves were performed and K_ds were determined. These results are consistent with the interpretation that the A ring can accommodate structural bulk off the 2 and 3 positions. The alkyl groups may help optimize binding orientation to give the enhanced affinity. The effects of polar groups are less clear. Polar groups such as bromo, ethylidene, hydroxymethylene or 2-oxa resulted in very low binding affinities. 2-Fluoro-DHT bound with 51% of the DHT affinity. The polar effect does not seem to relate to resonance effects on the 3-ketone, as conjugated Δ^1-bonds do not significantly affect binding. In the case of Δ^4-bonds, there are minor affinity effects but these are explained by steric changes brought about by the absence of the 5α-hydrogen. The 10β-methyl group in many examples also contributed to high ABP affinity. Finally, the 5α-hydrogen configuration was preferred over the 5β-hydrogen or no hydrogen (Δ^4- or Δ^5-double bond). This suggests that even though ABP appears to bind steroids from the beta face, it requires a *trans* A–B ring junction if it is to make optimum bonding with the critical C-3 position.

The D ring

The D ring offered another perspective on binding[7]. No D-ring modification was found that significantly enhanced ABP binding. A double bond at Δ^{14} (17β-hydroxy-7α-methylestra-4,14-diene-3-one) had high affinity for ABP, while a Δ^{16}-compound which lacked the 17-hydroxyl (5α-androst-16-en-3-one) bound poorly. Methyl and ethinyl groups at 17α were acceptable on good binding frameworks such as DHT or testosterone. On poor binding frameworks no enhancement of affinity was seen.

The 17β-hydroxyl was a key factor in separating the affinities of steroids for ABP from AR. Here it was seen that a methoxy or a bulky benzyloxy group could be substituted for hydroxy without dramatic inhibition of ABP affinity. Esters such as enanthate or glucuronide were not tolerated by ABP. From this it was learned that ABP had a requirement for a polar hydrogen bond accepting functionality at 17β but did not need a hydrogen bond donor. (Epitestosterone with a 17α-hydroxyl bound poorly.) When the polar hydrogen bond accepting fluorine was substituted for hydroxyl, the binding was not as good, suggesting that the protein prefers an oxygen at 17β, although a hydroxyl group is not essential. From these studies it is clear that ABP recognizes the D-ring binding component of a steroid, but it is not as important a contributor as the A ring to affinity.

Substitutions at C-7 and C-11

Methyl substitutions at C-7 had little effect on ABP affinity of the seven analogues tested[7]. It is well known in the literature that 7α-methyl substitutions greatly enhance the potency of androgens, but here, too, there was little or no enhancement of androgen receptor affinity[7]. The range of affinity changes went from 0 to 20% affinity difference between structural pairs, which is unlikely to be biologically significant. This suggests that the potency effects of 7α-methyl substitutions probably are derived from effects on metabolism rather than from changes in affinity for receptor or transport proteins.

In the C ring the effects of 11β-hydroxyl and 11-ketones were examined[7]. Affinity to ABP was greatly reduced by the addition of the polar 11-ketone and the axial 11β-hydroxyl groups. Interestingly, when the 3-ketone was absent, the presence of an 11β-hydroxyl allowed 33% binding even though the parental binding was not detectable. Why the hydroxyl should be helpful is not clear, although some stability must be derived from two-point bonding over a single point. No other examples of enhanced binding have been observed following polar substitutions in any ring, with the exception of the A-ring fused heterocyclic steroids and the irreversible inhibitors.

A-ring fused heterocycles

During ABP binding studies with clinically interesting steroids, it was discovered that one A-ring fused pyrazole and an A-ring fused isoxazole had unexpectedly high ABP binding affinity[7]. Some compounds in this class have been reported to possess potent anabolic and weak androgenic properties. A series of A-ring fused heterocyclic steroids was prepared to (1) determine their ABP affinity; (2) determine their SAR; and (3) determine whether their SAR was consistent with the binding model for non-heterocyclic steroids[8]. Examples of several heterocyclic steroids studied are found in Table 3. In general, it was found that the 5'-methyl and unsubstituted pyrazoles bound well to ABP and poorly to TeBG. The androstenoisoxazoles in most cases bound well to ABP and poorly to TeBG. Unsubstituted A-ring fused oxazoles, imidazoles, thiazoles and triazoles bound to ABP with low to medium affinity, depending on the case, and poorly to TeBG. In all cases alkyl-substituted heterocyclics had little or no affinity to ABP or TeBG (Lobl et al., unpublished data). These studies demonstrate a

Table 3 Selected binding affinities for A-ring fused heterocyclic steroids to ABP[8]

Structure			Rat ABP relative binding affinity to DHT
Dihydrotestosterone			90
	R	R'	
	H	H	90
	H	CH$_3$	84
	CH$_3$	H	0
			90
			0

unique ABP binding pocket adjacent to the steroid A-ring site that is not present in either AR or hTeBG. The pocket sterically allows the binding of unsubstituted 5-membered heterocyclic rings but alkylated rings do not bind optimally. In the best case ABP binds with almost four times the affinity of DHT. These data are consistent with the SAR determined for the non-heterocyclic steroids, with the extension of the site size to accommodate the extra ring. They also explain why the 2-alkyl groups are acceptable in ABP but not AR and TeBG.

NON-STEROIDAL COMPETITIVE INHIBITORS

One of the questions that were raised by the unexpected tolerances of ABP for the A-fused heterocycles is to what extent could the binding site accept non-steroidal structures. In the androgen receptor area flutamide, RU 23 908, AA560 and cimetidine bind to the androgen cytoplasmic receptor (AR) and act as antiandrogens, presumably by competitive inhibition[9]. In the oestrogen series non-steroidal compounds such as diethyl stilboestrol and nafoxidine act as agonists and antagonists, respectively. The interest in non-steroidal ABP binding agents centred on the hopefully improved biological profile of such compounds over steroids and whether or not competitive antagonists to androgen transport by ABP would lead to inhibition of male fertility. In an effort to find such non-steroidal compounds, Rousseau and colleagues discovered a series of dicyclohexane derivatives that inhibited both ABP binding[10] and hormone-stimulated aromatase activity in Sertoli cells[11]. The structures and ABP binding affinities of several of these compounds are given in Table 4. The compounds have the chemical skeleton of saturated diethyl stilboestrol, where the A and D rings of the natural steroidal androgen are replaced by two cyclohexane rings and the B and C rings by an ethane linker. The binding affinities of these compounds are not as good as those of natural androgens or some of the analogues mentioned earlier, but they are extremely important for several reasons. First, they demonstrate that a non-steroid can bind well to ABP and the active site is permissive. Second, they provide a series of competitive antagonists for ABP that cannot be metabolized to known androgens or antiandrogens. With these antagonists the physiological role of ABP can be explored independently. Finally, they allow further exploration of the nature of the ABP active site, provide new opportunities for active-site-directed irreversible inhibitors, and additional compounds for the study of binding differences between the receptor, ABP and hTeBG (SAR).

Table 4 ABP binding affinity of several dicyclohexane derivatives[11]

Structure	Symbol*	ABP inhibition constant, K_i (nM)
	a	160
	b	240
	c	390
	d	600

* a = D,1-3,4-bis(4-oxocyclohexyl)hexane;   b = D,1-3-(4-oxocyclohexyl)-4(*cis*-4-hydroxycyclohexyl)hexane;   c = meso-3,4-bis(4-hydroxycyclohexyl)hexane;   d = D,1-3-(*cis*-4-hydroxycyclohexyl)-4-(*trans*-4-hydroxycyclohexyl)hexane

ACTIVE-SITE-DIRECTED IRREVERSIBLE INHIBITORS

Active-site-directed irreversible inhibitors are chemicals which have affinity for the active or binding sites of enzymes or receptor proteins. Such irreversible inhibitors bind to the active site using structural and chemical properties mimicking natural binders and then are irreversibly bound by light, nucleophilic or electrophilic methods of activation. Once a substrate is irreversibly bound, the labelled protein can be characterized and the amino acids in and adjacent to the active site identified. Several active-site-directed irreversible inhibitors are known for ABP and AR.

In 1980 Danzo and colleagues reported that Δ^6-testosterone could photo-affinity label rat ABP[12]. They demonstrated that the protein was irreversibly labelled in the normal dihydrotestosterone binding site. This result confirms the previous SAR work with competitive binders showing that the steroidal 3,4,6,7 edge plays an active role in protein binding. The labelled ABP was shown to be composed of two dissimilar subunits in a ratio of three heavier to one light, each with a binding site for steroid[12, 13]. Photo-affinity labelling of rabbit ABP showed it to be composed of two dissimilar subunits in a 1:1 ratio[14]. Studies with photoaffinity labels will continue to be useful in elucidating the structure, function and regulation of ABP.

Affinity labels have greatly facilitated the purification of the cytoplasmic androgen receptor. In this case the androgen was labelled with a bromo-acetate which could react with neighbouring nucleophiles. Androgen receptor instability (rapidly denatures when not ligand bound) had proved to be a major difficulty in receptor purification procedures. Rat prostate, steer seminal vesicle and rat kidney androgen receptor purifications have been facilitated by using affinity-labelled androgen[15–18]. Again the design of these bromoacetate affinity labels was facilitated by the known interaction of the androgen receptor at the 17β position.

The main disadvantage with affinity labels is that, to date, they react irreversibly to the protein. Accordingly, the labelled protein can be purified and thoroughly characterized but is not biologically active. Nevertheless, active-site-directed irreversible affinity labels are powerful tools for the protein chemist and their design is facilitated by knowledge of binding site SAR.

DIFFERENCES IN STEROID RELATIVE AFFINITY TO ABP, AR AND TeBG

The SAR studies allow the construction of a conceptual model for the binding of steroids to ABP[20]. ABP appears to prefer the steroid beta face and C-4,6,7,15 edge. The site is shaped so that the alpha face of the A ring can be sensed while the alpha faces of the B and D rings are tangentially sensed. The 3-ketone forms a strong protein association and the 17β-hydroxyl contributes a weak polar association. Other areas of the steroid make hydrophobic and/or steric contributions. An artist's cartoon of the ABP binding site is shown in Figure 1. Such models are always tenuous and subject to revision based on new information. This one has proved valuable in helping predict active ABP binding structures.

Although the scope of this review focuses on the SAR studies of ABP, it is instructive to show that similar analyses of the binding affinities to AR and hTeBG have also yielded distinctly different topological preferences for

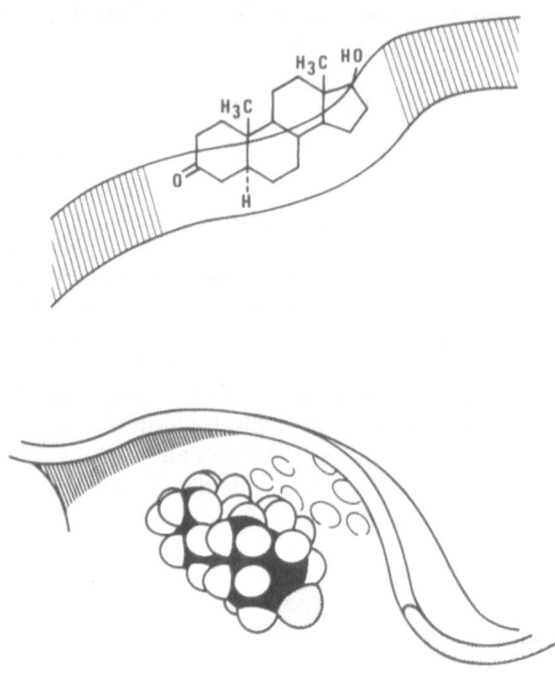

ABP BINDING POCKET

Figure 1   Conceptual view of how androgens bind to ABP[2]. The shaded surface is meant to represent a stylized protein binding pocket

steroids. Table 5 illustrates the variety of differential steroidal affinities found for ABP, hTeBG and AR. These compounds provide unique research tools to study the contributions of androgen transport proteins independently or collaboratively with other combined activity.

Table 5   Relative binding affinity (RBA) differences of various steroids to ABP, AR and hTeBG. The RBA is determined relative to DHT*

Compound	ABP	AR	hTeBG
17β-Methoxy-2α-methyl-5α-androstan-3-one	263†	2†	0
17β-Methoxy-17-methyl-5α-1'H-androstano(3,2-c)pyrazole	375†	0†	0
17α-Ethinyl-3,3-difluoro-5α-androstano-17-ol	⩾100	17	83
17α-Ethinyl-17-hydroxy-5α-androstan-3-one	⩾100	15	⩾100
17β-Hydroxy-4-methyl-4-androsten-3-one	⩾100	73	⩾100
17β-Hydroxy-5α-androst-1-en-3-one	84	73	98
17β-Hydroxy-4-methyl-4-estren-3-one	79	96	42
3α-Methyl-5α-androstane-3β,17β-diol	28	0	81
17α-Ethyl-17-hydroxy-4-estren-3-one	7	92	3

* Some of the data reported in this table can be found in References 7 and 22
† From full displacement curves

CONTRACEPTIVE HYPOTHESES AND PRELIMINARY BIOLOGICAL RESULTS

It was initially observed by Tindall *et al.* that compounds such as flutamide, BOMT and cyproterone acetate bound well to the androgen receptor but poorly to ABP[6]. They reasoned that it should be possible to find compounds that bound well to ABP but poorly to the androgen receptor. A compound with such properties should be a competitive antagonist to transport of androgen by ABP, and the weak androgenic activity of the compound itself would deprive androgen-dependent tissues in the testis and reproductive tract of the high concentrations of androgen thought to be essential for spermatogenesis and sperm maturation. Such a compound would not be concentrated in other tissues and would not interfere with androgen action in those tissues. Several compounds with the desired set of binding affinities were found during our SAR studies. One compound, MMA (17β-methoxy-2α-methyl-5α-androstan-3-one), was tested under several contraceptive protocols[19]. MMA has 2.6 times the affinity to ABP of dihydrotestosterone and 8% the affinity to AR. When proven fertile male rats were given MMA, 1–30 mg/kg, for 69 days and killed on day 70, only minor effects were seen on the testis, seminal vesicles and prostate (Table 6). Surprisingly, by 21 days after the last treatment there were remarkable effects on testis and epididymal weights and histology (Table 6). At no time

Table 6 The effect of MMA on testis, epididymal and seminal vesicle weights following 69 daily treatments and 69 daily treatments and 21 days' non-treatment. The data are presented as a percentage of control[19]

MMA treatment (mg kg^{-1} day^{-1})	Day	Testis weight	Epididymis weight	Seminal vesicle weight
3	69	98	96	71*
10	69	101	99	68†
30	69	89	95	102
3	90	95	93	87
10	90	92	86*	68†
30	90	53†	82†	67†

* $p \leqslant 0.01$
† $p \leqslant 0.001$

during the dosing period were the treated males infertile. The lack of a clear efficacy with MMA during the treatment period and a clear compound-related post-treatment effect suggested that we may have been administering the drug too frequently. In a second series of experiments rats were given MMA for 21 consecutive days (loading period) and then administered MMA once every 5 days until day 49. In this case the testis, epididymis, prostate and seminal vesicles all showed significant weight reductions and the animals in the 20 and 30 mg/kg groups were infertile (Lobl *et al.*, unpublished data). It is concluded from these and other studies that MMA does not act by a mechanism typical for androgens such as DHT. These preliminary biological results show that MMA did not induce functional sterility, as expected, but had some antifertility and antispermatogenic activity.

Another compound in this series, 17β-methoxy-17-methyl-(5α)-$1'$-H-androstano(3,2-c)pyrazole (U-57965), with a greater difference in ABP and AR affinities (3.75 times and less than 0.1 times, respectively) than MMA, was tested in rats to learn whether the results seen earlier were a general property of compounds with large affinity differences. No change in testicular weight was observed in 90-day-old rats treated with 0.1, 1.0 or 10 mg/kg of U-57965, although fertility may have been reduced by the lowest dose. Further studies are needed to determine whether these novel activities are due to these compounds' unique affinity differences for ABP and AR.

SUMMARY, CONCLUSIONS AND FUTURE RESEARCH NEEDS

Androgen binding protein is the natural androgen carrier protein in the testis and epididymis. Its presence in serum and the ability to distinguish it from TeBG in animals that produce both proteins stimulates many questions about its physiological role. It clearly is involved in maintaining the high intratubular androgen concentrations in the testicular and epididymal tubular lumina. It may protect androgen from metabolism similarly to the hypothesized role for TeBG. Finally, it may play a critical role in the male reproductive system. It was this last notion that stimulated the structure activity study of ABP binding ligands. Several hundred steroidal and non-steroidal structures have been evaluated for binding affinity to ABP by several research groups. High-affinity competitive antagonists and photo-affinity labels have been identified, and two of these compounds were studied in preliminary biological experiments. They did not induce functional sterility or inhibit sperm maturation, as female rats bred to treated males were fertile. Unusual effects not typical of androgens such as DHT were seen on testicular histology following treatment with the competitive antagonist—MMA. Additional research is needed to see whether these novel effects are due to intrinsic properties of MMA or to the desired competitive antagonism of ABP transport of androgen.

Two important questions need to be addressed if studies are to continue on the possible involvement of ABP in male reproduction. First, it should be determined whether MMA inhibits the transport of androgens in the testis and from the testis to the epididymis and whether it is able to lower intraluminal or tissue androgens. Second, it needs to be determined whether hABP has a different SAR from that of hTeBG. The first question will answer the issue of whether or not the hypothesized mechanism has been achieved by MMA. If it is able to do these things, then it may not be possible to induce functional sterility with ABP competitive antagonists. If it is not able to inhibit the transport of androgens, then another way must be found to test the hypothesis. Still open to question is how to utilize these activities in antispermatogenic approaches. The second question is important if the concept is to work in humans. Ideally it would be desirable for testicular function to be inhibited (via ABP) without inhibiting the transport of androgen by TeBG. Future studies of SARs of androgens will be important in order to elucidate the mechanisms of androgen action in the male reproductive system.

ACKNOWLEDGEMENTS

We thank D. Squires and T.C. Britton for helping prepare several of the steroids mentioned in this manuscript. We also thank K.T. Kirton for help with some of the biological studies with MMA.

REFERENCES

1. Hansson, V., Reusch, E., Trygstad, O., Torgersen, O., Ritzen, E.M. and French, F.S. (1973). FSH stimulation of testicular androgen binding protein. *Nature New Biol.*, **246**, 56
2. Lobl, T.J. (1981). Androgen transport proteins: physical properties, hormonal regulation, and possible mechanism of TeBG and ABP action. *Arch. Androl.*, **7**, 133
3. Hsu, A-F. and Troen, P. (1978). An androgen binding protein in the testicular cytosol of human testis. *J. Clin. Invest.*, **61**, 1611
4. Ritzen, E.M., French, F.S., Weddington, S.C., Nayfeh, S.N. and Hansson, V. (1974). Steroid binding in polyacrylamide gels. *J. Biol. Chem.*, **249**, 6597
5. Gunsalus, G.L., Musto, N.A. and Bardin, C.W. (1978). Immunoassay of androgen binding protein in blood: a new approach for the study of the seminiferous tubule. *Science, N.Y.*, **200**, 65
6. Tindall, D.J., Cunningham, G.R. and Means, A.R. (1978). 5α-Dihydrotestosterone binding to androgen binding protein. *J. Biol. Chem.*, **253**, 166
7. Cunningham, G.R., Tindall, D.J. and Means, A.R. (1979). Differences in steroid specificity for rat androgen binding protein and the cytoplasmic receptor. *Steroids*, **33**, 261
8. Britton, T.C., Lobl, T.J., Campbell, J.A., Tindall, D.J., Cunningham, G.R. and Means, A.R. (1980). The synthesis and affinity of A-ring fused heterocyclic steroids to rat androgen binding protein and rat cytoplasmic androgen receptor. In *Proceedings of the 179th National Meeting of the American Chemical Society*, March 24-27, Houston, Texas, Medi 7
9. Tindall, D.J., Chang, C.H., Lobl, T.J. and Cunningham, G.R. (1984). Androgen antagonists in androgen target tissues. In *Pharmacol. Therap.*, **24**, 367
10. Rousseau, G.G., Quivy, J.I., Colas, G., Delpech, S., Hochereau-de Reviers, M.T. and Laporte, P. (1981). Nonsteroidal inhibitors of androgen binding to ABP: synthesis, binding properties and effects on male fertility. *Int. J. Androl. Suppl*, **3**, 50
11. Verhoeven, G., Cailleau, J., Quivy, J.I. and Rousseau, G.G. (1983). Dicyclohexane derivatives that bind to androgen-binding protein (ABP) also inhibit hormone stimulated aromatase activity in rat Sertoli cells. *J. Steroid Biochem.*, **18**, 127
12. Taylor, C.A. Jr., Smith, H.E. and Danzo, B.J. (1980). Characterization of androgen-binding protein in rat epididymal cytosol using a photoaffinity ligand. *J. Biol. Chem.*, **255**, 7769
13. Larrea, F., Musto, N., Gunsalus, G. and Bardin, C.W. (1981). The microheterogeneity of rat androgen-binding protein from the testis, rete testis fluid, and epididymis, as demonstrated by immunoelectrophoresis and photoaffinity labeling. *Endocrinology*, **109**, 1212
14. Danzo, D.J., Taylor, C.A. Jr. and Eller, B.C. (1982). Some physicochemical characteristics of photoaffinity-labeled rabbit androgen-binding protein. *Endocrinology*, **111**, 1270
15. Chang, C.H., Rowley, D.R., Lobl, T.J. and Tindall, D.J. (1982). Purification and characterization of androgen receptor from steer seminal vesicle. *Biochemistry*, **21**, 4102
16. Chang, C.H., Rowley, D.R. and Tindall, D.J. (1983). Purification and characterization of the androgen receptor from rat ventral prostate. *Biochemistry*, **22**, 6170
17. Chang, C.H., Lobl, T.J., Rowley, D.R. and Tindall, D.J. (1984). Affinity labeling of the androgen receptor in rat prostate cytosol with 17β-((bromoacetyl)oxy)-5α-androstan-3-one. *Biochemistry*, **23**, 2527
18. Mainwaring, W.I.P. and Johnson, A.D. (1980). Use of affinity label 17β-bromoacetoxy-testosterone in the purification of androgen receptor proteins. In Bresciani, F. (ed.) *Perspectives in Steroid Receptor Research*, pp. 89-97. (New York: Raven Press)
19. Lobl, T.J., Frielink, R.D., Kirton, K.T. and Campbell, J.A. (1980). The effects of 17β-methoxy-2α-methyl-5α-androstan-3-one on spermatogenesis, hormones and fertility in the male rat. In *Proceedings Fifth Annual Meeting, American Society of Andrology*, March 11-14, Chicago, Illinois

20. Lobl, T.J., Campbell, J.A., Tindall, D.J., Cunningham, G.R. and Means, A.R. (1980). A model for the mechanism of androgen binding, transport, and translocation to the nucleus. In Steinberger, A. and Steinberger, E. (eds.) *Testicular Development, Structure and Function*, pp. 323–330. (New York: Raven Press)
21. Kirchhoff, J., Soffie, M. and Rousseau, G.G. (1979). Differences in the steroid-binding site specificities of rat prostate androgen receptor and epididymal androgen-binding protein (ABP). *J. Steroid Biochem.*, **10,** 487
22. Cunningham, G.R., Tindall, D.J., Lobl, T.J., Campbell, J.A. and Means, A.R. (1981). Steroid structural requirements for high affinity binding to human sex steroid binding protein (SBP). *Steroids*, **38,** 243

6
Male contraception with LHRH agonists

A. BELANGER, F. LABRIE, Y. TREMBLAY, A. DUPONT and
R. ST-ARNAUD

INTRODUCTION

Stimulated by the unexplained lack of success of LHRH and its agonists in
the treatment of infertility in men[1], we investigated in detail the effect of
acute and chronic administration of these peptides on testicular functions
in experimental animals. We then made the observation that short-term
administration of an LHRH agonist to adult male rats leads to a loss of
testicular LH and prolactin receptors, as well as to decreased serum testosterone levels accompanied by inhibition of ventral prostate, seminal vesicle
and testis weight[2-5]. It is of great interest that, among the species so far
studied, man is the most sensitive to the inhibitory effect of treatment with
LHRH agonists on testicular steroidogenesis[5, 6]. In fact, while, in the rat,
treatment with LHRH agonists increases 5α-reductase activity and formation of 3α-androstanediol as well as 5α-dihydrotestosterone, which can
partially counteract the inhibitory effect on testosterone production[5, 7], no
such effect is seen in man, where androgen biosynthesis can be completely
inhibited and medical castration is thus achieved relatively easily with
no secondary effect other than those related to low circulating androgen
levels[5, 8, 9].

CASTRATION LEVELS OF SERUM ANDROGENS IN MAN

As mentioned above, man is the most sensitive of all species studied to the
inhibitory effect of LHRH agonists[4-6]. In fact, a single intranasal administration of a potent LHRH agonistic analogue decreases circulating levels
of testosterone and its precursors in normal men for up to 2 days[6]. It has
also been shown that chronic treatment of adult men with cancer of the
prostate with LHRH agonists can rapidly achieve medical castration[7-12].

Following the preliminary observation showing that twice daily intranasal administration of the LHRH agonist [D-Ser(TBU)⁶]-LHRH ethylamide led to a marked inhibition of serum testosterone levels[5], a detailed study
of the effect of the same LHRH agonist was performed at various doses by

the intranasal and subcutaneous routes[17]. The effect of chronic treatment with the LHRH agonist administered by nasal spray (200 or 500 μg, twice daily) or subcutaneously (50 μg daily) for periods up to 8 months was studied on serum sex steroid and LH levels in 18 patients with cancer of the prostate at stage A or B who had been treated surgically by prostatectomy and had no sign of active disease. Basal serum testosterone concentration decreased to 71.1 ± 18.3 (NS) and $28.6 \pm 9.3\%$ ($p < 0.01$) of control in patients receiving the 200 and 500 μg doses by nasal spray, respectively (Figure 1). In patients treated subcutaneously at the 50 μg dose, a more

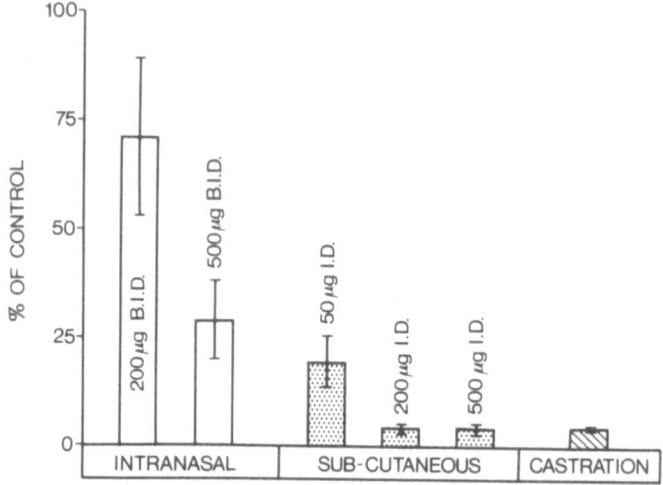

Figure 1   Effect of increasing doses of the LHRH agonist [D-Ser-(TBU)⁶, des-Gly-NH₂¹⁰]-LHRH ethylamide administered for 1 month by the intranasal route (200 or 500 μg) twice a day or once daily subcutaneously at the doses of 50, 200 or 500 μg. Measurements were performed at 08.00 and compared with the values observed after surgical castration

rapid inhibition of serum testosterone levels to $19.6 \pm 6.4\%$ of control ($p < 0.01$) was observed[17]. A more complete and rapid inhibition of serum testosterone levels to 5–8% of control (castrated levels) is achieved with the daily 200 or 500 μg dose subcutaneously[8-16] (Figure 1). Elegant studies by Crowley et al.[18] have shown the potent antisteroidogenic activity of another LHRH agonist in patients with precocious puberty. Similar inhibition of serum androgen levels has been obtained with all the other currently available potent LHRH agonists[19-21].

Since spermatogenesis can be stimulated by androgens, it is thus clear that maximal inhibition of testicular androgen secretion must be achieved. For this purpose, the intranasal route is clearly unacceptable and 200 μg or more of the peptide administered by the subcutaneous route is required (Figure 1). However, while this figure shows the serum steroid concentrations at 08.00, 24 h after last subcutaneous administration of the peptide, it is essential to measure serum steroid levels at shorter time intervals in order to detect any early increase in serum androgens. Such an example can be seen in Figure 2, which illustrates an incomplete blockade of testosterone secretion following treatment for 1 month with the daily 50 μg subcutaneous

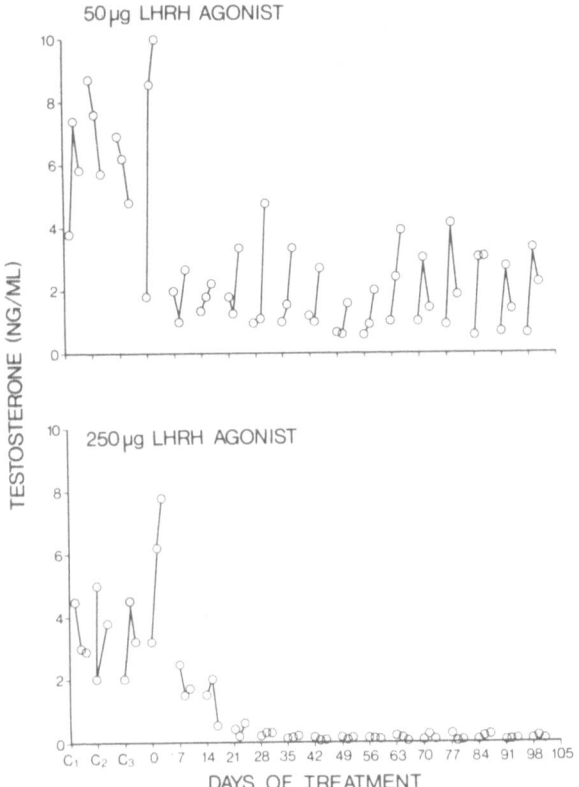

Figure 2 Serum levels of testosterone measured at 08.00, 13.00 and 18.00 in patients with prostate cancer (stage A treated by prostatectomy) and receiving daily (30th day) subcutaneous injections of 50 μg or 250 μg of the LHRH agonist [D-Ser(TBU)⁶, des-Gly-NH₂¹⁰]-LHRH ethylamide

dose, while it shows that a complete inhibition is obtained with the 250 μg daily dose. Measurements of serum testosterone performed 24 h after injection of LHRH agonists do not detect this early but important elevation in serum testosterone which could have stimulatory effects on spermatogenesis.

A series of biological parameters, including complete blood count, sequential multiple analyser (SMA-12) and urinalysis, were performed at monthly intervals, and the symptomatology was evaluated weekly. No side-effect that could be attributed to treatment with the LHRH agonist was noticed up to 3 years of treatment, except those related to decreased androgen formation, such as a gradual decrease in potency in the small proportion of men who were sexually active at the start of treatment. Hot flushes were noticed in approximately 50% of subjects.

MECHANISMS OF ACTION

Our findings of low serum 17-hydroxyprogesterone and testosterone levels in the presence of normal progesterone and pregnenolone concentrations suggest that treatment of men with LHRH agonists inhibits the steroidogenic pathway at the level of 17-hydroxylase and 17,20-desmolase activities during the first 2–3 weeks of treatment with LHRH agonists. These sites of enzymatic blockage are identical with those described after similar treatment in experimental animals[6, 7, 22, 23].

However, under long-term treatment conditions, a different pattern is seen. In fact, in the presence of a more than 95% inhibition of serum testosterone and dihydrotestosterone levels, serum LH measured by radio-immunoassay can remain normal or be only slightly decreased[17]. Since we had previously found a discrepancy between serum LH measured by radio-immunoassay and bioassay in rhesus monkeys treated with a high dose of an LHRH agonist[24], we have performed a similar study in men. It was then found that while the values of serum LH measured by radio-immunoassay and by bioassay (mouse Leydig cell assay) were parallel during the first 2 weeks of treatment, a progressive and marked loss of bioactivity was measured at later time intervals. Thus, after 1 month of treatment, the LH bioactivity was reduced to approximately 5% of control, while the radio-immunoassayable LH was reduced by only 40–50%[25] (Figure 3). These data indicate that the loss of LH bioactivity, rather than testicular desensitization, is the major factor responsible for the almost complete inhibition of testicular steroidogenesis during chronic treatment with LHRH agonists in man. LHRH agonists thus achieve a medical hypophysectomy selective for gonadotropes.

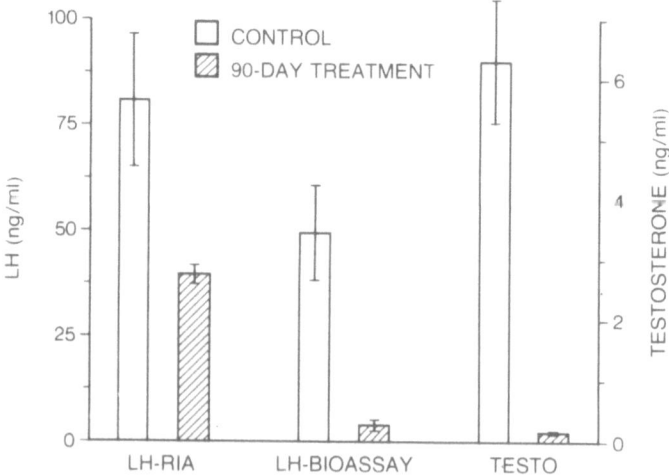

Figure 3 Effect of one-month treatment with an LHRH agonist (500 μg/day, subcutaneously) and a pure antiandrogen on serum LH measured by radio-immunoassay and by the mouse Leydig cell bioassay as well as on serum testosterone concentration in patients with advanced cancer of the prostate

INHIBITION OF SPERMATOGENESIS

Since the marked loss of testis weight following treatment with the LHRH agonist[4, 26] was probably due to some defect in spermatogenesis, it seemed important to investigate the cellular changes occurring in rat testis during chronic administration of [D-Ala[6]]-LHRH ethylamide. When the LHRH agonist was administered at the dose of 1 μg every second day, degenerative changes were observed after 4 weeks in almost all seminiferous tubules. In about 20-30% of tubules, both germinal and Sertoli cells were almost completely absent.

Although long-term treatment with LHRH agonists in male rats causes degenerative changes in a large proportion of the seminiferous tubules with a complete loss of spermatozoa in most tubules, the inhibitory effects are never complete. This is probably due to the fact that, in this species, LHRH agonist treatment increases 5α-reductase activity[5, 27], which, as mentioned earlier, counteracts the inhibitory effect resulting from the almost complete inhibition of testosterone production. Although the rat was the first species in which the inhibitory effects of treatment with LHRH agonists were described on both androgen biosynthesis[2, 3] and spermatogenesis[26] and studies in this species have been essential for understanding some of the mechanisms involved[4, 5], it is not the best model for the human. In fact, in man there is no stimulatory effect of LHRH agonist treatment on 5α-reductase activity and a parallel inhibitory effect is observed on both testosterone and 5α-dihydrotestosterone formation[5-13]. Our current studies in the dog indicate that this species is a more appropriate model for studying the antifertility effects of LHRH agonists. The pattern of serum steroid levels observed after LHRH agonist treatment in man and in dog is very similar. Histology of the testis after chronic treatment of dogs with [D-Ser(TBU)[6]]-LHRH ethylamide shows a marked atrophy of the tubules and a complete inhibition of sperm formation. That treatment with LHRH agonists can inhibit spermatogenesis in men has been shown by the study of Linde et al.[12].

INHIBITION OF TESTICULAR STEROIDOGENESIS IN THE DOG

Since the dog shows testicular steroidogenic changes similar to those found in man following chronic treatment with LHRH agonists, we have studied in detail the effect of chronic administration of a potent LHRH agonist on testicular steroidogenesis in this species.

Figure 4 shows that the chronic administration of an LHRH agonist in the dog causes a marked inhibition of plasma testosterone as well as dihydrotestosterone levels. A maximal decrease in serum testosterone levels is already reached at 2 weeks of treatment, at a time when dihydrotestosterone concentration is reduced by approximately 50%. The maximal inhibitory effect on dihydrotestosterone is delayed to 6 weeks. However, treatment with the LHRH agonist causes no change of plasma 17-hydroxyprogesterone and progesterone levels (Figure 4). It is also of interest to mention that the concentration of plasma androstane-3α,17β-diol remains unchanged after castration as well as after administration of LHRH agonist (data not shown). Measurement of plasma steroid levels in dogs castrated for 12 weeks shows that plasma progesterone and 17-hydroxyprogesterone levels also remain unchanged, while testosterone and dihydrotestosterone concentrations are inhibited to levels comparable with those in animals treated with LHRH agonist.

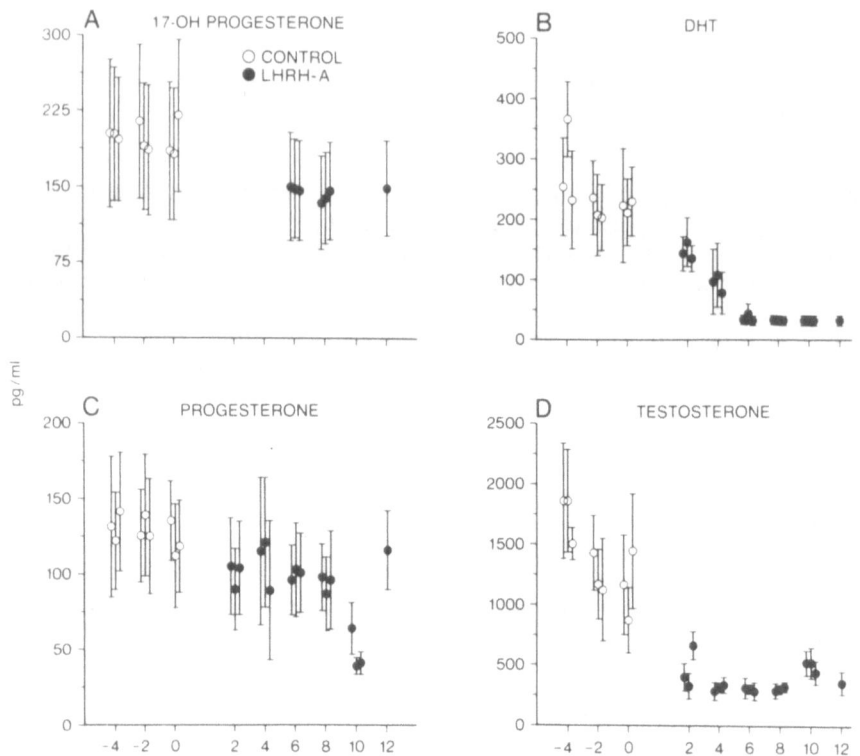

Figure 4 Serum levels of (A) 17-hydroxyprogesterone, (B) dihydrotestosterone (DHT), (C) progesterone and (D) testosterone (T) in adult male dogs ($n = 6$) receiving daily subcutaneous administration of 25 µg of [D-Ser(TBU)^6, des-Gly-NH$_2$^{10}]-LHRH ethylamide. Blood samples were collected at 08.00, 11.00 and 15.00 on three control pretreatment days (-4, -2 and 0) and then on a single day once every 2 weeks during the 12 weeks of treatment

The present data indicate that, in the dog, the major steroids of the testicular steroidogenic pathway are dramatically inhibited after repeated administration of LHRH agonist without any sign of change of 5α-reductase activity. In fact, the suppression of plasma steroid levels observed in these dogs is comparable with that obtained after castration, thus explaining the marked and rapid reduction of prostate weight[28].

The present data could suggest that decreased synthesis of pregnenolone and its metabolites, induced by treatment with LHRH agonist, is due to a blockade in the steroidogenic pathway before pregnenolone formation. In fact, in addition to the effect observed on testicular 17-hydroxylase and 17,20-desmolase activities, it is known that single administration of a high dose of hCG in the rat causes a reduction in the activity of the enzymatic system involved in cholesterol formation. Although radio-immunoassayable and bioactive LH were not measured in this study, the apparent lack of effect of treatment with LHRH agonist on testicular 17-hydroxylase, 17,20-desmolase and 5α-reductase activities suggests that pituitary desensitization is probably responsible for the almost complete inhibition of testicular steroidogenesis.

INHIBITION AND RECOVERY OF SPERMATOGENESIS IN THE DOG

After 4 months of chronic treatment with LHRH agonist, we have observed that the testicular and prostate weights are reduced by 65% and 87%, respectively. However, 6 months after cessation of treatment, the weight of these glands had returned to normal values.

Figure 5 illustrates the individual responses of semen parameters to the

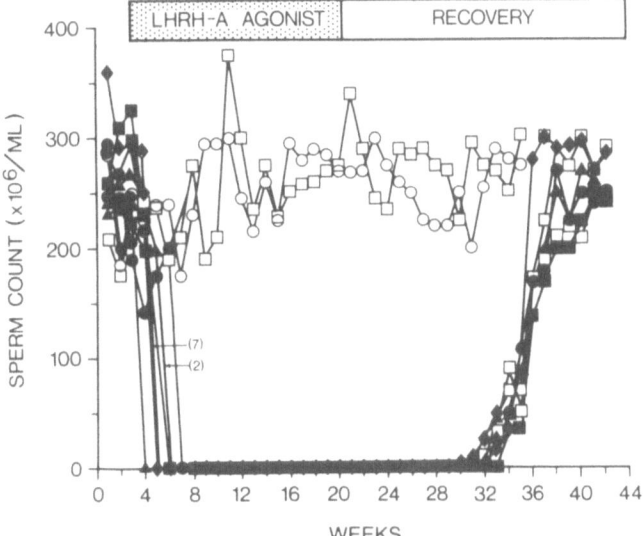

Figure 5 Inhibitory effect of chronic treatment with an LHRH agonist (25 μg/day, subcutaneously) on sperm count in the dog

chronic treatment with the LHRH agonist. It can be seen that between 4 and 7 weeks a marked reduction is observed on the sperm count. In fact, no ejaculate as well as no erection can be obtained in treated dogs after this time interval. On the other hand, a complete recovery of the volume of ejaculate and of the sperm count is achieved 4 months after cessation of treatment.

As shown in Figure 6, treatment with the agonistic analogue induces a dramatic inhibition of plasma testosterone and dehydroepiandrosterone levels (from 1671 ± 247 and 807 ± 19 to 128 ± 12 and 28 ± 15 pg/ml, respectively); while androst-5-ene-3β, 17β-diol concentration is only reduced from 231 ± 25 to 98 ± 15 pg/ml ($p < 0.01$), thus suggesting that dog adrenals are also able to secrete such C-19 steroids. A rapid lowering of plasma dihydrotestosterone and androstane-3β, 17β-diol levels is also obtained and remains constant for the treatment period (data not shown). However, in agreement with previous observations in the human[2], chronic administration of the LHRH agonist does not cause a change in plasma androstane-3α, 17β-diol levels. As can be seen from Figure 6, complete recovery of plasma steroid levels is achieved at 3 months following cessation of treatment. However, there is

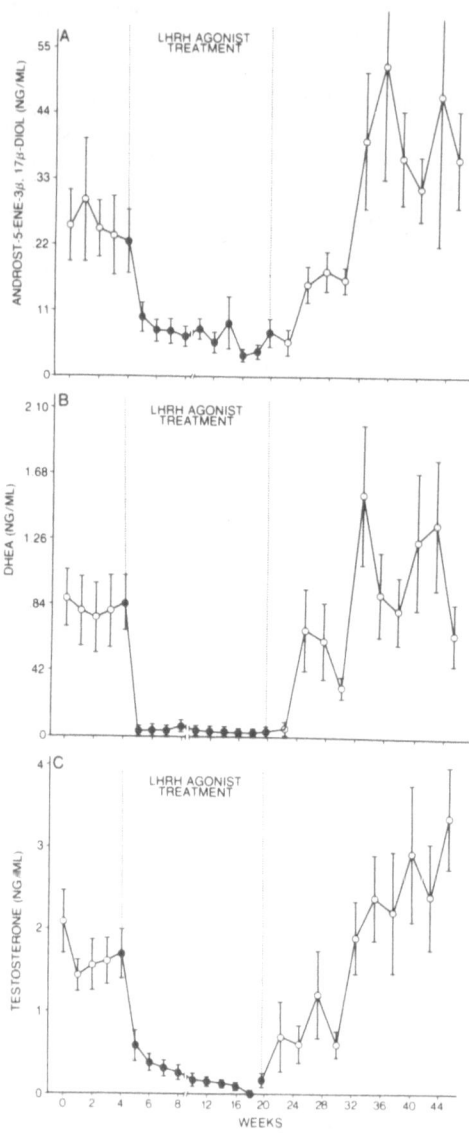

Figure 6 Serum levels of androst-5-ene-3β,17β-diol, dehydroepiandrosterone (DHEA) and testosterone in adult male dogs ($n=6$) receiving daily subcutaneous administration of 1.5 μg/kg body weight of LHRH-A. Blood samples were collected at 08.00 on four control pretreatment weeks and then on a single day once every 2 weeks during the treatment and recovery periods

a tendency for plasma androst-5-ene-3β, 17β-diol and testosterone levels to be slightly higher than the normal levels.

COMBINED TREATMENT WITH AN LHRH AGONIST AND TESTOSTERONE

In order to maintain normal volume of the ejaculate and libido in dogs treated with the LHRH agonist, testosterone was administrated per-cutaneously (Laboratoires Besins-Iscovesco). The volume of ejaculate is not reduced in dogs receiving the combined treatment, while a complete inhib-ition is observed in dogs treated with LHRH agonist (Figure 7). More interesting is the observation that while the libido and normal volume of ejaculate can be maintained in dogs receiving both drugs, the sperm count in animals that are treated with testosterone was not different from that of the animals receiving LHRH agonist alone (complete inhibition).

The present data demonstrate clearly that the volume of ejaculate in dogs treated with LHRH agonist can be completely reversed by the combined administration of an androgen.

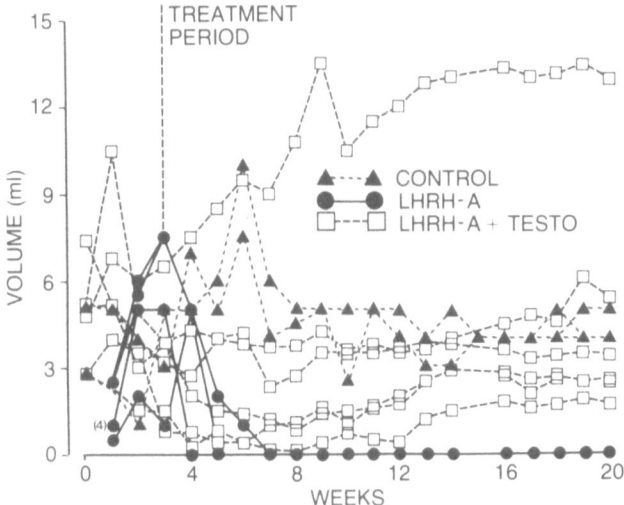

Figure 7 Inhibitory effect of chronic treatment with an LHRH agonist on the volume of ejaculate in the dog. The volume of the ejaculate was maintained by percutaneous administration of testosterone

CONCLUSIONS

Although the rat was the first species in which the inhibitory effects of treatment with LHRH agonists on both androgen biosynthesis and sperm-atogenesis were described[4, 26] and studies in this species have been essen-tial for understanding some of the mechanisms involved[2-7], it is not the best model for the human. In fact, the present study clearly indicates that the dog is a more appropriate model for studying the antifertility effects of LHRH agonists. The pattern of serum steroid levels observed after LHRH agonist treatment in man and in the dog is very similar. In both cases we have observed a medical hypophysectomy selective for gonadotropes which led to azoospermia. Moreover, as we have observed in man, a change in androgen action may lead to a marked inhibition of adrenal C-19 steroid formation, an effect of potential major importance for the treatment of androgen-dependent diseases.

REFERENCES

1. Krabbe, S. and Shakkeback, N.E. (1977). Gonadotropin-releasing hormone (LHRH) and human chorionic gonadotropin in the treatment of two boys with hypogonadotrophic hypogonadism. *Acta Paediatr. Scand.*, **66**, 361
2. Auclair, C., Kelly, P.A., Labrie, F., Coy, D.H. and Schally, A.V. (1977). Inhibition of testicular luteinizing hormone receptor levels by treatment with a potent luteinizing hormone-releasing hormone agonist or human chorionic gonadotropin. *Biochem. Biophys. Res. Commun.*, **76**, 855
3. Auclair, C., Kelly, P.A., Coy, D.H., Schally, A.V. and Labrie, F. (1977). Potent inhibitory activity of [D-Leu^6, des-Gly-NH$_2$^{10}] LHRH ethylamide on LH/hCG and PRL testicular receptor levels in the rat. *Endocrinology*, **101**, 1890
4. Labrie, F., Auclair, C., Cusan, L., Kelly, P.A., Pelletier, G. and Ferland, L. (1978). Inhibitory effects of LHRH and its agonists on testicular gonadotropin receptors and spermatogenesis in the rat. In Hansson, V. (ed.) *Endocrine Approach to Male Contraception*, pp. 303–308. (*Int. J. Androl.*, Suppl. 2)
5. Labrie, F., Bélanger, A., Cusan, L., Séguin, C., Pelletier, G., Kelly, P.A., Lefebvre, F.A., Lemay, A. and Raynaud, J.P. (1980). Antifertility effects of LHRH agonists in the male. *J. Androl.*, **1**, 209
6. Bélanger, A., Labrie, F., Lemay, A., Caron, S. and Raynaud, J.P. (1980). Inhibitory effects of a single intranasal administration of [D-Ser(TBU)^6, des-Gly-NH$_2$^{10}]LHRH agonist on serum steroid levels in normal adult men. *J. Steroid Biochem.*, **13**, 123
7. Bélanger, A., Cusan, L., Auclair, C., Séguin, C., Caron, S. and Labrie, F. (1980). Effect of an LHRH agonist and hCG on testicular steroidogenesis in the adult rat. *Biol. Reprod.*, **22**, 1094
8. Labrie, F., Dupont, A., Bélanger, A., Cusan, L., Lacoursière, Y., Monfette, G., Laberge, J.G., Emond, J.P., Fazekas, A.T.A., Raynaud, J.P. and Husson, J.M. (1982). New hormonal therapy in prostatic carcinoma: combined treatment with an LHRH agonist and an antiandrogen. *J. Clin. Invest. Med.*, **5**, 267
9. Labrie, F., Dupont, A., Bélanger, A., Lacoursière, Y., Raynaud, J.P., Husson, J.M., Gareau, J., Fazekas, A.T.A., Sandow, J., Monfette, G., Girard, J.G., Emond, J. and Houle, J.G. (1983). New approach in the treatment of prostate cancer: complete instead of only partial withdrawal of androgens. *Prostate*, **4**, 579
10. Labrie, F., Dupont, A., Bélanger, A., Lefebvre, F.A., Cusan, L., Raynaud, J.P., Husson, J.M. and Fazekas, A.T.A. (1983). New hormonal therapy in prostate cancer: combined use of a pure antiandrogen and an LHRH agonist. *Horm. Res.*, **18**, 18
11. Labrie, F., Dupont, A., Bélanger, A., Lefebvre, F.A., Cusan, L., Monfette, G., Laberge, J.G., Emond, J.P., Raynaud, J.P., Husson, J.M. and Fazekas, A.T.A. (1983). New hormonal treatment in cancer of the prostate: combined administration of an LHRH agonist and an antiandrogen. *J. Steroid Biochem.*, **19**, 999
12. Linde, R., Doelle, G., Alexander, N., Kirchner, F., Vale, W., Rivier, J. and Rabin, D. (1981). Reversible inhibition of testicular steroidogenesis and spermatogenesis by a potent gonadotropin-releasing hormone agonist in normal men. *N. Engl. J. Med.*, **305**, 663
13. Labrie, F., Bélanger, A., Carmichael, R., Séguin, C., Lefebvre, F.A., Faure, N. and Dupont, A. (1983). Inhibition of the testicular steroidogenic pathway in experimental animals and men. In D'Agata, R., Lipsett, M.B. and Van der Molen, H.J. (eds.) *Recent Advances in*

Male Reproduction: Molecular Basis and Clinical Implications, pp. 239–248. (New York: Raven Press)

14. Labrie, F., Dupont, A., Bélanger, A., Labrie, C., Lacoursière, Y., Raynaud, J.P., Husson, J.M., Emond, J., Houle, J.G., Girard, J.G., Monfette, G., Paquet, J.P., Vallières, A., Bossé, C. and Delisle, R. (1985). Combined antihormonal treatment in prostate cancer, a new approach using an LHRH agonist or castration and an antiandrogen. In *Hormones and Cancer*. (New York: Raven Press) (In press)

15. Labrie, F., Dupont, A., Bélanger, A., Labrie, C., Lacoursière, Y., Emond, J., Monfette, G., Houle, J.G., Girard, J.G., Vallières, G., Bossé, C. and Delisle, R. (1985). Dramatic response of prostate cancer to complete antihormonal treatment. *Acta Med.* (In press)

16. Labrie, F., Dupont, A., Bélanger, A., Emond, J. and Monfette, G. (1984). Pure antiandrogens permit to take advantage of the well-tolerated LHRH agonists for the treatment of prostate cancer. *Proc. Natl. Acad. Sci. USA*, **81**, 3861

17. Faure, N., Labrie, F., Lemay, A., Bélanger, A., Gourdeau, Y., Laroche, B. and Robert, G. (1982). Inhibition of serum androgen levels by chronic intranasal and subcutaneous administration of a potent luteinizing hormone-releasing hormone (LHRH) agonist in adult men. *Fertil. Steril.*, **37**, 416

18. Crowley, W.F. Jr., Comite, F., Vale, W., Rivier, J., Loriaux, D.L. and Cutler, G.B. Jr. (1981). Therapeutic use of pituitary desensitization with a long-acting LHRH agonist: a potent new treatment for idiopathic precocious puberty. *J. Clin. Endocrinol.*, **52**, 370

19. Walker, K.J., Turkes, A.O., Nicholson, R.I., Turkes, A. and Kriffiths, K. (1983). Therapeutic potential of the LHRH agonist, ICI 118630, in the treatment of advanced prostatic carcinoma. *Lancet*, 413

20. Warner, B., Worgul, T.J., Drago, J., Demers, L., Dufau, M., Max, D., Santen, R.J. and members of the Abbott Study Group (1973). Effect of very high dose D-Leucine[6]-gonadotropin-releasing hormone proethylamide on the hypothalamic-pituitary testicular axis in patients with prostatic cancer. *J. Clin. Invest.*, **71**, 1842

21. Ahmed, S.R., Shamet, S.M., Brooman, P.J.C., Howell, A. and Blacklock, N.J. (1983). Treatment of advanced prostate cancer with LHRH analogue ICI 118630: clinical response and hormonal mechanisms. *Lancet*, 415

22. Bélanger, A., Auclair, C., Séguin, C., Kelly, P.A. and Labrie, F. (1979). Down-regulation of testicular androgen biosynthesis and LH receptor levels by an LHRH agonist: role of prolactin. *Mol. Cell. Endocrinol.*, **13**, 47

23. Bélanger, A., Auclair, C., Ferland, L. and Labrie, F. (1980). Time-course of the effects of treatment with a potent LHRH agonist on testicular steroidogenesis and gonadotropin receptor levels in the adult rat. *J. Steroid Biochem.*, **13**, 191

24. Resko, J., Bélanger, A. and Labrie, F. (1982). Effects of chronic treatment with a potent LHRH agonist on serum LH and steroid levels in the male rhesus monkey. *Biol. Reprod.*, **26**, 378

25. Kelly, S., Labrie, F. and Dupont, A. (1983). Loss of LH bioactivity in men treated with an LHRH agonist and an antiandrogen. In *Proceedings of the 65th Annual Meeting of the Endocrine Society*, p. 81

26. Pelletier, G., Cusan, L., Auclair, C., Kelly, P.A., Désy, L. and Labrie, F. (1978). Inhibition of spermatogenesis in the rat by treatment with [D-Ala[6], des-Gly-NH$_2$[10]]LHRH ethylamide. *Endocrinology*, **103**, 641

27. Carmichael, R., Bélanger, A., Cusan, L., Séguin, C., Caron, S. and Labrie, F. (1980). Increased testicular 5α-androstane-3α,17β-diol formation induced by treatment with [D-Ser(TBU)[6],des-Gly-NH$_2$[10]]LHRH ethylamide in the rat. *Steroids*, **36**, 383

28. Vickery, B.H., McRae, G.I. and Bonash, H. (1981). Effect of prolonged systemic administration of an LHRH agonist upon prostatic size and function in geriatric dogs. *J. Androl.*, **2**, 30

7
The epididymis as a target for contraception: role of testosterone metabolism

M. MOTTA, S. ZOPPI and L. MARTINI

INTRODUCTION

Until recently the epididymis was considered as a 'passive channel' through which the spermatozoa could leave the seminiferous tubules in order to be stored before being ejaculated. Recently the recognition that during the time of their passage through the epididymis the spermatozoa change from functionally immature cells unable to fertilize an egg to cells with full fertilizing capacity, thus achieving complete maturation[1-3], has assigned to this organ a crucial role in the physiology of male reproduction. Because of this primary function, the epididymis must now be considered as an 'active structure', highly involved in the post-testicular maturation of spermatozoa. This observation has focussed interest on the epididymis as a possible target for pharmacological male contraception.

The process of sperm maturation requires a co-operative interaction between the sperm and the epididymal epithelium. The morphological and biochemical modifications occurring in the spermatozoa seem to be mediated by secretory products of the epididymis[3]. The possible role of epididymal proteins in promoting sperm maturation has been stressed by the results of Orgebin-Crist and Jahad[4]. These workers have shown that the maturation of rabbit spermatozoa in cultured epididymal tubules was prevented by the addition to the media of protein synthesis inhibitors.

A number of epididymal secretory glycoproteins have been identified in the epididymal tissue and fluid of the rat[5-7], rabbit[8], hamster[8] and bull[9]. After being produced in the caput segment of the epididymis[10], these proteins interact with and remain attached to spermatozoa, as these cells are transported along the duct[8, 11, 12]. It is interesting to note that protein synthesis shows regional differences, which parallel the morphological changes occurring in the luminal sperm[13]. The greatest activity of the protein synthesis machinery is present in the initial segment of the epididymis, where the spermatozoa undergo the most dramatic morphological and biochemical changes.

METABOLISM OF TESTOSTERONE IN THE EPIDIDYMIS

A considerable body of data has accumulated indicating that the epididymis is an androgen-dependent target tissue. In agreement with current theories on steroid hormone action, high-affinity cytoplasmic and nuclear receptors for androgens have been demonstrated in the epididymis; also, the transfer of the 'activated' cytoplasmatic receptors to the nuclear compartment has been shown to occur in this structure[14, 15]. However, the study of the mechanism of action of androgens must also take into account the possibility that testosterone and other androgens may be transformed into their 'active' metabolites.

As with the majority of androgen-dependent structures, many *in vitro* and *in vivo* studies have shown that in the epididymis testosterone undergoes intensive enzymatic transformations[16-19]. It has been demonstrated that this structure is able to metabolize testosterone into dihydrotestosterone (DHT) and 5α-androstane-3α,17β-diol (3α-diol)[17, 20-23]. It has also been reported that the epididymis is able to form 5α-androstane-3β,17β-diol (3β-diol), Δ_4-androstenedione, 5α-androstanedione and androsterone. The enzymes responsible for these conversions (5α-reductase-3-hydroxysteroid-dehydrogenase and 17β-oxidoreductase) have been shown by a number of investigators[17, 23, 24] to be present in the epididymis.

DHT and 3α-diol are the predominant steroids found in the epididymal tissue of different species, including man[25-28]. The ability of the epididymis to convert testosterone into DHT and 3α-diol is only second to that of the prostate[17]. In addition, the amounts of these metabolites differ in the different segments of the epididymis (caput, corpus and cauda). It has been shown in the authors' laboratory that, when these different segments are incubated *in vitro* separately with [14C]-testosterone as a substrate, the highest concentrations of both DHT and 3α-diol are formed in the caput (Figure 1). This means that the highest 5α-reductase-3-hydroxysteroid-dehydrogenase activity is found in this epididymal segment. This result is in agreement with previously reported data[18, 29-32].

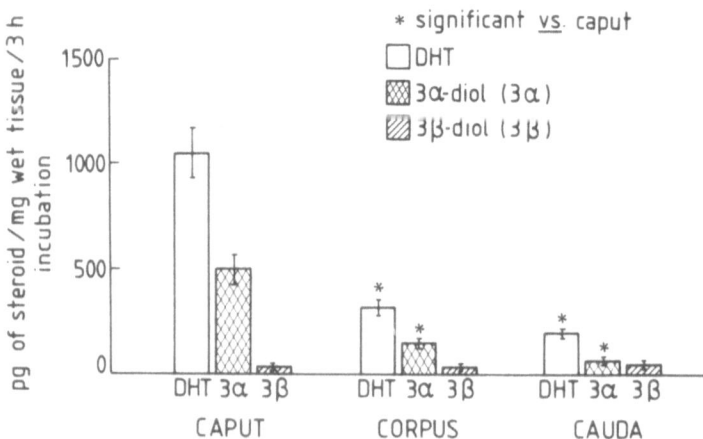

Figure 1 *In vitro* metabolism of testosterone in the different sections of the epididymis of normal rats

It is interesting to underline that the highest enzymatic activity is found in the caput, where the highest concentration of receptor sites binding androgen molecules has also been detected[14]. Klinefelter and Amann[33] have observed that the 5α-reductase-3-hydroxysteroid-dehydrogenase activity appears to be exclusively localized in the principal cells of the epididymis, indicating a specific distribution of these enzymes. It is, then, possible that these cells (where presumably the androgen receptors are localized and where the androgen-induced synthesis of new protein occurs) have a major role in sperm maturation.

ROLE OF ANDROGENS IN THE CONTROL OF EPIDIDYMAL FUNCTION AND SPERM MATURATION

The epididymis is critically dependent upon a continuous supply of androgens for its growth and function[34, 35]. Furthermore, the protein secretory activity of this structure is strongly influenced by the androgen element present in the organ[1-3, 36].

A rapid regression of the secretory epithelium occurs upon castration[37, 38]; this is accompanied by a significant depletion of the intracellular components directly linked to the mechanism of action of androgens. For instance, specific androgen receptors[14] and the testosterone-metabolizing enzyme 5α-reductase[22, 23, 37, 39] appear to be decreased after orchidectomy. The secretory function of the epididymis is restored by the administration of androgens[36, 40-42].

The acquisition of the fertilizing activity of the spermatozoa in the epididymis is also dependent upon androgens in various species of animals and possibly in humans[43-45]. It has been shown that the androgen-induced maturation of spermatozoa in cultured epididymal tissue may be prevented by the presence of anti-androgens[4].

The 5α-reduced metabolites of testosterone (DHT and 3α-diol) have been implicated as the steroids primarily responsible for maintaining epididymal functions, and consequently these metabolites appear to be necessary for maintaining the viability of the spermatozoa and for inducing sperm maturation[3, 18, 44-46]. After castration, the fertilizing capacity of epididymal spermatozoa can be maintained only after substitution therapy performed with testosterone, DHT and 3α-diol[3]. In addition, the administration of 5α-reductase inhibitors to castrated testosterone-pretreated mice induces *in vitro* a decrease in the fertilizing capacity of spermatozoa, followed by a reduction in sperm number and mobility[47, 48].

CONTRIBUTION OF SYSTEMICALLY CIRCULATING ANDROGENS AND INTRALUMINALLY TRANSPORTED ANDROGENS IN THE CONTROL OF EPIDIDYMAL 5α-REDUCTASE-3-HYDROXYSTEROID-DEHYDROGENASE ACTIVITY

Androgens reach the epididymis either through the general circulation or directly through the rete testis fluid. Although androgens are important for the functional integrity of the epididymis as well as for the maturation of epididymal spermatozoa, as previously described, and may modify the activity of the 5α-reductase-3-hydroxysteroid-dehydrogenase system (References 22, 29; Zoppi *et al.*, unpublished), the evidence available does not permit of an answer to the question as to whether the effective androgens are those present in the general circulation or those reaching the epididymis via the rete testis.

In order to investigate the relative contribution of systemic and intraluminal androgens in the regulation of the 5α-reductase-3-hydroxysteroid-dehydrogenase activity of the epididymis, the following experiments have been performed in the authors' laboratory. The experimental model selected has been that of the unilateral ligation of the efferent ducts of adult male rats. In this model the vasculature to the testis and to the epididymis is left intact. Consequently, the ipsilateral epididymis (that of the ligated side) receives androgen supply only from the general circulation; the contralateral epididymis remains obviously exposed to both systemic and intraluminal androgens. Animals submitted to unilateral ligation and to sham operation were sacrificed 3, 7, 14 and 28 days after the operation. The weights of both testes and epididymes were recorded; afterwards both the ipsilateral (ligated) and contralateral epididymes were removed and incubated *in vitro* in the presence of [^{14}C]-testosterone, and the amounts of 5α-reduced metabolites of testosterone were determined.

The unilateral ligation of the efferent ducts induces a significant and progressive decrease in the weight of the ipsilateral testis and epididymis, when compared with the contralateral testis and epididymis. This decrease is due to the ligation itself, since no significant variations are observed in the sham-operated rats. The histological analysis of the testis of the ligated side shows changes in the morphology of the seminiferous tubules, without any modifications in the interstitial cell compartment. That the Leydig cells are normally functioning is also suggested by the presence of normal physiological serum levels of testosterone recorded in these rats (Zoppi and Motta, unpublished). The decrease in weight of the testis of the ligated side and the morphological changes observed are similar to those described in the dog after ligation of the epididymis at the level of the cauda[49] and in the rat after ligation of the efferent ducts[25]. The degenerative changes are probably due to an initial increase of intraluminal pressure and to blood stasis[49]. The decrease in the weight of the epididymis is probably the consequence of lack of testicular fluid content and of the disappearance of spermatozoa.

After unilateral ligation, the formation of DHT and 3α-diol in the ipsilateral epididymis is significantly decreased 3, 7 and 14 days after the operation, in comparison with that of the contralateral epididymis (Figures 2 and 3). However, at 28 days the formation of both DHT and 3α-diol is almost identical in both the ipsilateral and contralateral epididymes. In contrast, the formation of Δ_4-androstenedione and of its 5α-reduced metabolite (5α-androstenedione) does not show any significant variation in the epididymis of the ligated side up to 7 days; subsequently, a significant decrease is observed at 14 and 28 days after the operation (data not shown).

These results indicate that the contribution of intraluminal androgens in the control of the epididymal 5α-reductase-3-hydroxysteroid-dehydrogenase activity exceeds that of the systemic androgens, at least in the first weeks

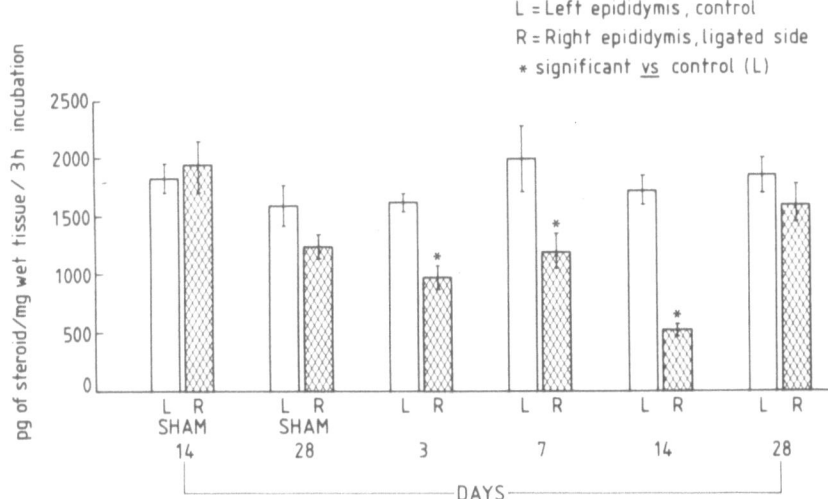

Figure 2 Effect of unilateral ligation of the efferent ducts on the *in vitro* formation of 5α-dihydrotestosterone (DHT) in the rat epididymis

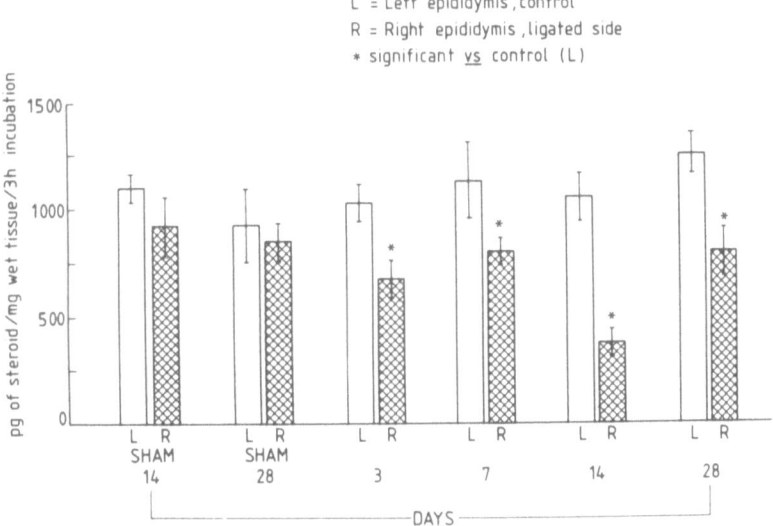

Figure 3 Effect of unilateral ligation of the efferent ducts on the *in vitro* formation of 5α-androstane-3α,17β-diol (3α-diol) in the rat epididymis

after the operation. The data show, in addition, that later there is a recovery of the enzymatic activity in the epididymis of the ligated side; this suggests the possibility that androgens reaching the epididymis through the systemic or local circulation might compensate for the lack of intraluminal testosterone later.

The observed decrease of 5α-reductase-3-hydroxysteroid-dehydrogenase activity at the level of the ipsilateral epididymis after interruption of the intraluminal fluid transport of androgens is equivalent to that produced by unilateral castration (Zoppi *et al.*, unpublished).

CONCLUSIONS

Androgens appear to be of pivotal importance in the process of epididymal sperm maturation. The 5α-reduced metabolites of testosterone (mainly DHT and 3α-diol) seem to be responsible for the spermatozoa reaching full fertilizing capacity. The present results confirm that the process of 5α-reduction of testosterone occurring in the epididymis, which provides this structure with the necessary amounts of DHT and 3α-diol, is under androgenic control. Moreover, the present data show that the epididymal 5α-reductase-3-hydroxysteroid-dehydrogenase system is particularly influenced by the androgenic quota coming directly from the testis via the rete testis fluid.

The relevance of this study to fertility control in males is obvious. The availability of agents which interfere with the fertilizing capacity of spermatozoa by modifying the metabolism of testosterone at the epididymal level and which leave substantially unaltered the plasma androgen concentration would produce an antifertility effect devoid of undesirable side-effects (loss of libido, etc.). Therefore, knowledge of the mechanisms controlling the enzymatic conversion of testosterone into its active metabolites in the epididymis is a basic prerequisite for developing drugs which change the activity of the androgen-metabolizing enzymes. In the light of these observations, it is possible to postulate that inhibitors of the 5α-reductase might represent an important tool for the control of fertility in the male.

ACKNOWLEDGEMENTS

The experiments carried out in the authors' laboratory and described in this chapter were supported by grant of the Consiglio Nazionale delle Ricerche through the programme 'Medicina Preventiva e Riabilitativa', Rome, Italy. All such support is here gratefully acknowledged. Thanks are also due to Mrs Ornella Mornati for her skilful technical assistance.

REFERENCES

1. Bedford, J.M. (1975). Maturation, transport and fate of spermatozoa in the epididymis. In Greep, R.O. and Hamilton, D.W. (eds.) *Handbook of Physiology*. Section 7, *Endocrinology*. Vol. 5, *Male Reproductive System*, pp. 303-319. (Washington DC: American Physiological Society)
2. Hamilton, D.W. (1975). Structure and function of the epithelium lining the ductuli efferentes, ductus epididymidis, and ductus deferens in the rat. In Hamilton, D.W. and Astwood, E.B. (eds.) *Handbook of Physiology*. Section 7, *Endocrinology*. Vol. 5, *Male Reproductive System*, pp. 259-301. (Washington DC: American Physiological Society)
3. Orgebin-Crist, M.C., Danzo, B.J. and Davies, J. (1975). Endocrine control of the development and maintenance of sperm fertilizing ability in the epididymis. In Hamilton,

D.W. and Astwood, E.B. (eds.) *Handbook of Physiology*. Section 7, *Endocrinology*. Vol. 5, *Male Reproductive System*, pp. 319-338. (Washington DC: American Physiological Society)

4. Orgebin-Crist, M.C. and Jahad, N. (1978). Maturation of rabbit epididymal spermatozoa in organ culture-inhibition by antiandrogens and inhibitors of ribonucleic acid and protein synthesis. *Endocrinology*, **103**, 46

5. Cameo, M.S. and Blaquier, J.A. (1976). Androgen-controlled specific proteins in rat epididymis. *J. Endocrinol.*, **69**, 47

6. Faye, J.D., Duguet, L., Mazzuca, M. and Bayard, F. (1980). Purification, radioimmunoassay, and immunohistochemical localization of a glycoprotein produced by rat epididymis. *Biol. Reprod.*, **23**, 423

7. Lea, O.A., Petrusz, P. and French, F.S. (1978). Purification and localization of acidic epididymal glycoprotein (AEG): A sperm coating protein secreted by the rat epididymis. *Int. J. Androl., Suppl.*, **2**, 592

8. Moore, H.D.M. (1980). Localization of specific glycoproteins secreted by the rabbit and hamster epididymis. *Biol. Reprod.*, **22**, 705

9. Vierula, M. and Rajaniemi, N. (1980). Radioiodination of surface proteins of bull spermatozoa and their characterization by dodecyl sulphate polyacrylamide gel electrophoresis. *J. Reprod. Fertil.*, **58**, 483

10. Kohane, A.C., Cameo, M.S., Pineiro, L., Garberi, J.C. and Blaquier, J.A. (1980). Distribution and site of production of specific proteins in the rat epididymis. *Biol. Reprod.*, **23**, 181

11. Kohane, A.C., Gonzales Echeverria, F., Pineiro, L., Cameo, M.S. and Blaquier, J.A. (1980). Interaction of proteins of epididymal origin with spermatozoa. *Biol. Reprod.*, **23**, 737

12. Voglmayr, J.K., Fairbanks, G., Jackowitz, M.A. and Colella, J.R. (1980). Post-testicular developmental changes in the ram sperm cell surface and their relationship to luminal fluid proteins of the reproductive tract. *Biol. Reprod.*, **22**, 655

13. Flickinger, C.J. (1981). Regional differences in synthesis, intracellular transport and secretion of protein in the mouse epididymis. *Biol. Reprod.*, **25**, 871

14. Pujol, A. and Bayard, F. (1979). Androgen receptors in the rat epididymis and their hormonal control. *J. Reprod. Fertil.*, **56**, 217

15. Tezon, J.G., Vazquez, M.H. and Blaquier, J.A. (1982). Androgen-controlled subcellular distribution of its receptor in the rat epididymis: 5alpha-dihydrotestosterone-induced translocation is blocked by antiandrogens. *Endocrinology*, **111**, 2039

16. Djøseland, O., Hansson, V. and Haugen, H.N. (1973). Androgen metabolism by rat epididymis. 1. Metabolic conversion of ^{3}H-testosterone in vivo. *Steroids*, **21**, 773

17. Gloyna, R.E. and Wilson, J.D. (1969). A comparative study of the conversion of testosterone to 17beta-hydroxy-5alpha-androstan-3-one (Dihydrotestosterone) by prostate and epididymis. *J. Clin. Endocrinol. Metab.*, **29**, 970

18. Hastings, C.D. and Djøseland, O. (1979). Androgen metabolism by rat epididymis: metabolic conversion of ^{3}H-dihydrotestosterone in vivo and in vitro. *Arch. Androl.*, **2**, 215

19. Inano, H., Ayoka, M. and Tamaoki, B.I. (1969). In vitro metabolism of steroid hormones by cell-free homogenates of epididymides of adult rats. *Endocrinology*, **84**, 997

20. Danzo, B.J. and Eller, B.C. (1976). Nuclear binding of ^{3}H-androgens by the epididymis of sexually mature castrated rabbits. *J. Steroid Biochem.*, **7**, 733

21. Danzo, B.J. and Eller, B.C. (1978). Androgen metabolism by and binding to mature rabbit epididymal tissue: Studies on cytosol. *J. Steroid Biochem.*, **9**, 209

22. Danzo, B.J. and Eller, B.C. (1980). Androgen metabolism by mature rabbit epididymal tissue: the effects of castration and androgen replacement. *J. Steroid Biochem.*, **13**, 661

23. Robaire, B., Ewing, L.L., Zirkin, B.R. and Irby, D.C. (1977). Steroid Δ_4-5α-reductase and 3α-hydroxysteroid-dehydrogenase in the rat epididymis. *Endocrinology*, **101**, 1379

24. Robaire, B. and Zirkin, B.R. (1981). Hypophysectomy and simultaneous testosterone replacement: effects on male rat reproductive tract and epididymal Δ_4-5α-reductase and 3α-hydroxysteroid-dehydrogenase. *Endocrinology*, **109**, 1225

25. Aafjes, J.H. and Vreeburg, J.H.M. (1972). Distribution of 5α-dihydrotestosterone in the epididymis of bull and boar, and its concentration in rat epididymis after ligation of efferent testicular ducts, castration and unilateral gonadectomy. *J. Endocrinol.*, **53**, 85

26. Leinonen, P., Hammond, G.L. and Vihko, R. (1980). Testosterone and some of its precursors and metabolites in the human epididymis. *J. Clin. Endocrinol. Metab.*, **51**, 423

27. Sulcova, J. and Starka, L. (1973). The metabolism of androgens in normal human testis and epididymis in vitro. *Endocrinol., Exp. (Bratislava)*, **7**, 113

28. Zoppi, S., Motta, M. and Martini, L. (1984). Effects of three aromatase inhibiting steroids on the 5α-reduction of androgens in the prostate. *J. Endocrinol. Invest.*, **7** (Suppl. 1), 162

29. Hastings, C.D. and Djøseland, O. (1977). Androgen metabolism by rat epididymis. 6. Metabolic conversion of 5α-androstane-3α,17β-diol in vitro. *Steroids*, **30**, 531

30. Monsalve, A. and Blaquier, J.A. (1977). Partial characterization of epididymal 5α-reductase in the rat. *Steroids*, **30**, 41

31. Pujol, A. and Bayard, F. (1978). 5α-Reductase and 3α-hydroxysteroid oxidoreductase enzyme activities in epididymis and their control by androgen and the rete testis fluid. *Steroids*, **31**, 485

32. Saksena, S.K., Lan, I.F. and Chang, M.C. (1976). The inhibition of the conversion of testosterone into 5α-dihydrotestosterone in the reproductive organs of the male rat. *Steroids*, **27**, 751

33. Klinefelter, G.R. and Amann, R.P. (1980). Metabolism of testosterone by principal cells and basal cells isolated from the rat epididymal epithelium. *Biol. Reprod.*, **22**, 1149

34. Blaquier, J.A. (1971). Selective uptake and metabolism of androgens by rat epididymis. The presence of a cytoplasmic receptor. *Biochem. Biophys. Res. Commun.*, **45**, 1076

35. Scheer, H. and Robaire, B. (1980). Steroid Δ_4-5α-reductase and 3α-hydroxysteroid-dehydrogenase in the rat epididymis during development. *Endocrinology*, **107**, 948

36. Iusem, N.D., Larminat De, M.A., Tezon, J.G., Blaquier, J.A. and Belocopitow, E. (1984). Androgen dependence of protein N-glycosylation in rat epididymis. *Endocrinology*, **114**, 1448

37. Setty, B.S., Riar, S.S. and Kar, A.B. (1977). Androgenic control of epididymal function in rhesus monkey and rabbit. *Fertil. Steril.*, **28**, 674

38. Moore, H.D.M. (1981). Effects of castration on specific glycoprotein secretions of the epididymis in the rabbit and hamsters. *J. Reprod. Fertil.*, **61**, 397

39. Larminat De, M.A., Monsalve, A., Charreau, E.H., Calandra, R.S. and Blaquier, J.A. (1978). Hormonal regulation of 5α-reductase activity in rat epididymis. *J. Endocrinol.*, **79**, 157

40. Jehan, Q. and Setty, B.S. (1977). Influence of sex steroids on the secretory function of the epididymis in castrated rats. *Endokrinologie*, **3**, 281

41. Jones, R., Brown, C.R., Von Glos, K.I. and Parker, M.G. (1980). Hormonal regulation of protein synthesis in the rat epididymis. Characterization of androgen-dependent and testicular fluid-dependent proteins. *J. Biochem.*, **188**, 667

42. Kohane, A.C., Pineiro, L. and Blaquier, J.A. (1983). Androgen-controlled synthesis of specific proteins in the rat epididymis. *Endrocrinology*, **112**, 1590

43. Bedford, M.J. (1966). Development of the fertilizing ability of spermatozoa in the epididymis of the rabbit. *J. Exp. Zool.*, **163**, 319

44. Lubicz-Nawrocki, C.M. (1976). The effect of metabolites of testosterone on the development of fertilizing ability by spermatozoa in the epididymis of castrated hamsters. *J. Exp. Zool.*, **197**, 89

45. Orgebin-Crist, M.C., Jahad, N. and Hoffman, L.H. (1976). The effects of testosterone, 5α-dihydrotestosterone, 3α-androstanediol and 3β-androstanediol in the maturation of rabbit epididymal spermatozoa in organ culture. *Cell. Tissue Res.*, **167**, 515

46. Orgebin-Crist, M.C. and Hoffman, L.H. (1976). The effect of testosterone and testosterone metabolites on epididymal function. In Spilman, C.H., Lobl, T.J. and Kirton, K.T. (eds.) *Regulatory Mechanisms of Male Reproductive Physiology*, pp. 141–158. (Amsterdam: Excerpta Medica)

47. Cohen, J., Ooms, M.P. and Vreeburg, J.T.M. (1981). Reduction of fertilizing capacity of epididymal spermatozoa by 5α-steroid-reductase inhibitors. *Experientia*, **37**, 1031

48. Lau, I.F., Saksena, S.K. and Chang, M.C. (1979). Antifertility effect of 3-oxo-4-androstene-17β-carboxylic acid in male mice. *Arch. Androl.*, **2**, 179

49. Vare, A.M. and Bansal, P.C. (1974). The effects of ligation of cauda epididymidis on the dog testis. *Fertil. Steril.*, **25**, 256

8
Effect of 6 month treatment with a gonadotrophin releasing hormone agonist analogue on endocrine and histological features of human testis tissue

I. HUHTANIEMI, H. NIKULA, M. PARVINEN and S. RANNIKKO

INTRODUCTION

The paradoxical antigonadotrophic effects of highly potent GnRH ana-logues (for a recent review, see Reference 1) have provided a new tool for inhibition of the pituitary–gonadal function. Besides certain diseases where inhibition of the pituitary–gonadal function is the goal of treatment (e.g. sex-hormone-dependent malignancies and precocious puberty), the same effect may be desirable in the development of new contraceptive methods in the male, in combination with treatment with testosterone (T) to prevent the loss of libido and impotence[2, 3]. Apart from decreased circulating gon-adotrophin and gonadal hormone levels, very little is known in the human about the gonadal effects of GnRH agonists in the long term. We found it of importance to assess the specific effects of long-term GnRH agonist treatment on morphology and hormonal function of human testis tissue. Such information may appear useful in assessment of the feasibility of GnRH agonists for the development of male contraception. The prelimi-nary data of this study are reported here.

MATERIALS AND METHODS

Patients

Eight patients (aged 63–77 years) with advanced prostate carcinoma, con-firmed by biopsy, were studied. None of the patients had received any prior treatment for prostatic cancer, and the previous history of the patients revealed no hormonal disturbances. Consent was obtained after the thera-peutic options available had been explained. The patients were told that buserelin treatment was available only for 6 months, after which one of the currently available routine treatments had to be chosen (orchidectomy or oestrogen therapy). The study was approved by the ethical committee of the hospital.

Treatments

Five of the patients were orchidectomized subcapsularily as the first therapeutic measure. Three patients were treated with the GnRH agonist analogue buserelin (D-Ser, TBU[6], des-Gly[10],-GnRH,N-ethylamide; Hoechst AG, Frankfurt am Main, FRG) for 6 months, after which period these patients were orchidectomized. The buserelin treatment was initiated with a 7 day treatment of 500 μg subcutaneously every 8 h, and followed for the rest of the treatment period with intranasal administration of 600 μg of the agonist three times daily. The antigonadal effect of the buserelin treatment was followed by frequent measurements of serum gonadotrophin and T levels. These data, and the methods and results of the clinical part of this study, will be reported later.

Testis tissue

The testis tissues were transported on crushed ice within 20 min after removal to the laboratory and processed immediately for the histological and biochemical measurements.

Small fragments (1–2 mm³) of testicular tissue were fixed in 4% formaldehyde + 1% glutaraldehyde in 0.2 M phosphate buffer (pH 7.4) at 4°C, postfixed in 1% OsO_4, and embedded in Epon. Sections of 1 μm thickness were cut with an LKB-Huxley ultramicrotome (LKB, Bromma, Sweden), and stained with toluidine blue for light microscopic observation.

The testis fragments contained 5–16 tubular cross-sections that were evaluated by the score-count method described by Johnsen[4]. Scores from 1 to 10 correspond with histological findings, in short, 1 indicating the presence of no cells in tubular sections, and 10 indicating complete spermatogenesis with many spermatozoa and germinal epithelium organized in a regular thickness, leaving an open lumen.

The endogenous T levels of the tissues were measured as described in Reference 5. Other tissue pieces were incubated for measurement of T production in the absence and presence of hCG stimulation, as described in Reference 6. T released to the medium was measured by radio-immunoassay after extraction with diethylether.

Other pieces of the testis tissues were snap-frozen in liquid nitrogen and stored at −70°C until used for measurements of LH and FSH receptors. The receptor measurements were carried out as described for human testis tissue in References 5–7, [125I]-hCG and [125I]-hFSH being used as ligands.

Statistical analysis of the results was performed using Student's t test.

RESULTS

Steroid and receptor measurements in the testis tissues

The endogenous levels of T, and the basal and hCG-stimulated production of this androgen in testicular slices *in vitro*, are presented in Table 1. The concentrations of receptors in the testis tissues are shown in Table 2.

Table 1 Endogenous testosterone concentration and *in vitro* testosterone production (basal and hCG-stimulated) of the testis tissue from prostatic cancer patients orchidectomized as the first therapeutic manoeuvre (controls) or after treatment for 6 months with buserelin (mean ± SE)

(n)	*Endogenous testosterone* (ng/g *wet tissue*)	*Testosterone production* in vitro	
		Basal (ng/g × 3 h)	*% stimulation by hCG*
Controls (5)	524 ± 83	910 ± 138	44 ± 11
Buserelin (3)	17 ± 3*	44 ± 10*	62 ± 27

* $p < 0.01$ *vs.* control

Table 2 LH and FSH receptors in the testis tissue from prostatic cancer patients orchidectomized as the first therapeutic manoeuvre (controls) or after treatment for 6 months with buserelin (mean ± SE)

	(n)	*LH receptors* (pmol/g)	*FSH receptors* (pmol/g)
Controls	(5)	0.21 ± 0.045	0.52 ± 0.12
Buserelin	(3)	0.21 ± 0.047	0.16 ± 0.058*

* $p < 0.05$ *vs.* control

Histological picture of the testis tissues

Light microscopic pictures of testis tissues representing the control and buserelin treatment groups are shown in Figures 1 and 2. Although the number of maturation phase spermatids was reduced in all patients, an otherwise normal histological picture of the seminiferous tubules was seen in the control samples, with presence of all germ cell types. In contrast, severe atrophy of the seminiferous tubules was seen in testis tissue of the patients treated with buserelin. Many of the tubules showed only Sertoli cells, and the cells of the seminiferous epithelium were frequently absent. An increase of phagocytosed material was seen within the tubules, probably originating from the degenerating cells not able to enter meiosis and obviously degenerating at the late spermatogonial steps or at the preleptotene stage of the prophase of meiosis. The number of Leydig cells appeared to be similar to that in the controls.

The histological scoring of the seminiferous tubules according to Johnsen (see above) revealed a clear arrest of spermatogenesis by buserelin treatment. The mean score in the control tissues was 5.6 ± 0.49 (SE), and only 2.3 ± 0.70 ($p < 0.01$) after the buserelin treatment.

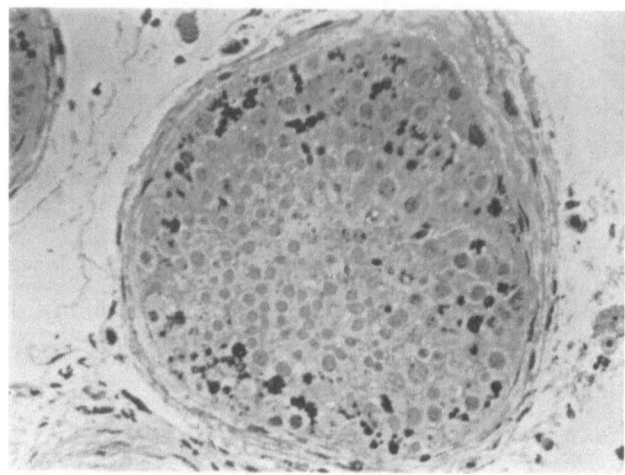

Figure 1 An example of the histological structure of the testis of a patient with prostatic carcinoma (no previous treatment), showing a pattern with score 8 of the seminiferous epithelium. All germ cell types are present, but only few spermatozoa (maturation phase spermatids) are present. The tubular lumen is not open. Staining, toluidine blue; magnification × 230

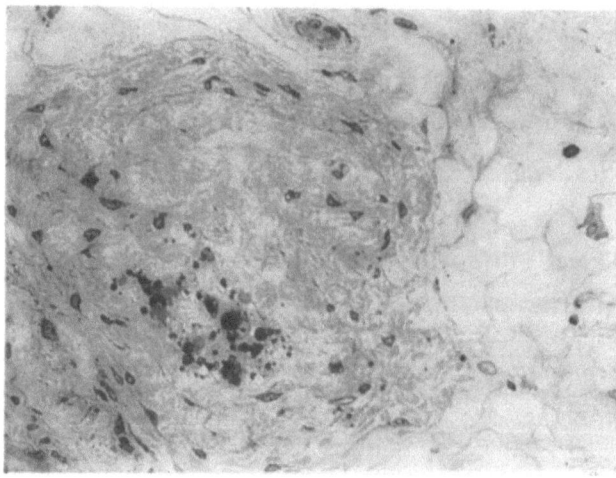

Figure 2 Histological structure of the testis tissue from a prostatic cancer patient treated for 6 months with buserelin. Few spermatogonia and Sertoli cells with phagocytosed degenerative material are seen in the centre of the fibrotic seminiferous tubules (score 3). Leydig cells are few in number. Staining, toluidine blue; magnification × 230

DISCUSSION

As shown by a number of recent studies, treatment with high doses of GnRH agonist analogues inhibits human testicular androgen production, and the treatment can successfully be used as a form of 'chemical castration' in prostatic cancer. Besides blockade of Leydig cell steroidogenesis, the inhibition of the seminiferous tubular function and spermatogenesis provides a potential tool for male contraception. The unavoidable side-effects accompanying the decrease of T production are impotence and loss of libido. These can be eliminated by simultaneous T treatment[3], but the antispermatogenic effect remains, because of persistent decrease of FSH secretion.

The GnRH agonist treatment effectively inhibited T production in our patients, since only about 5% of the endogenous T and of the T-producing capacity remained after the 6 months treatment. The same effect was reflected by the circulating T levels that remained after 3 weeks of therapy in the castrate range, below 0.5 ng/ml (results not shown). It was interesting to note that the stimulability of T production by hCG *in vitro* was not affected by buserelin treatment. A similar low stimulability of about 50% was found in both groups of tissues.

It was of particular interest to note that the concentration of LH receptors was not affected by the agonist treatment, despite the clearly decreased levels of circulating gonadotrophins (by over 70-80%). This suggests that, in keeping with results from experimental animals[8], the testicular LH receptors may not be regulated by the homologous hormone. Prolactin is unequivocally shown to be the regulating tropic hormone in rodents[9, 10], but, owing to apparent absence (or very low level) of prolactin receptors in the human testis[7], the role of this pituitary hormone, and, in general, the nature of the LH receptor regulating factor, still remains open.

In contrast to the LH receptors, those for FSH decreased by about 70% during the buserelin treatment. Since circulating FSH also decreases, this finding may suggest that these receptor sites are more closely dependent on circulating levels of the homologous hormone. It is also possible that normal intratesticular androgen level is required for maintenance of these receptor sites. Nevertheless, the clear decrease of the FSH binding and the deleterious effects on seminiferous tubules are in good agreement, whereas reasons for the disparity between the severely reduced androgen production and the persistence of normal LH receptor levels remain obscure.

In the study reported here the histological changes in the seminiferous tubules after the GnRH agonist treatment were so great that their full reversibility may be questionable. This obviously limits the applicability of GnRH agonists in development of an acceptable male contraceptive method. Since spermatogonia were seen in the buserelin-treated cases, the reversibility of the tubular alterations is possible. Whether a more suitable, possibly lower dose, treatment will prove effective in inhibiting spermatogenesis with less severe changes in the tubular histology remains to be solved.

ACKNOWLEDGEMENTS

This study was supported by the Finnish Cancer Fund, The Medical Research Council of The Academy of Finland and The University of Helsinki. The skilful technical assistance of Ms Marjatta Vallas is gratefully acknowledged. Buserelin was supplied by Hoechst AG (Frankfurt, FRG).

REFERENCES

1. Sandow, J. (1983). Clinical applications of LHRH and its analogues. *Clin. Endocrinol.*, **18**, 571
2. Heber, D. and Swerdloff, R.S. (1981). Gonadotropin-releasing hormone analog and testosterone synergistically inhibit spermatogenesis. *Endocrinology*, **108**, 2019
3. Doelle, G.C., Alexander, A.N., Evans, R.M., Linde, R., Rivier, J. and Rabin, D. (1983). Combined treatment with LHRH agonist and testosterone in man. *J. Androl.*, **4**, 298
4. Johnsen, S.G. (1970). Testicular biopsy score count—a method for registration of spermatogenesis in human testes: Normal values and results in 335 hypogonadal males. *Hormones*, **1**, 2
5. Huhtaniemi, I., Leinonen, P., Hammond, G.L. and Vihko, R. (1980). Effect of oestrogen treatment on testicular LH/hCG receptors and endogenous steroids in prostatic cancer patients. *Clin. Endocrinol.*, **13**, 561
6. Huhtaniemi, I., Bolton, N., Leinonen, P., Kontturi, M. and Vihko, R. (1982). Testicular luteinizing hormone receptor content and in vitro stimulation of cyclic adenosine 3′,5′-monophosphate and steroid production: A comparison between man and rat. *J. Clin. Endocrinol. Metab.*, **55**, 882
7. Wahlström, T., Huhtaniemi, I., Hovatta, O. and Seppälä, M. (1983). Localization of luteinizing hormone, follicle-stimulating hormone, prolactin and their receptors in human and rat testis using immunohistochemistry and radioreceptor assay. *J. Clin. Endocrinol. Metab.*, **57**, 825
8. Huhtaniemi, I.T., Stewart, J.M., Channabasavaiah, K., Fraser, H.M. and Clayton, R.N. (1984). Effect of treatment with GnRH antagonist, GnRH antiserum and bromocriptine on pituitary-testicular function of adult rats. *Mol. Cell. Endocrinol.*, **34**, 127
9. Aragona, C., Bohnet, H. and Friesen, H.G. (1977). Localization of prolactin binding in prostate and testis: the role of serum prolactin concentration on the testicular LH receptors. *Acta Endocrinol. (Copenh.)*, **84**, 402
10. Huhtaniemi, I.T. and Catt, K.J. (1981). Induction and maintenance of gonadotropin and lactogen receptors in hypoprolactinemic rats. *Endocrinology*, **109**, 483

9
The future of plant-derived chemicals as contraceptive agents

N. R. FARNSWORTH and A. S. BINGEL

INTRODUCTION

Most scientific efforts designed to discover new drugs from plants are not generally viewed with enthusiasm by those heavily involved in drug development programmes. This is both unusual and unfortunate, since it is a fact that current widely employed drugs that are still extracted from plants are used to treat amoebic dysentery (emetine), asthma (ephedrine, pseudoephedrine), cancer (etoposide, teniposide, vinblastine, vincristine), cardiac arrhythmias (quinidine), cardiac insufficiency (digitoxin, digoxin, lanatosides A,B and C, ouabain), constipation (sennosides A and B), coughs (codeine, narcotine), glaucoma (physostigmine, pilocarpine), gout (colchicine), hypertension (deserpidine, rescinnamine, reserpine, protoveratrines A and B), leukoderma and vitiligo (xanthotoxin), malaria (quinine), pain (codeine, morphine), parkinsonism (L-dopa), post-partum haemorrhage (sparteine), stomach ulcers (atropine, hyoscyamine, scopolamine), or otherwise are used as analeptics (α-lobeline, picrotoxin), antiemetics (Δ^9-tetrahydrocannabinol), coronary vasodilators (khellin) and skeletal muscle relaxants ((+)-tubocurarine), to mention only a few.

Virtually the entire spectrum of pharmacological effects is covered by useful agents still extracted from higher plants. Further, one cannot neglect the fact that plants provide the pharmacologist with a number of biodynamic agents that have been useful as pharmacological probes or tools, such as strychnine, swainsonine, bicuculline, mescaline, forskolin, lectins and other agents. Plant-derived active principles also provide the chemist with templates for use in synthesizing new drugs by molecular modification.

In spite of this panorama of drugs from plants, examples of useful contraceptive agents remain to be discovered. Most published reports concerning contraceptive plants and their active principles have been the subject of recent reviews[1-12]. Plant oestrogens have also been reviewed, but will not be discussed at this time[13-15]. Sparteine and its enantiomer pachycarpine are the only two plant constituents that are currently used in humans for any condition related to fertility regulation, i.e. as oxytocics[16-19].

It should be stated at this point that the interest of our research group in the area of plants and fertility regulation has been due to an affiliation with the Task Force on Plants for Fertility Regulation within the World

Health Organization Special Programme of Research, Development and Research Training in Human Reproduction. This programme has been described in some detail in recent publications[20-23], and more will be said of this later.

THE WHO SPECIAL PROGRAMME OF RESEARCH IN HUMAN REPRODUCTION TASK FORCE ON PLANTS FOR FERTILITY REGULATION

In response to the demand of its member states that the World Health Organization take a more active role in research concerned with family planning, the Special Programme of Research, Development and Research Training in Human Reproduction was established more than 10 years ago. A decision was made in 1976 to establish within the Special Programme a Task Force on Plants for Fertility Regulation having two major objectives: first, to develop safe, effective and acceptable fertility-regulating agents of plant origin; and second, to strengthen resources in developing countries so that the latter could undertake research in this area. Major emphasis is currently placed on identifying non-steroidal, orally effective agents for use by women on a 'morning after' or 'post-coital' basis, or 'after missed menses', and on plants that could be used by men for fertility regulation.

A majority of the resources of the Task Force have been invested in a network of collaborating centres, each being identified as having botanical, chemical and biological expertise within, or in close proximity to, the same institution. The Steering Committee of the Task Force is of the opinion that, because of the multidisciplinary nature of the research involved in the network of collaborating centres, effective communication must be maintained among personnel in all three disciplines comprising the research groups. At present, the network includes centres at the Chinese University of Hong Kong, Department of Biochemistry, Hong Kong; the Natural Products Research Institute, Seoul National University, Republic of Korea; the University of Peradeniya, Department of Pharmacology, Sri Lanka; the Central Drug Research Institute, Lucknow, India; the Shanghai Institute of Planned Parenthood Research, Shanghai, and the Family Planning Research Institute, Wuhan Medical College, Wuhan, People's Republic of China; and the University of Illinois at Chicago, Health Sciences Centre, Program for Collaborative Research in the Pharmaceutical Sciences, Chicago, USA.

Each centre within the network has a project leader and three co-principal investigators (i.e. in botany, chemistry and biology), as well as technical support personnel. The research groups have been equipped to carry out all aspects of research required to identify promising fertility-regulating activity of specific types, and have been provided with special botanical, chemical and bioassay protocols. When necessary, there is also an exchange of personnel between centres for the purpose of gaining experience with the various protocols used in the programme. Additional details of the organization and work carried out in the centres have been published[20-23].

Specific plants thought to be promising as a source of fertility-regulating agents are assigned to each centre on the basis of the world literature on this subject, which has been collected and analysed[23]. Assignment of plants is also based on their availability in the country where each centre is located, as well as on other factors.

Although more than 4500 species of plants have been identified through a systematic literature search as having an alleged or experimentally derived effect on mammalian reproduction, only about 1500 species appear to have the possibility of being useful as 'morning after', 'post-coital' or 'after missed menses' drugs. The major pharmacological categories of fertility-regulating activity that are related to these modalities are listed in Table 1, with the estimated number of species for which information seems to be pertinent.

Table 1 Number of plant species with potential and/or reported fertility-regulating activity

Reported activity	Ethnomedical	Experimental
Antifertility (unspecified)	44	14
Abortifacient	307	16
Uterotonic	2	119
Embryotoxic	0	4
Labour induction (ecbolic)	309	1
Menstrual induction	541	2
Anti-implantation	0	34
Oestrous cycle disruption	0	3
Oestrogenic	59	98
Antiprogesterone	0	4
Total	1262	295

A large number of chemical substances of known composition have been reported to have 'antifertility', abortifacient and/or anti-implantation activity when tested in laboratory animals or in humans. These are presented in Table 2. Most of these chemical substances appear to be candidates for further studies, especially to determine those which may be orally active as anti-implantation agents. A number of these would obviously have marked pharmacological effects that would preclude their being considered as generally safe and useful, orally effective, fertility-regulating agents in humans.

Montañoa tomentosa AND ZOAPATANOL

Perhaps the most promising non-steroid plant-derived substance being developed for use by women as a fertility-regulating agent is zoapatanol, an unusual oxepane diterpene isolated from the zoapatle plant, *Montañoa tomentosa* (Compositae)[48, 92-96].

Most of the work on this plant has been carried out at the Ortho Pharmaceutical Corporation in the US and in Mexico[97-101]. Recent reviews are available that document the current status of work on this plant[4, 6, 95, 96, 102], which has a long history of use in Mexico as a menstrual inducer and/or abortifacient[95-97,104]. Landgren et al.[103] administered a tea

Table 2 Plant-derived substances of known composition reported to have antifertility, abortifacient and/or anti-implantation activity

Compound name	Chemical class	Type of activity	Species	Route*	Reference(s)
Albitocin	triterpene glycoside	abortifacient	guinea-pig	s.c.	24
Angelicin	furocoumarin	abortifacient	mouse	p.o.	25
Apiol	phenylpropanoid	abortifacient	guinea-pig	p.o.	26
			rabbit	p.o.	26
Aristolic acid	phenanthrene	abortifacient	rabbit	p.o.	27
			mouse	p.o.	28
		anti-implantation	mouse	p.o.	28,29
Aristolic acid methyl ester	phenanthrene	abortifacient	mouse	p.o.	30
		antifertility†	mouse	p.o.	31
Brevicolline	carboline alkaloid	abortifacient	guinea-pig	i.m.	32
Byakangelicin	coumarin	anti-implantation	rat	i.p.	33
Coronaridine	indole alkaloid	anti-implantation	rat	p.o.	34
p-Coumaric acid	phenylpropanoid	abortifacient	mouse	p.o.	35
Demecolcine	alkaloid	abortifacient	mouse	p.o.	36
Dubinidine	furoquinoline alkaloid	abortifacient	rat	p.o.	37
Embelin	benzoquinone	anti-implantation	rat	p.o.	38,39
Euphol	triterpene	abortifacient	goat	i.a.	40
Gossypol	sesquiterpene	anti-implantation	rat	i.p.	41
(+)-Gossypol	sesquiterpene	antifertility	rat	i.p.	42
Guaiazulene	sesquiterpene	abortifacient	mouse	i.p.	43
p-Hydroxypropiophenone	phenylpropanoid	abortifacient	guinea-pig	s.c.	44
Isothankunoside	triterpene	antifertility	mouse	p.o.	45
Maytansine	ansamacrolide	abortifacient	mouse	i.p.	46
α-Momorcharin	proteid	abortifacient	mouse	i.p.	47
Montanol	diterpene	abortifacient	guinea-pig	i.p.	48,49
Pachycarpine	quinolizidine alkaloid	labour inducer	human	i.m.,i.v.	19
α-Peltatin	lignan	anti-implantation	mouse	i.p.	50
β-Peltatin	lignan	anti-implantation	mouse	i.p.	50
Perforine	alkaloid	abortifacient	rat	p.o.	37
Phaseolus vulgaris lectin	proteid	abortifacient	mouse	i.p.,i.m.	51
Pinellin	proteid	abortifacient	mouse	s.c.	52
Piperine	piperidine alkaloid	abortifacient	mouse	i.p.,p.o.	53
			monkey	i.p.	53
		anti-implantation	mouse	p.o.	53

Plumbagin	naphthoquinone	abortifacient	rat	i.p.	54
		antifertility	rat	p.o	55
		abortifacient	rat	i.p.	56
Podophyllotoxin	lignan	anti-implantation	mouse	s.c.	57
Pseudolaric acid B	diterpene	abortifacient	rat	p.o.	58
Reserpine	indole alkaloid	anti-implantation	mouse	i.p.	59
Sambucus nigra lectin	proteid	abortifacient	mouse	s.c.	60
(12S)-3,12-Seco-ishwaran-12-ol	sesquiterpene	anti-implantation	mouse	p.o.	61
Simplexin	diterpene	abortifacient	monkey	i.a.	62
Skimmianine	quinoline alkaloid	abortifacient	rat	p.o.	37
Solanine	steroid alkaloid	abortifacient	mouse	i.p.	63
Sparteine	quinolizidine alkaloid	labour inducer	human	i.m.,i.v.	16–19
Sphaerophysine	guanidine base	labour inducer	human	i.v.	64
Stigmast-5-ene-3β,7α-diol	steroid	anti-implantation	mouse	p.o.	65
Stigmast-5-ene-3β,7β-diol	steroid	antifertility	mouse	p.o.	66
Trichosanthin	proteid	abortifacient	human	i.a.,i.m.	67–75
α-Trichosanthin	proteid	abortifacient	mouse	i.p.	47
(+)-Usnic acid	benzofuran	anti-implantation	mouse	p.o.	57
Vasicine	quinazoline alkaloid	abortifacient	guinea-pig	i.p.	76, 77
			rabbit	i.m.	78
			human	i.m.,i.v.	79,80
Vincaleukoblastine	bisindole alkaloid	abortifacient	rat	i.v.	81
			hamster	i.v.	82
m-Xylohydroquinone	simple phenol	antifertility	mouse	p.o.	83
			rat	p.o.	83
Yuanhuacine	diterpene	abortifacient	human	p.o.	84,85
Yuanhuadine	diterpene	abortifacient	human	i.a.	86–88
Yuanhuafine	diterpene	abortifacient	human	i.a.	89
Zoapatanol	diterpene	abortifacient	monkey	i.a.	90,91
			guinea-pig	i.p.	92–94
				p.o.	95

* i.a., intra-amniotic; i.m., intramuscular; i.p., intraperitoneal; i.v., intravenous; p.o., oral; s.c., subcutaneous

† Generally meant to prevent conception. The testing procedure did not allow of interpretation of the mechanism

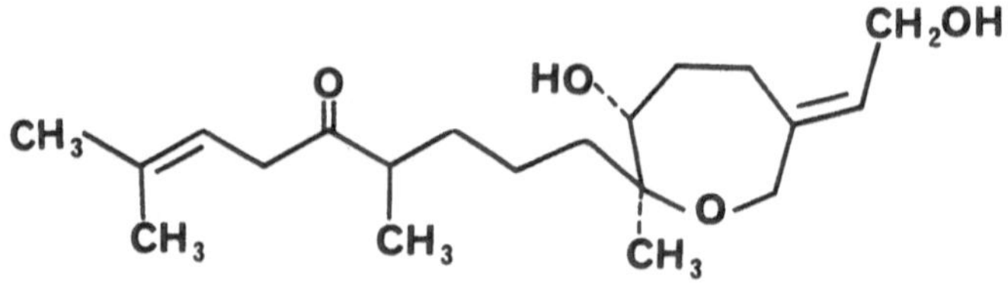

Figure 1 Structure of zoapatanol

prepared from the leaves of *M. tomentosa* orally to six volunteer women hospitalized for early pregnancy (6–7 weeks) termination. Maximum doses approved by the Swedish Drug Regulatory Agency were administered three times daily for 2 days. There was a significant dilation of the cervix in all six subjects and all reported menstrual-like cramps. Four of the six subjects showed some bleeding. No abortions as a result of the tea occurred, and thus standard cervical dilation and vacuum extraction procedures were carried out to terminate each pregnancy. No adverse reactions were experienced by the six women included in the study. Perhaps early abortifacient effects may be demonstrated if higher and/or more frequent doses of *M. tomentosa* tea are administered.

At high doses extracts of *M. tomentosa* leaves are reported to have anti-implantation activity in the rat and mouse, and abortifacient activity in the hamster. Using the 22 day pregnant guinea-pig model, crude and semi-purified extracts of *M. tomentosa* showed abortifacient activity, following oral and/or intraperitoneal administration. Zoapatanol, isolated from this plant, is active in the guinea-pig model, following oral and intraperitoneal administration[95].

Although present evidence seems to point to the fact that zoapatanol is the major active principle in this plant, a Mexican group has reported *in vitro* uterotonic activity for extracts of *M. tomentosa* and other *Montanoa* species, showing that the diterpene kauradienoic acid has this effect[99, 101].

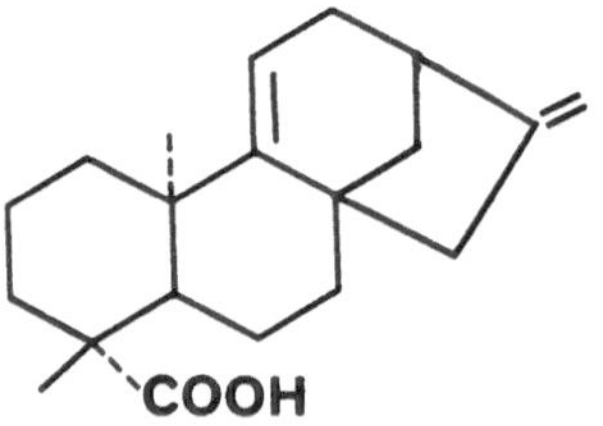

Figure 2 Structure of kauradienoic acid

The intensity of interest in *M. tomentosa* by the Ortho Pharmaceutical Corporation is demonstrated somewhat by the number of patents that have been assigned to them on the fertility-regulating activity of extracts from this plant and its active constituents, including their work on the semi-synthesis and total synthesis of zoapatanol[49, 92–94, 105–138]. The synthesis of zoapatanol has been independently reported by Nicolaou *et al.*[139].

DIFFICULTIES IN INTERPRETING PUBLISHED DATA ON FERTILITY-REGULATING PLANTS

As can readily be seen from a review of the literature, numerous plant extracts have already been tested in laboratory species, most commonly rats and mice, for post-coital antifertility activity. Nevertheless, it frequently remains unclear as to whether or not a given extract does indeed possess such activity. Such uncertainty extends beyond the simple question as to whether equivocal results might indeed have been positive if a higher dose had been administered. Rather, the uncertainty stems largely from the poor experimental designs persistently employed by a number of groups engaged in such research. These investigators ostensibly purport to identify effective fertility-regulating plants, presumably so that ultimately their active constituents could be developed for practical use. Close examination of their data, however, reveals that their testing often has been inadequate either to support or to negate the possibility that the plants examined might have fertility-regulating activity.

Lack of adequate numbers of properly treated vehicle controls is one major problem. Frequently there are no 'control' data of any sort presented; sometimes only totally *untreated* animals are mentioned. At other times, when more than one dosage regimen has been used (e.g. days 1 and 2 post coitum vs. days 3 and 4 post coitum), 'controls' have been treated on all 4 days. Complex statistical analyses, of course, can be used to ascertain the influence of multiple variables, when multiple variables are necessary or unavoidable. In the screening experiments being described, however, dosing the 'controls' in a manner unlike that for the experimentals can only represent poor experimental design on the part of the investigator.

Inadequate numbers of animals in given treatment groups (as few as four or five per group), worse yet often in the face of larger numbers of animals in other treatment groups (e.g. eight or ten per group), are another major problem. Since usually no mention has been made of toxicity to account for the smaller group sizes, one has to question an experimental design that leads to data such as 4/4 pregnant (0% activity) in one treatment group, 0/4 pregnant (100% activity) in a second group, and 3/9 pregnant (66.7% activity) in a third. Suppose that each group had contained 10 animals; could the data for all three groups have turned out to be 4/10 pregnant (60% activity)? Suppose, furthermore, that there had been a vehicle-treated control group in which 8/10 were pregnant (20% 'activity'). One hundred per cent fertility in a group of animals cannot be guaranteed; furthermore, one theoretically, at least, could encounter a plant that might *promote* fertility. That such poor experimental design *continues* to be employed suggests that perhaps the investigators do not really wish to determine *unequivocally* whether or not a given plant indeed possesses antifertility activity.

Aside from having difficulty in interpreting the practical *significance* of data reported in the literature, one may also have difficulty understanding what is *meant* by the data; for example, papers have been published in which antifertility effects were reported to be seen in 55.5%, 63.6% and 75% of groups containing *10* animals each.

If research of this type is to lead to the isolation of constituents possessing antifertility activity of potential, practical utility, greater care must be taken to ensure that experiments yield truly meaningful data, i.e. that truly inactive plants can be ruled out unequivocally as inactive, and that those possessing activity can, with confidence, be worked up towards a practical end.

SUMMARY AND CONCLUSIONS

It is clear that there is now, and will continue to be, a need for safe, effective, affordable and acceptable fertility-regulating agents for use by men as well as women. This need will be especially apparent in many developing countries of the world. Since plants are an abundant natural resource in most developing countries, it seems logical and prudent to initiate meaningful research programmes designed to study the flora of such countries for useful drugs, including effective agents for fertility regulation.

A brief resumé has been presented showing that obvious problems surround research involving the development of effective fertility-regulating agents from plants. Many of the problems can be overcome with assistance from organizations such as the Special Programme of Research, Development and Research Training in Human Reproduction of the World Health Organization. An ongoing activity of the WHO Special Programme, in the form of its Task Force on Plants for Fertility Regulation, has recently been established. This activity is target-oriented in having for its goal the development of safe, orally effective, plant-derived fertility-regulating agents for use by the male and by the female as well. In establishing a network of collaborating centres, primarily located in developing countries, to carry out the research required to accomplish this objective, a major effort has been made to strengthen research capabilities related to fertility regulation.

Evidence has been presented that plants do contain substances that are capable of affecting fertility, but further research and development is required and many questions remain to be answered.

Successful research and development programmes, whether situated in developed or developing countries and regardless of the type of biological activity being pursued, somehow seem to lack the understanding and support of decision makers who can adequately fund such programmes. Natural products research capability is a strength in most of the developing countries that is largely unnurtured, and encouragement, assistance and support must be provided when a need is demonstrated. However, the majority of developing countries do not have the financial resources single-handedly to initiate and sustain meaningful research programmes in the search for useful and effective plant-derived fertility-regulating agents that could improve health care in these countries.

An attempt has been made to illustrate that, on a global basis, plants historically and currently are a major source of drugs used to alleviate human suffering and improve health care. They represent an untapped reservoir of biodynamic agents. A WHO programme for research on plants to discover useful fertility-regulating agents has been described that must be characterized as limited, but can point to measurable successes. It can also serve as a model for the planning, organization and implementation of similar programmes in other developing countries.

Development of practical fertility-regulating agents from plants is a high-risk and expensive venture that, even with a modest international investment, has turned a great deal of attention to an untapped resource that could eventually produce great benefits.

REFERENCES

1. Farnsworth, N.R., Bingel, A.S., Cordell, G.A., Crane, F.A. and Fong, H.H.S. (1975). Potential value of plants as sources of new antifertility agents. I. *J. Pharm. Sci.*, **64**, 535
2. Farnsworth, N.R., Bingel, A.S., Cordell, G.A., Crane, F.A. and Fong, H.H.S. (1975). Potential value of plants as sources of new antifertility agents. II. *J. Pharm. Sci.*, **64**, 717
3. Farnsworth, N.R., Bingel, A.S., Soejarto, D.D., Wijesekera, R.O.B. and Perea-Sasiain, J. (1981). Prospects for higher plants as a source of useful fertility-regulating agents for human use. In Chang, C.-F., Griffin, D. and Woolman, A. (eds.) *Recent Advances in Fertility Regulation*, pp. 330-364. (Geneva: Atar)
4. Farnsworth, N.R., Fong, H.H.S. and Diczfalusy, E. (1983). New fertility regulating agents of plant origin. In Diczfalusy, E. and Diczfalusy, A. (eds.) *Research on the Regulation of Human Fertility*. Vol. II, pp. 776-809. (Copenhagen: Scriptor)
5. Farnsworth, N.R. and Waller, D.P. (1982). Current status of plant products reported to inhibit sperm activity and production. *Res. Front. Fertil. Reg.*, **2** (1), 1
6. Bingel, A.S. and Farnsworth, N.R. (1980). Botanical sources of fertility-regulating agents: Chemistry and pharmacology. In Briggs, M. and Corbin, A. (eds.) *Progress in Hormone Biochemistry and Pharmacology*, pp. 149-225. (Westmount, Quebec: Eden Press)
7. Chaudhury, R.R. and Haq, M. (1980). Review of plants screened for antifertility activity. I. *Bull. Med. Ethnobot. Res.*, **1**, 408
8. Chaudhury, R.R., Haq, M. and Gupta, U. (1980). Review of plants screened for antifertility activity. II. *Bull. Med. Ethnobot. Res.*, **1**, 420
9. Chaudhury, R.R. and Haq, M. (1980). Review of plants screened for antifertility activity. III. *Bull. Med. Ethnobot. Res.*, **1**, 542
10. Soejarto, D.D., Bingel, A.S., Slaytor, M. and Farnsworth, N.R. (1979). Fertility regulating agents from plants. *WHO Chron.*, **33**, 58
11. Rastogi, R.P. and Dhawan, B.N. (1982). Research on medicinal plants at the Central Drug Research Institute, Lucknow (India). *Indian J. Med. Res.*, **76** (Suppl.), 27
12. Kamboj, V.P. and Dhawan, B.N. (1981). Current status of plants investigated for fertility regulation in India. *Korean J. Pharmacog.*, **12**, 111
13. Doecke, F. (1981). Plant estrogens, antiestrogens and antigonadotrophins. *Veterinaermed. Endokrinol.*, **1981**, 647
14. Bickoff, E.M. (1963). Estrogen-like substances in plants. In Hisaw, F.L., Jr. (ed.) *Physiology of Reproduction*, pp. 93-118. (Corvallis, Oregon: Oregon State University Press)
15. Bickoff, E.M., Spencer, R.R., Witt, S.C. and Knuckles, B.E. (1969). *Studies on the Chemical and Biological Properties of Coumestrol and Related Compounds*. Tech. Bull. 1408, ARS, USDA, Washington, D.C.
16. Frascagh, G. (1948). The oxytocic action of sparteine sulfate in pregnancy, labor, and the puerperium. *Arch. Exp. Ginecol.*, **53**, 181
17. Gray, N.J. and Plentl, A.A. (1958). Sparteine: A review of its uses in obstetrics. *Obstet. Gynecol.*, **11**, 204
18. Newton, B.W., Benson, R.C. and McCorroston, C.C. (1966). Sparteine sulfate: A potent capricious oxytocic. *Am. J. Obstet. Gynecol.*, **94**, 234
19. Stubblefield, C.T., Barloon, J.H. and Keltner, R.O. (1968). Sparteine sulfate: A clinical evaluation of its use in 100 cases. *Obstet. Gynecol.*, **22**, 341
20. Spieler, J.M. (1981). World Health Organization, The Special Programme of Research, Development and Research Training in Human Reproduction, Task Force on Indigenous Plants for Fertility Regulation. *Korean J. Pharmacog.*, **12**, 94
21. Farnsworth, N.R. (1978). World Health Organization Program on Indigenous Plants for Fertility Regulation. *Proc. I.U.P.A.C. 11th International Symposium on the Chemistry of Natural Products*. Vol. 4, pp. 475-489
22. Soejarto, D.D., Bingel, A.S., Slaytor, M. and Farnsworth, N.R. (1978). Fertility regulating agents from plants. *Bull. WHO*, **56**, 343

23. Farnsworth, N.R., Loub, W.D., Soejarto, D.D., Cordell, G.A., Quinn, M.L. and Mulholland, K. (1981). Computer services for research on plants for fertility regulation. *Korean J. Pharmacog.*, **12**, 98

24. Lipton, A. (1967). Abortifacient and toxic actions of the glycoside 'albitocin' extracted from some *Albizia* species. *J. Pharm. Pharmacol.*, **19**, 792

25. Panashchenko, V.A. (1967). Furocoumarins as potential general contraceptives. *Farmakol. Alkaloidov Glikozidov*, **1967**, 226

26. Patoir, A., Patoir, G. and Bedrine, J. (1938). Experimental apiole poisoning. *Rev. Sud-Am. Endocrinol. Immunol. Quimioterap.*, **21**, 299

27. Pakrashi, A. and Chakrabarty, B. (1978). Antifertility effect of aristolic acid from *Aristolochia indica* in female albino rabbits. *Experientia*, **34**, 1377

28. Pakrashi, A. and Ganguly, T. (1982). Changes in uterine phosphatase levels in mice treated with aristolic acid during early pregnancy. *Contraception*, **26**, 635

29. Pakrashi, A. and Chakrabarty, B. (1978). Anti-oestrogenic and anti-implantation effect of aristolic acid from *Aristolochia indica*. *Indian J. Exp. Biol.*, **16**, 1283

30. Pakrashi, A. and Shaha, C. (1978). Effect of methyl ester of aristolic acid from *Aristolochia indica* on fertility of female mice. *Experientia*, **34**, 1192

31. Pakrashi, A. and Shaha, C. (1978). Short term toxicity study with methyl ester of aristolic acid from *Aristolochia indica* in mice. *Indian J. Exp. Biol.*, **17**, 437

32. Sizov, P.I. (1970). Influence of pachycarpine, brevicolline, and thalictrimine on the contractile ability of the uterus in rabbits. *Zaravookhr. Beloruss.*, **16**, 17

33. Pakrashi, A. (1967). Endocrinological studies on plant products. Part V. Effect of byakangelicin on female sex hormones and on fertility of rats. *Indian J. Exp. Biol.*, **5**, 75

34. Mehrotra, P.K. and Kamboj, V.P. (1978). Hormonal profile of coronaridine hydrochloride—an antifertility agent of plant origin. *Planta Med.*, **33**, 345

35. Pakrashi, A. and Pakrashi, P. (1973). Biological profile of *para*-coumaric acid isolated from *Aristolochia indica*. *Indian J. Exp. Biol.*, **16**, 1285

36. Didcock, K., Jackson, D. and Robson, J.M. (1956). The action of some nucleotoxic substances on pregnancy. *Br. J. Pharmacol.*, **11**, 437

37. Akhmedkhodzaev, J.S. (1978). Effect of *Haplophyllum* alkaloids on the estrous cycle and reproductive function of rats. *Farmakol. Prir. Veschestv*, **1978**, 51

38. Rathinam, K., Santhakumari, G. and Ramiah, N. (1976). Studies on the antifertility activity of embelin. *J. Res. Indian Med. Yoga Homeopathy*, **11**, 84

39. Krishnaswamy, M. and Purushothaman, K.K. (1980). Antifertility properties of *Embelia ribes*, (Embelin). *Indian J. Exp. Biol.*, **18**, 1359

40. Chen, X.-C. (1982). Preliminary studies on abortion-inducing constituents in *Euphorbia kansui*. *Yao Hsueh T'uang Pao*, **17**, 363

41. Yuan, Q.-X., Gao, D.-W. and Li, C.-Z. (1983). Antiimplantation effects of gossypol in female rats and its mechanism. *Sheng Chih Yu Bi Yun*, **3**, 25

42. Murthy, R.S.R., Basu, D.K. and Murti, V.V.S. (1981). Antifertility activity of (+)-gossypol on female albino rats. *Indian J. Pharmacol.*, **13**, 86

43. Caujolle, F. and Stanilas, E. (1951). Action of guaiazulene on uterine muscle. *C.R. Acad. Sci.*, **232**, 766

44. Benigno, P. and Serembe, M. (1952). Effect of *p*-hydroxypropiophenone on pregnancy. *Arch. Ital. Sci. Farmacol.*, **2**, 301

45. Dutta, T. and Basu, U.P. (1968). Crude extracts of *Centella asiatica* and products derived from its glycosides as oral antifertility agents. *Indian J. Exp. Biol.*, **6**, 182

46. Sieber, S.M., Wolpert, M.T., Adamson, R.H., Cysyk, R.L., Bono, V.H. and Johns, D.G. (1976). Experimental studies with maytansine—a new antitumor agent. *Comparative Leukemia Research 1975-1976*, 495

47. Law, L.-K., Tam, P.P.L. and Yeung, H.-W. (1983). Effect of alpha-trichosanthin and alpha-momorcharin on the development of peri-implantation mouse embryos. *J. Reprod. Fertil.*, **69**, 597

48. Levine, S.D., Adams, R.E., Chen, R., Cotter, M.L. Hirsch, A.F., Kane, V.V., Kanojia, R.M., Shaw, C., Wachter, M.P., Chin, E., Huettemann, R., Ostrowski, P., Mateos, J.L., Noriega, L., Guzman, A., Mijarez, A. and Tovar, L. (1979). Zoapatanol and montanol, novel oxepane diterpenoids from the Mexican plant zoapatle (*Montanoa tomentosa*). *J. Am. Chem. Soc.*, **101**, 3404

49. Kanojia, R.M., Wachter, M. and Chen, R.H.K. (1978). Oxepane derivatives useful as uteroevacuating agents. German patent 2,751,396

50. Jackson, H. (1959). Antifertility agents. *Pharmacol. Rev.*, **11**, 135
51. Huang, C.-K. and Chang, C.-Y. (1980). Proteins from *Phaseolus vulgaris* for abortion. *Chiang-su I Yao*, **6**, 13
52. Tao, Z.-J., Xu, Q.-Y., Wu, K.-Z., Lian, S.-H. and Sun, D. (1981). Isolation, crystallization, biological activities and some chemical characteristics of pinellin. *Sheng Wu Hua Hsueh Yu Sheng Wu Wu Li Hsueh Pao*, **13**, 77
53. Piyachaturawat, P., Glinsukon, T. and Peugvicha, P. (1982). Postcoital antifertility effect of piperine. *Contraception*, **26**, 625
54. Cho, D. (1933). Action of plumbagin, the effective element of *Plumbago zeylanica*. *Jap. J. Obstet. Gynecol.*, **16**, 254
55. Azad Chowdhury, A.K., Sushanta, K.C. and Khan, A.K. (1982). Antifertility activity of *Plumbago zeylanica* Linn. root. *Indian J. Med. Res. Suppl.*, **76**, 99
56. Thiersch, J.B. (1963). Effect of podophyllin (P) and podophyllotoxine (PT) on the rat litter *in utero*. *Proc. Soc. Exp. Biol. Med.*, **113**, 124
57. Wiesner, R.P. and Yudkin, J. (1955). Control of fertility by antimitotic agents. *Nature (London)*, **176**, 249
58. Wang, W.-C., Lu, R.-F., Zhao, S.-X. and Zhu, Y.-Z. (1982). Antifertility effect of pseudolaric acid B. *Chung-kuo Yao Li Hsueh Pao*, **3**, 188
59. Kendle, K.E. and Bennett, J.P. (1969). Studies upon the mechanism of reserpine induced arrest in egg transport in the mouse oviduct. II. Comparative effects of some agents with actions on smooth muscle and tissue amines. *J. Reprod. Fertil.*, **20**, 435
60. Elzbieta, P. (1976). Effect of phytohaemagglutinin (pha) from the bark of *Sambucus nigra* on embryonic and foetal development in mice. *Folia Biol. (Cracow)*, **24**, 213
61. Pakrashi, A. and Shaha, C. (1977). Anti-implantation and anti-oestrogenic activity of a sesquiterpene from the roots of *Aristolochia indica*. *Indian J. Exp. Biol.*, **15**, 1197
62. Wang, Q.-R., Huang, W.-J., Han, J., Lin, C.-M., Zhu, M.-L. and Chang, C.-H. (1981). Isolation and characterization of simplexin, an antifertile principle of *Wikstroemia chamaedaphne*. *Yao Hsueh T'ung Pao*, **16**, 51
63. Bell, D.P., Gibson, J.G., McCarrol, A.M. and McClean, G.A. (1976). Embryotoxicity of solanine and aspirin in mice. *J. Reprod. Fertil.*, **46**, 257
64. Naidenova, N.P. (1964). Stimulation of uterine contraction with spherophysine. *Akush Ginekol. (Sofia)*, **40**, 46
65. Pakrashi, A. and Basak, B. (1976). Abortifacient effect of steroids from *Ananas comosus* and their analogues on mice. *J. Reprod. Fertil.*, **46**, 461
66. Pakrashi, S.C., Achari, B. and Majumdar, P.C. (1975). Studies on Indian medicinal plants. Part XXXII. Constituents of *Ananas comosus* leaves. *Indian J. Chem.*, **13**, 755
67. Jin, Y.-C., Ho, C.-C., Wu, I.-E., Chen, Z.-R., Tong, S.-M., Zhou, Y.-F. and Wang, D.-Z. (1981). Trichosanthin, prostaglandin and traditional Chinese medicines for the termination of early pregnancy. *Sheng Chi Yu Bi Yun*, **1**, 19
68. Ding, G.-S. (1980). Trials of some Chinese medicinal herbs. *Proceedings US-China Pharmacology Symposium*, 29-31 October 1979, pp. 103-121. (Washington, DC: National Academy of Sciences)
69. Yang, P.-Y., Wang, S.-X., Zan, L.-J., Kuo, J.-C., Mang, W.-C. and Wang, W.-L. (1980). Kinetic, morphological and functional changes of placenta by trichosanthin. *Reprod. Contracept.*, **1980**, 16
70. Liu, K.-W. and Liu, F.-Y. (1980). Study on the termination of early pregnancy by administration of combined trichosanthin in 304 cases. *Reprod. Contracept.*, **1980**, 11
71. Anon. (1976). Studies on the action mechanism of trichosanthin. *Chung-kuo K'o Hsueh*, **2**, 200
72. Anon. (1976). 200 cases of induced abortion by trichosanthin injection. *Natl. Med. J. China*, **56**, 215
73. Tso, J.-K., Liu, S.-F. and Liu, L.-Y. (1976). Serum hCG levels of women during and after abortion induced by trichosanthin. *T'ung We Hsueh Pao*, **22**, 166
74. Jiang, T., Gao, K., Zhou, G., Zhu, Y. and Cai, H. (1977). Changes in urinary pregnanediol and estriol excretions during second trimester abortion induced by trichosanthin — a protein extracted from radix trichosanthes. *T'ung Wu Hsueh Pao*, **23**, 243
75. Tso, J.-K., Wang, Y.-P., Wang, M.-P. and Lin, Y.-F. (1978). Analysis of effects of trichosanthin on the function of syncytiotrophoblasts. *Acta Biol. Exp. Sin.*, **11**, 277
76. Chandhoke, N., Gupta, O.P. and Atal, C.K. (1978). Abortifacient activity of the alkaloid vasicine through the release of prostaglandin. *J. Steroid Biochem.*, **9**, 885

77. Gupta, D., Anad, K.K. and Ray Ghatak, B.J. (1978). Vasicine, alkaloid of *Adhatoda vasica*, a promising abortifacient. *Indian J. Exp. Biol.*, **16**, 1075
78. Daftari P., Gupta, S., Chandhoke, N., Gupta, O.P. and Atal, C.K. (1980). Abortifacient activity of vasicine in different species of laboratory animals. *Indian J. Pharmacol.*, **12**, 58
79. Atal, C.K. (1980). *Chemistry and Pharmacology of Vasicine—A New Oxytocic and Abortifacient*. (Jammu, India: Regional Research Laboratory)
80. Wakhloo, R.L., Kaul, G. and Gupta, O.P. (1980). Safety evaluation in human subjects of vasicine hydrochloride, a promising oxytocic and abortifacient agent. *Indian J. Pharmacol.*, **12**, 58
81. Lacher, M.J. (1964). Vinblastine. *Lancet*, **1964**, 1390
82. Ferm, V.H. (1963). Congenital malformations in hamster embryos after treatment with vinblastine and vincristine. *Science, N.Y.*, **141**, 426
83. Batra, B.K. and Hakim, S. (1956). The effect of metaxylohydroquinone on mice and rats. *J. Endocrinol.*, **14**, 228
84. Sanyal, S.N. (1954). Temporary sterility effect of *Pisum sativum* (Linn.). A comparative study. *Int. Med. Abstr. Rev.*, **16**, 91
85. Sanyal, S.N. (1960). Ten years of research on an oral contraceptive from *Pisum sativum*. *Sci. Cult.*, **25**, 661
86. Anon. (1979). Clinical observations on 201 cases of mid-term abortion induced by yuanhuacine. *Chung-hua Fu Chan K'o Tsa Chih*, **14**, 287
87. Liang, Y.-G. (1979). Morphological observations of placenta in 56 cases of mid-term abortion induced by yuanhua preparations. *Chung-hua Fu Chan K'o Tsa Chih*, **14**, 290
88. Yang, B.-Y., Lin, Z.-M., Wang, X.-X. and Yang, S.-Z. (1981). Mechanism of the action of yuanhuacine to induce labor during mid-pregnancy. *Chung-hua I Hsueh Tsa Chih (Beijing)*, **61**, 613
89. Wang, C.-R., Chen, Z.-X., Ying, B.-P., Zhou, B.-N., Liu, J.-S. and Pan, B.C. (1981). Studies on the active principles of the root of yuan-hua (*Daphne genkwa*). II. Isolation and structure of a new antifertility diterpene, yuanhuadine. *Hua Hsueh Hsueh Pao*, **39**, 421
90. Wang, C.-G., Huang, H.-Z., Xu, R.-S., Dou, Y.-Y., Wu, X.-C. and Li, Y. (1982). Isolation and structure of a new diterpeneorthoester yuanhuafine. *Yao Hsueh T'ung Pao*, **17**, 46
91. Wang, C.-G., Huang, H.-Z., Xu, R.-S., Dou, Y.-Y., Wu, X.-C. and Li, Y. (1982). Isolation and structure of a new diterpeneorthoester, yuanhuafine. *Yao Hsueh T'ung Pao*, **17**, 174
92. Kanojia, R.M. (1977). Isolation of utero-evacuant substances from plant extracts. US patent 4,086,882
93. Wachter, M.P. and Kanojia, R.M. (1978). Purification of utero-evacuant extracts from plant substances. US patent 4,086,358
94. Chen, R.H.K. and Kanojia, R.M. (1978). Isolation of uteroevacuant substances from plant extracts. US patent 4,127,651
95. Hahn, D.W., Erickson, E.W., Lau, M.T. and Prost, A. (1981). Antifertility activity of *Montanoa tomentosa* (zoapatle). *Contraception*, **23**, 133
96. Hahn, D.W., McGuire, J.L. and Chang, M.C. (1980) Contragestational agents. *Res. Front. Fertil. Reg.* **1**, 362
97. Gallegos, A.J. (1983). The Zoapatle. 1. A traditional remedy from Mexico emerges to modern times. *Contraception*, **27**, 211
98. Estrada, A.V., Enriquez, R.G., Lozoya, X., Bejar, E., Giron, H., Ponce-Monter, H. and Gallegos, A.J. (1983). The Zoapatle. II. Botanical and ecological determinants. *Contraception*, **27**, 227
99. Ponce-Monter, H., Giron, H., Lozoya, X., Enriquez, R.G., Bejar, E., Estrada, A.V. and Gallegos, A.J. (1983). The Zoapatle. III. Biological and uterotonic properties of aqueous plant extract. *Contraception*, **27**, 239
100. Southam, L., Pedron, N., Ponce-Monter, H., Giron, H., Estrada, A., Lozoya, Z., Enriquez, R.G., Bejar, E. and Gallegos, A.J. (1983). The Zoapatle. IV. Toxicological and clinical studies. *Contraception*, **27**, 255
101. Lozoya, X., Enriquez, R.G., Bejar, E., Estrada, A.V., Giron, H., Ponce-Monter, H. and Gallegos, A.J. (1983). The Zoapatle. V. The effect of kauradienoic acid upon uterine contractility. *Contraception*, **27**, 267
102. Fong, H.H.S. (1984). Current status of gossypol, zoapatanol and other plant derived

fertility regulating agents. In Krogsgaard-Larsen, P., Brogger Christensen, S. and Kofod, H. (eds.) *Natural Products and Drug Development* (Alfred Benzon Foundation Symposium 20), pp. 355–370. (Copenhagen: Munksgaard)

103. Landgren, B.M., Aedo, A.R., Hagenfeldt, K. and Diczfalusy, E. (1979). Clinical effects of orally administered extracts of *Montanoa tomentosa* in early human pregnancy. *Am. J. Obstet. Gynecol.*, **135**, 480

104. Gallegos, A.J. and Cortes-Gallegos, V. (1977). Compositions and methods for fertility control. US patent 4,006,227

105. Anon. (1978). Isolation of utero-evacuant substances from plant extracts. Canadian patent 1,500,518

106. Chen, R.H.K. (1978). Isolation of uteroevacuant substances from plant extracts. US patent 4,112,078

107. Chen, R.H.K. (1979). Isolation of uteroevacuant substances from plant extracts. US patent 4,112,079

108. Kanojia, R.M. (1977). Isolation of uteroevacuant substances from plant extracts. US patent 4,046,882

109. Kanojia, R.M. (1977). Isolation of uteroevacuant substances from plant extracts. US patent 4,060,604

110. Kanojia, R.M. and Huettemann, R.E. (1976). Isolation of uteroevacuant substances from plant extracts. US patent 3,986,952

111. Kanojia, R.M. and Levine, S.D. (1977). Isolation of uteroevacuant substances from plant extracts. US patent 4,061,739

112. Mateos, J.L. and Noriega, L. (1979). Uteroevacuant extracts from plant substances. Canadian patent 1,063,941

113. Mateos, J.L., Noriega, L., Huettemann, R.E. and Kanojia, R.M. (1976). Purification of uteroevacuant extracts from plant substances. US patent 3,996,132

114. Mateos, J.L., Noriega, L., Huettemann, R., Kanojia, R.M. and Wachter, M. (1976). Isolation of uteroevacuant substances from plant extracts. South African patent 7,502,305

115. Mateos, J.L., Noriega, L., Huettemann, R.E. and Kanojia, R.M. (1978). Uteroevacuant extracts from plant substances. US patent 4,076,805

116. Wachter, M.P. and Kanojia, R.M. (1978). Chemical products and methods. US patent 4,130,556

117. Wachter, M.P. and Kanojia, R.M. (1979). Isolation of uteroevacuant substances from plant extracts. Canadian patent 1,048,040

118. Kanojia, R.M., Wachter, M.P. and Chen, R.H.K. (1978). Oxepanes. US patent 4,102,895

119. Chen, R.H.K. (1979). Total synthesis of the uteroevacuant substance D,L-zoapatanol. US patent 4,177,194

120. Chen, R.H.K. (1980). Total synthesis of the uteroevacuant substance D,L-zoapatanol. US patent 4,182,717

121. Chen, R.H.K. (1980). Total synthesis of the uteroevacuant substance D,L-zoapatanol. US patent 4,221,717

122. Chen, R.H.K. (1980). Total synthesis of the uteroevacuant substance D,L-zoapatanol. US patent 4,222,937

123. Chen, R.H.K. (1980). Total synthesis of (IRS,4SR,5RS)-4-(4,8-dimethyl-5-hydroxy-7-nonenyl)-4-methyl-3,8-dioxabicyclo(3.2.1)octane-1-acetic acid. US patent 4,237,054

124. Chen, R.H.K. and Hajos, Z.G. (1980). Total synthesis of (IRS,4SR,5RS)-4-(4,8-dimethyl-5-hydroxy-7-nonenyl)-4-methyl-3,8-dioxabicyclo(3.2.1)octane-1-acetic acid. US patent 4,215,048

125. Hajos, Z.G. (1981). Total synthesis of IRS,4SR,5RS-4-(4,8-dimethyl-5-hydroxy-7-nonen-1-yl)-4-methyl-3,8-dioxabicyclo(3.2.1)octane-1-acetic acid and related compounds. US patent 4,284,565

126. Hajos, Z.G. and Levine, S. (1981). Total synthesis of IRS,4SR,5RS-4-(4,8-dimethyl-5-hydroxy-7-nonen-1-yl)-4-methyl-3,8-dioxabicyclo(3.2.1)octane-1-acetic acid. US patent 4,277,401

127. Hajos, Z.G. and Wachter, M.P. (1981). Synthesis of dioxabicyclo(3.2.1)-octanes and oxepanes. European patent 38,696

128. Hajos, Z.G. and Wachter, M.P. (1981). Synthesis of dioxabicyclo(3.2.1)-octanes and oxepanes. US patent 4,276,216.

129. Hajos, Z.G. and Wachter, M.P. (1982). Dioxabicyclo(3.2.1)octanes and oxepanes. European patent 45,631

130. Hajos, Z.G. and Wachter, M.P. (1980). Synthesis of IRS,4SR,5RS-4-(4,8-dimethyl-5-

hydroxy-7-nonen-1-yl)-4-methyl-3,8-dioxabicyclo(3.2.1)octane-1-acetic acid. US patent 4,237,055

131. Kane, V.V. (1981). Uteroevacuant substance D,L-zoapatanol. US patent 4,296,035
132. Kane, V.V. (1980). Total synthesis of the uteroevacuant substance D,L-zoapatanol. US patent 4,237,053
133. Kane, V.V. (1980). Total synthesis of the uteroevacuant substance D,L-zoapatanol. US patent 4,239,689
134. Wachter, M.P. (1981). Chemical intermediates in the preparation of oxepane compounds. US patent 4,256,644
135. Kane, V.V. and Doyle, D.L. (1981). Total synthesis of (DL)-zoapatanol: a stereoselective synthesis of a key intermediate. *Tetrahedron Lett.*, **22**, 3027
136. Kane, V.V. and Doyle, D.L. (1981). Total synthesis of (DL)-zoapatanol. *Tetrahedron Lett.*, **22**, 3031
137. Jiang, J.B., Urbanski, M.J. and Z.H. Hajos (1983). Total synthesis of dioxane analogues related to zoapatanol. *J. Org. Chem.*, **48**, 2001
138. Wani, M.C., Vishnuvajjala, B.R., Swain, W.E. Jr., Rector, D.H., Cook, C.E., Petrow, V., Reel, J.R., Allen, K.M. and Levine, S.G. (1983). Synthesis and biological activity of zoapatanol analogues. *J. Med. Chem.*, **26**, 426
139. Nicolaou, K.C., Claremon, D.A. and Barnette, W.F. (1980). Total synthesis of (DL)-zoapatanol. *J. Am. Chem. Soc.*, **102**, 6611

10
Gossypol—the male fertility-regulating agent

N. R. KALLA

INTRODUCTION

The discovery of the activity of gossypol as a male antifertility agent has aroused considerable interest among students of reproductive biology[1], and constitutes a major lead in the search for methods of regulation of fertility in males. In 1957 the Chinese scientist Liu-Bao-Shu reported in a local medical journal of Shanghai that in places where crude cottonseed oil was consumed in cooking there were usually more cases of infertility[2]. It was only in early 1970 that a systematic study established that the active ingredient in cottonseed oil responsible for the induction of infertility is gossypol $(C_{30}H_{30}O_8)$, a polyphenol.

METABOLISM OF GOSSYPOL

The metabolic fate of gossypol has been studied after the administration of a single oral dose of $[^{14}C]$-gossypol to pigs and rats (for details see References 3-5). Identification of metabolites was carried out by IR, mass spectrometry, thin layer chromatography, UV, etc. The possible sequence of reactions is decarbonylation of gossypol resulting in the formation of apogossypol and CO_2; oxidation of gossypol leads to the formation of gossypolone, which is subsequently transformed to gossypolonic acid. Further oxidation of gossypolonic acid leads to the formation of demethylated gossic acid. Abou-Dania and his associates[3-5] have reported water-soluble glucuronides, sulphates and hybrids of derivatives of the metabolites of gossypol (Figure 1). Systematic information on the effect of metabolites of gossypol on testis function is lacking. Recently Waller and his associates have observed that apogossypol inhibits the respiratory enzymes associated with mitochondria isolated from rat testis and liver (unpublished). Further research is necessary into the physiological effects of metabolites of gossypol, particularly on the male reproductive system.

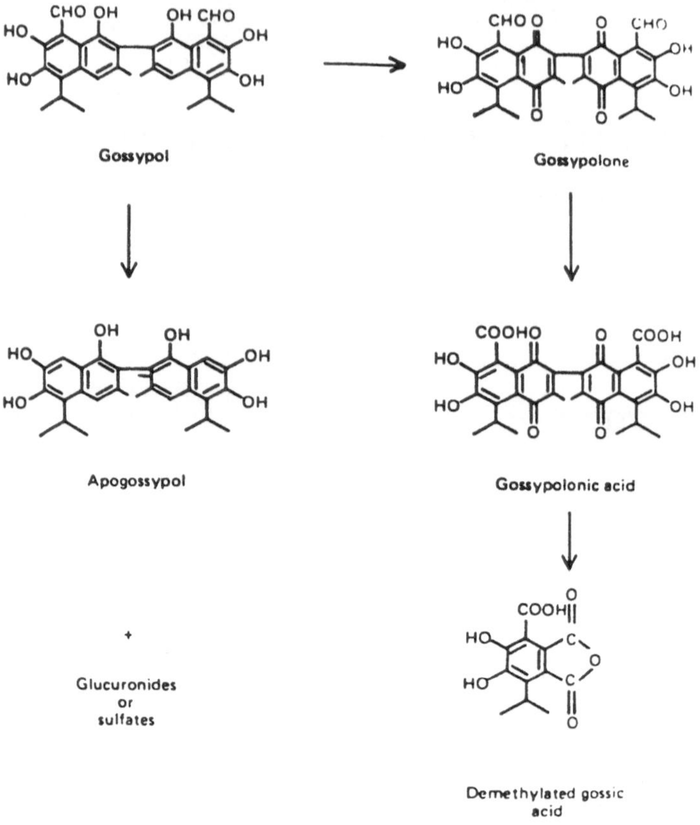

Figure 1 The metabolic pathway of gossypol

LD$_{50}$ OF GOSSYPOL

LD$_{50}$ studies of gossypol have been made in several species of animal (Table 1). The LD$_{50}$ of gossypol formic acid is much higher than that of gossypol acetic acid (in the rat LD$_{50}$ of gossypol formic acid is 4.623 mg/kg). Dogs appear to be quite sensitive to the toxic effect of gossypol. Repeated oral doses of 10–200 mg/kg per day have been reported to be fatal in less than a month; even smaller doses of 2–4 mg/kg per day for 2–3 months have been reported to be fatal. Chickens are also sensitive to gossypol[5].

Table 1 Single dose oral LD$_{50}$ of gossypol

Animal species	Route	Dose	LD$_{50}$ dose (mg/kg body weight)
Mouse	oral	single	500– 950
Rat	oral	single	2400–3340
Rabbit	oral	single	350– 600
Guinea-pig	oral	single	280– 300
Pig	oral	single	550

PHARMACOKINETICS OF GOSSYPOL

The absorption, distribution and excretion of gossypol have been reported in the rat, mouse, rabbit, swine, dog, rhesus monkey and chicken. After the administration of a single dose of [^{14}C]-gossypol to mice (40 mg/kg), dogs (2 mg/kg), rats (15 mg/kg) and monkeys (2 mg/kg), the biological half-life of gossypol in blood was 45, 31, 16.5 and 11 h, respectively[6]. The major route of removal of gossypol from the body is through the faeces (94.6% in 20 days in swine and 76.5% in 9 days in rats); excretion through urine, CO_2 and perspiration is marginal[7]. Excretion of gossypol in the bile established circulation of gossypol between liver and intestine.

GENERAL PHARMACOLOGICAL EFFECTS OF GOSSYPOL

Chinese workers have reported pharmacological effects of gossypol in different animal species. Dose and duration of gossypol treatment elicited different physiological effects. In isolated rabbit heart brief perfusion with Lock solution containing gossypol (1 mg/ml) has been reported to induce loss of K content of the left ventrical myocardium[8]. In the dog abnormal heart electric activity as reflected by ECG together with severe myocardial damage has been observed[9]. Increase in blood serum level of glutamic-pyruvic-transaminase after gossypol treatment is suggestive of impairment of liver function[10]. Gossypol inhibits the detoxification function of the liver as detected by pentobarbital sleeping time[11]. The renal functions have been reported to be normal after gossypol treatment[12, 13]. A high dose of gossypol (100 mg/kg for 7 days) has been reported to impair the adrenocortical function[14]; 25 mg/kg per day for 4 months induced ultrastructural changes in the rat adrenal gland[15]. At lower doses no effect on the adrenal gland was noted. The function of the autonomic nervous system has been investigated, the male cat being used as an experimental model. Gossypol showed an anticholinergic effect and weakened intestinal contraction[16]. In the rat gossypol has been reported to block neuromuscular transmission without affecting nerve conduction[17].

ANTIFERTILITY EFFECT OF GOSSYPOL

Using the rat as an experimental animal model, we have observed that onset of infertility after gossypol treatment is dose- and duration-dependent, the minimum dose required to induce infertility being 7.5 mg/kg for approximately 12 weeks. Doses below 7.5 mg/kg do not induce infertility in rats[18]. At an antifertility dose, cellular damage to the seminiferous epithelium develops sequentially; spermatids were most susceptible, followed by pachytene spermatocytes. At higher doses exfoliation of germ cells has been observed after 2–4 weeks.

It has been reported that mice and rabbits do not respond to the antifertility effects of gossypol[19, 20]. In these studies gossypol was given orally to the animals. In order to investigate the relationship between the route of administration and the antifertility effect of gossypol, we have administered gossypol to adult male Swiss mice by three different routes—orally, subcutaneously and intraperitoneally. When administered intraperitoneally, gossypol was quite toxic, as all the animals died after 4 weeks' drug treatment (Table 2). Whatever the route of administration, gossypol did not exhibit antifertility effects in mice (data for the subcutaneous route are not shown in the table but the results were similar to those for the other two routes). Recently species differences in the antifertility effects of gossypol have been reported[21].

Table 2 Mortality in mice after gossypol treatment

Treatment	No. of animals	Weight of animals	Treatment (weeks)			
			1	2	3	4
Control						
Oral intubation	5	18.66 ± 0.34	×	×	×	×
Intraperitoneal	5	18.00 ± 0.50	×	×	×	×
2.5 mg/kg						
Oral intubation	5	17.60 ± 0.80	×	×	×	×
Intraperitoneal	5	18.50 ± 0.50	×	×	×	(2) (3) 23 25
5.0 mg/kg						
Oral intubation	5	18.00 ± 1.65	×	(1) 10	×	×
Intraperitoneal	5	19.00 ± 0.40	×	×	×	(2) 24
10.0 mg/kg						
Oral intubation	5	18.25 ± 1.20	×	×	×	(1) (2) 27 29
Intraperitoneal	5	18.50 ± 1.20	×	(2) 10	(1) 16	(2) 25
20.0 mg/kg						
Oral intubation	5	18.50 ± 1.20	×	×	(4) 15	(1) 26
Intraperitoneal	5	18.80 ± 0.63	(2) 7	(2) 10	(1) 15	—

Numbers in parentheses indicate the number of animals that died
The lower number indicates the day on which these animals died
× indicates that none of the animals died in the group

Rats and mice have shown species specificity for the antifertility effect of gossypol. The hamster has been reported to be a better animal model in terms of reproducibility and consistency of the experimental data[22].

In order to establish the efficacy of gossypol as a male antifertility agent in primate models, we have undertaken a short-term study using the bonnet monkey, *Macaca radiata*, as an experimental animal[23]. Gossypol (4 mg/kg on 5 days a week) was given to male bonnet monkeys by the oral route for 3 months. Marked reduction in the sperm count/ejaculate and sperm motility were observed after gossypol treatment; both motility and sperm count/ejaculate returned to the normal level 8–10 weeks after termination of gossypol treatment (Figures 2 and 3). The sperm morphology was normal

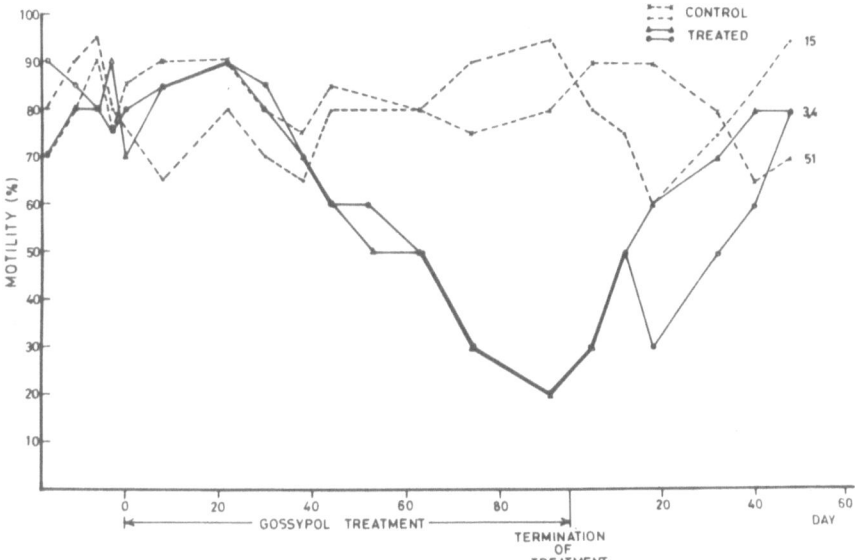

Figure 2 The effect of gossypol on sperm motility in the bonnet monkey

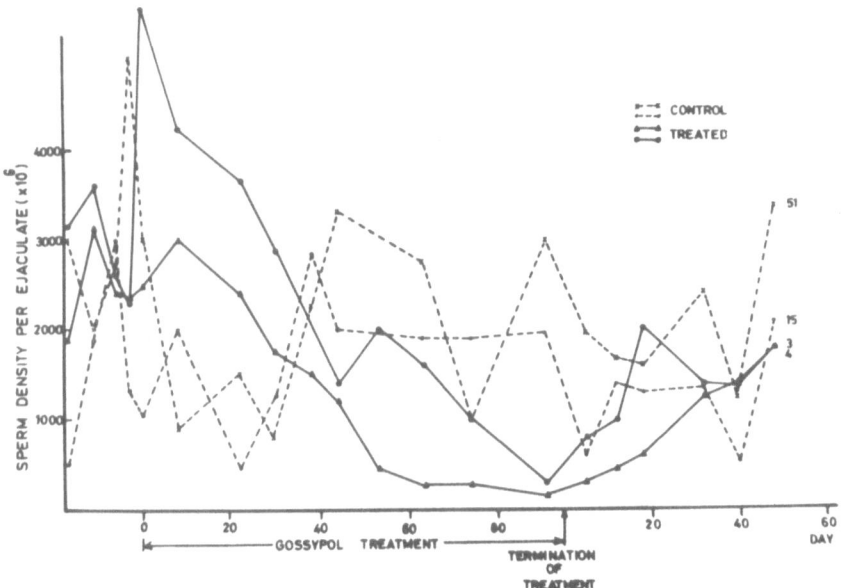

Figure 3 The effect of gossypol on sperm density in the bonnet monkey

in gossypol-treated animals. Ultrastructural changes in the mitochondrial and plasma membrane of the spermatozoa have been observed after gossypol treatment. The citric acid and fructose levels in the semen of gossypol-treated animals did not differ from those of the controls. No haematological changes have been observed after gossypol treatment[24].

EFFECT OF GOSSYPOL ON THE ENDOCRINE SYSTEM

The effect of gossypol on the hypothalamic–pituitary axis and sexual behaviour has been investigated in detail by several workers.

Blood hormone levels

Gossypol treatment (7.5–40 mg/kg for 4–12 weeks) did not have any significant effect on the circulating levels of LH, FSH and testosterone[25, 26]. In clinical studies, both in the People's Republic of China and outside China, gossypol has not been reported to produce any effect on the circulating levels of gonadotrophins, testosterone and prolactin in both loading and maintenance phase[1, 22, 27].

In vitro studies on testicular steroidogenesis

Dym and his associates have observed that gossypol inhibits the hCG-stimulated production of testosterone by isolated Leydig cells[28]. We have, however, observed that gossypol did not alter testosterone production when present in incubates at concentrations ranging from 3.5×10^{-5} M to 3.5×10^{-4} M. Preincubation of testis homogenate with gossypol (7×10^{-6}–3.5×10^{-4} M) for 1–4 h did not alter subsequent hCG-induced testosterone production[28]. In agreement with our observations, no alterations in Leydig cell survival, morphology and testosterone production have been observed during 3 days of culture of Leydig cells in the presence of gossypol; however, with higher concentrations of gossypol in the medium, a reduction in the cell survival has been reported[29]. The decreased level of testosterone in hCG-stimulated Leydig cell assay is not due to decreased production of testosterone but to reduction in the Leydig cell number. No ultrastructural changes have been observed in Leydig cells after gossypol treatment[30].

GONADOTROPHIN RECEPTOR BINDING

In order to investigate the effect of gossypol on [^{125}I]-hCG binding to testis hCG receptors, rat testis homogenate was incubated with [^{125}I]-hCG in the presence of gossypol. No appreciable effect of gossypol on [^{125}I]-hCG binding was observed[25]. Similarly, no difference in [^{125}I]-FSH binding to rat testis homogenate after gossypol treatment was observed[25]. However, gossypol has been reported to inhibit ABP production *in vitro*. Ultrastructural changes in Sertoli cells have also been observed after gossypol treatment *in vitro*[29]. In our preliminary study we did not observe any change in immunocytochemical localization of ABP in rat testis after gossypol treatment, nor have we observed any ultrastructural changes in rat Sertoli cells after gossypol treatment. It is quite possible that the response of Sertoli cells to gossypol treatment *in vivo* may differ from the response *in vitro*. It is quite important to note that decreased ABP production by Sertoli cells after gossypol treatment can be used as a sensitive marker of gossypol action, thus offering a new method of screening gossypol and its analogues for antifertility activity.

ANDROGEN RECEPTOR BINDING

It has been reported that gossypol administration causes reduction of the ventral prostate weight of the immature rat[31]. An antiandrogenic effect of gossypol has also been suggested[20]. The impairment of prostate function, if any, after gossypol treatment could be due to inhibition in the testosterone release/synthesis mechanism or to a direct effect of gossypol on the prostate. We have incubated a cytosol fraction containing androgen receptors from the prostate of castrated male rats with different concentrations of gossypol in vitro. At no concentration did gossypol inhibit the binding of [3H]-DHT to androgen receptors of the prostate. Gossypol administration to immature rats also failed to inhibit the binding of [3H]-DHT to androgen receptors[31]. Weights of androgen-sensitive organs such as the seminal vesicles and the prostate have been reported to be in the normal range after gossypol treatment. No effect on the secretory products of the accessory sex organs was observed[23]. These studies suggest that the androgenic status of animals is not impaired by gossypol treatment[25, 26].

MECHANISM OF ACTION OF GOSSYPOL

A considerable amount of data on the effects of gossypol on the testis has accumulated in recent years. However, the precise mechanism of action of gossypol is not known. The Chinese workers have reported the involvement of prostaglandins in the induction of infertility by gossypol. According to Qian, the antispermatogenic action of gossypol may be brought about through two separate mechanisms: a direct effect on the germinal epithelium and enhancement of gonadal prostaglandin biosynthesis[32]. In a similar study we have also observed that aspirin, a prostaglandin synthetase inhibitor, counteracted the gossypol-induced enhancement of prostaglandin biosynthesis and consequently protected spermatozoa from the deleterious effect of gossypol to some extent. In the rat administration of gossypol at a dose of 40 mg/kg per day for 4 weeks almost completely immobilized the vas deferens spermatozoa; if aspirin (300 mg/kg per day) was given orally together with gossypol, at least 40% of the spermatozoa were motile (Kalla et al., unpublished). Similar results have been observed by Chinese workers[33]. Potassium deficiency has been reported to further augment the effect of gossypol. It will be worth while measuring the levels of prostaglandins in the testis after gossypol treatment, to assign a role to prostaglandins in the mechanism of action of gossypol.

In order to establish the specific lesion in the testis–epididymis complex after gossypol treatment, a number of enzymes have been studied. We have reported inhibition of ATPase associated with spermatozoa after gossypol treatment. Activities of glucose-6-phosphatase, fructose 1,6-diphosphatase, glucose-6-phosphate isomerase, amylase, succinic dehydrogenase, glucuronidase, acid phosphatase, alkaline phosphatase, kinases, aldolase, NADP-isocitrate dehydrogenase, glycerophosphate dehydrogenase and lactic dehydrogenase-X in the testis have been investigated after gossypol treatment. LDH-X, a testis-specific enzyme, has been implicated in the mechanism of action of gossypol[34, 35].

FUTURE PROSPECTS

From the available literature it would appear that gossypol is perhaps the only candidate for large-scale clinical trial as a male contraceptive agent. Discovery of a more potent analogue and separation of (−)-gossypol from racemic gossypol will add new dimensions in the development of gossypol as a male contraceptive pill.

REFERENCES

1. National Coordinating Group on Male Fertility Agents (1978). Gossypol a new antifertility agent for males. *Chinese Med. J.*, **4**, 417
2. Liu, B.S. (1957). Suggestions of feeding cottonseed oil for contraception. *Shanghai Acta Med.* **6**, 43
3. Abou-Dania, M.B., Lyman, C.M. and Dickert, J.W. (1970). Metabolic fate of gossypol: The metabolism of ^{14}C gossypol in rats. *Lipids*, **5**, 938
4. Abou-Dania, M.B. and Dickert, J.W. (1975). Metabolic fate of gossypol: The metabolism of ^{14}C gossypol in swine. *Toxicol. Appl. Pharmacol.*, **31**, 32
5. Abou-Dania, M.B. (1976). Physiological effects and metabolism of gossypol. *Residue Rev.*, **61**, 125
6. Tang, X.C., Zhu, M. and Shi, Q.S. (1980). Comparative studies on the absorption, distribution and excretion of ^{14}C gossypol in four species of animals. *Acta Pharmacol. Sin.*, **15**, 212
7. Xue, S.P., Liu, Y., Han, S.M. and Su, S.Y. (1975). The pharmacokinetics of ^{14}C gossypol acetic acid in rats. II. Quantitative studies on the kinetics of the distribution, excretion and metabolism of ^{14}C gossypol in the rat body. *Acta Biol. Exp. Sin.*, **12**, 275
8. Qian, S.Z., Xu, Y. and Jing, G.W. (1969). Potassium depleting effect of gossypol on isolated rabbit heart and its possible mechanism. *Yao Hsueh Pao*, **14**, 116
9. Xue, S.P. (1980). Studies on the antifertility effect of gossypol, a new contraceptive for males. Presented at Soochow *Conference on Gossypol*
10. Anon. (1980). Effect of gossypol on serum transaminase of rats. *Shan Hsi Hsi I Yao*, **9**, 46
11. Lei, H.P., Chen, C.C., Wang, L.K. and Kowan, M.C. (1980). Effect of gossypol on liver. *Chung-hua I Hsueh Tso Chih*, **59**, 402
12. Shieh, S.P., Liang, D.C., Shao, T.S., Wu, Y.W., Liu, Y., Zho, Z.H. and Wang, N.Y. (1979). Study on the effect of gossypol on the metabolism of potassium-42 in rats. *Chieh Pou Hsueh Pao*, **10**, 80
13. Fai, Y., Liang, D., Gou, Y., Liu, Y., Gor, X., Chow, C. and Xue, S. (1982). Effect of gossypol on the activity of renal cell membrane, sodium, potassium ATPase of rat and guinea pigs. *Shengzhi Yu Piyun*, **2**, 42
14. Yuan, D.X., Liu, X.Y., Cao, Y.C., Wang, J.Y. and Fu, Z.L. (1980). Histochemical observation of the effect of gossypol on pituitary, adrenal cortex and hypothalamus. *Chieh Pou Hsueh Pao*, **11**, 331
15. Ma, R.H., Jiang, C.S., Li, F. and Wu, X.R. (1980). Effects of gossypol on some functions of the autonomic nervous system. *Wuhan I Hsueh Yuan Hsueh Pao*, **9**, 65
16. Shu, H.D., Yang, Q.Z. and Xue, K. (1982). Effect of gossypol acetic acid on neuromuscular transmission. *Acta Pharmacol. Sin.*, **3**, 17
17. Shu, H., Yang, Q. and Xue, K. (1982). Effects of gossypol acetate on the nervous system. *Zhongguo Yaoli Xuebao*, **13**, 27
18. Kalla, N.R. (1982). Gossypol—the male antifertility agent. *IRCS Med. Sci.*, **10**, 766
19. Hahn, D.W., Rusticus, C., Probst, A., Hahn, R. and Johnson, A.N. (1981). Antifertility and endocrine activities of gossypol in rodents. *Contraception*, **24**, 97
20. Coulson, P.B., Snell, R.L. and Parise, C. (1980). Short term metabolic effect of the antifertility agent gossypol on various reproductive organs of male mice. *Int. J. Androl.*, **3**, 507
21. Hunt, S. and Mittwoch, U. (1984). Effect of gossypol on sperm counts in two inbred strains of mice. *J. Reprod. Fertil.*, **70**, 341

22. Prasad, M.R.N. and Diczfalusy, E. (1983). Gossypol. In Benagiano, G. and Diczfalusy, E. (eds.) *Endocrine Mechanism in Fertility Regulation*, pp. 233–248. (New York: Raven Press)

23. Kalla, N.R., Foo, J.T.W., Hurkadli, K.S. and Sheth, A.R. (1983). Studies on the male antifertility agent gossypol acetic acid. VI. Effect of gossypol acetic acid on the fertility of the bonnet monkey, *Macaca radiata*. *Andrologia*, **16**, 244

24. Kalla, N.R., Foo, J.T.W., Hurkadli, K.S. and Sheth, A.R. (1984). Effect of gossypol on the fertility of male bonnet monkeys, *Macaca radiata*. In Segal, S.S. (ed.) *Gossypol*. (New York: Plenum Press) (In press)

25. Kalla, N.R., Foo, J.T.W. and Sheth, A.R. (1982). Studies on the male antifertility agent gossypol acetic acid. V. Effect of gossypol acetic acid on the fertility of male rats. *Andrologia*, **14**, 492

26. Weinbauer, G.F., Rovan, E. and Frick, J. (1982). Antifertility efficiency of gossypol acetic acid in male rats. *Andrologia*, **14**, 270

27. Frick, J., Danner, Ch., Kohle, R. and Kunit, G. (1980). Male fertility regulation. In Cortes-Prieto, J., Campas da Paz and Neves-e-Castro, M. (eds.) *Research on Fertility and Sterility*, pp. 291–304 (Lancaster: MTP)

28. Kalla, N.R., Rovan, E., Weinbauer, G. and Frick, J. (1983). Effect of gossypol on testicular testosterone production in vitro. *J. Androl.*, **4**, 331

29. Zhuang, L.Z., Philips, D.M., Gunsalus, G.L., Bardin, C.W. and Mather, J.P. (1983). Effects of gossypol on rat Sertoli and Leydig cells in primary culture and established cell lines. *J. Androl.*, **4**, 336

30. Rovan, E., Weinbauer, G.F., Frick, J. and Adam, H. (1983). Ultrastructural analysis of rat testis after gossypol acetic acid treatment. *Urol. Res.*, **11**, 75

31. Kalla, N.R., Rovan, E., Weinbauer, G.F. and Frick, J. (1984). The effect of gossypol on prostate androgen receptors in male rats. In Segal, S.S. (ed.) *Gossypol* (New York: Plenum Press) (In press)

32. Qian, S.Z. and Wang, Z.G. (1984). Gossypol: A potential antifertility agent for male. *Ann. Rev. Pharmacol.*, **24**, 329

33. Qian, S.Z. (1981). Effect of gossypol on potassium and prostaglandin metabolism and mechanism of action of gossypol. In Chang, C.F., Griffin, D. and Woolman, A. (eds.) *Recent Advances in Fertility Regulation*, pp. 152–159 (Geneva: Atar)

34. Lee, C.Y. and Malling, H.V. (1981). Selective inhibition of sperm specific LDH-X by an antifertility agent, Gossypol. *Fed. Proc.*, **40**, 718

35. Lee, C.Y.G., Moon, Y.S., Yuan, J.H. and Chen, A.F. (1982). Enzyme inactivation and inhibition by gossypol. *Mol. Cell. Biochem.*, **47**, 65

11
Cottonseed oil for birth control

G.-Z. LIU

THE DISCOVERY OF GOSSYPOL'S ANTIFERTILITY PROPERTY

The earliest account of infertility caused by consumption of cottonseed oil which contained gossypol was by a traditional herb doctor, Liu Bao-shan[1], who in 1957 reported that more than 30 families in a village in south-east China became sterile as a result of the consumption of cottonseed oil.

'Around 10-25 years before the outbreak of Japanese aggression of China in 1937,' wrote Liu Bao-shan, 'a village situated at the juncture of Wu-xi, Jiang-yin and Chang-shu counties in the Jiang-su province was called the Wang Village. In the spring of 1929, I accompanied my school mate Wang Yin-min to pay a visit to that village. I discovered that the 30 some families in that village were quite well to do owing to their diligence and thriftiness. All the people there ate and clad economically. They chose to consume cotton seed oil as their cooking oil because it was much cheaper than other kinds of cooking oil. As a result, within the 10-15 years while taking cotton seed oil, not a single child, be it a boy or a girl, was born to any of the 30 families. For quite a period of time, no-body knew what was the matter, why all the families that were quite wealthy had had no childbirth? Many farmers tried to take a concubine, but still got no childbirth. Some farmers even tried to marry women who had given multiple births in the past, but when these women emigrated to Wang Village, they immediately became unable to conceive. After some time, some farmers became impatient and sent their concubines away to some neighbouring villages. To their surprise, these women promptly got pregnant when married to men in other villages. This puzzling phenomenon certainly made the farmers of Wang Village furious. They thought the almighty God was trying to exterminate the people in Wang Village on purpose.

'So, for at least 10 years, people in Wang Village were horrified because they thought they were going to be extinguished and did not know what to do.

'But the tragedy did not last indefinitely, up until the early forties. The mass production of soya-bean in the North-eastern provinces made the price of soya-bean oil so much cheaper than cotton seed oil. So the farmers in Wang Village quickly shifted from cotton seed oil to soya-bean oil for daily cooking. Quite unexpectedly, many of the wives in the 30 families began to conceive and have children.'

So Liu Bao-shan, the traditional doctor, was the first man to report the antifertility effect of cottonseed oil. In addition, he even speculated about the use of cottonseed oil for contraceptive purposes:

'I have not done any scientific research. ... I hope our scientists can strive to investigate ... because based on the experience in Wang Village, cotton seed oil is definitely effective in preventing conception. And whenever childbirth is desired again, just cease to take cotton seed oil. ... This looks to me a very simple and convenient way of contraception.'

Unfortunately, Liu Bao-shan's paper did not receive appropriate attention until the late 1960s, when many other parts of rural China experienced similar symptoms, with fatigue, burning sensation and infertility.

In the late 1960s many people in rural areas of China, such as the Hubei and Hebei provinces, complained of fatigue and of burning in the face, extremities and other exposed parts of their bodies. The farms in the areas raised cotton, but the afflicted people could not work in the fields. They hid in the shade, lying on rocks to get cool. Local doctors were puzzled. The disease had reached epidemic proportions, but the cause remained unknown. The peasants called their disease 'the burning fever'[2].

Burning fever was especially prevalent in Xingtai, a county in the Hebei province. The local doctors discovered that the peasants there consumed raw, home-made cottonseed oil. Commercially made cottonseed oil had been used in cooking for many years. Only in the 1960s, however, did the peasants begin to make oil from uncooked seeds, using their own pressing machines (Figure 1). Raw cotton seeds contain a substance called gossypol which is destroyed by heat. Unlike the commercial process, preparation of home-made oil does not include heating. Consequently gossypol remains

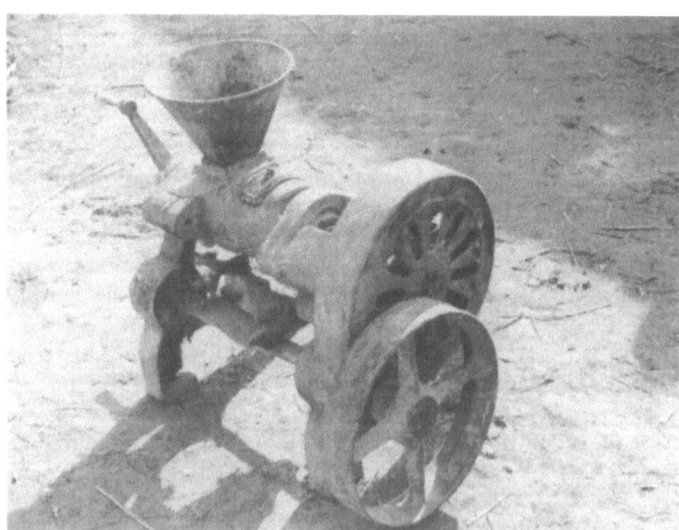

Figure 1   The pressing machine

dissolved in home-made oil. This substance was discovered to be the cause of the burning fever.

As soon as crude cottonseed oil was found to be the source of burning fever, Xingtai doctors advised their patients to stop pressing their own raw oil. The burning and fatigue disappeared; but several years later many couples were experiencing infertility problems (Figure 2). A large number of women suffered from amenorrhoea, but very few men recovered from their infertility and impotence despite continued examination, revealing azoospermia or oligospermia. In addition, some men noted a decrease in testicular size.

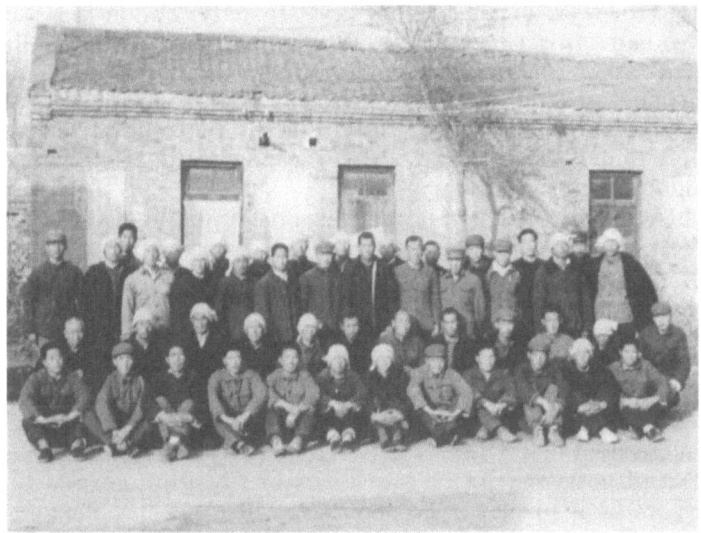

Figure 2   Patients suffering from infertility due to cottonseed oil

Medical and scientific research workers from universities and hospitals were sent to the area to investigate. They confirmed the findings of the local doctors. Infertility was prevalent, and women seemed to recover at a much higher rate than men.

Those men who did regain fertility were found to have had a lower total intake of cottonseed oil; both time and quantity played a part. This information naturally led people to wonder whether controlled doses of purified gossypol could be effectively used as a male fertility-control agent. Observational studies in the country had shown that burning fever, fatigue and infertility were the most common adverse effects of gossypol. Mortality was not observed as a result of burning fever. Because the rate of recovery from male infertility was dependent on the individual amount of cottonseed oil a man had consumed, scientists conjectured that infertility would, most likely, be reversible if the gossypol dosage could be limited. In other words, cessation of intake would allow the user to regain fertility.

PHARMACOLOGY AND TOXICOLOGY OF GOSSYPOL IN ANIMAL EXPERIMENTS

Although gossypol was found to have antifertility properties by the Chinese, the chemical was first discovered over 100 years ago by western scientists. In 1866 Longmore[3] was among the first chemists to make the discovery. However, the first isolation of a pure crystalline substance from cottonseed oil was accomplished by Marchlewski[4], who named the product gossypol.

For many decades scientists had spent much time and effort on trying to make use of cotton seeds as food material for humans and animals, since these materials contain vegetable protein and fat, and occur so abundantly in nature. However, owing to gossypol's toxicity, cotton seeds, especially uncooked, had proved harmful to most animals as well as poultry[5]. For instance, gossypol has been fed for long periods to cats and rabbits. The animals sooner or later developed weakness, loss of appetite and, in severe cases, paralysis, shortness of breath, cardiac hypertrophy, oedema of lungs, etc. Other animals, such as rats, cats, dogs and cattle, exhibit very similar symptoms and signs of poisoning.

Thus, the toxicity of gossypol was alarming, and attracted much attention in the West, research and study on gossypol being in progress for nearly a century. Although a voluminous literature had been published in connection with the pharmacology and toxicology of gossypol, the toxic effects on the genital systems of the animals had not been reported. Exhaustive search of the literature failed to reveal any mention of the inhibitory effect of gossypol on the testes and ovaries.

Liu Bao-shan's classical description of infertility caused by consumption of cotton seeds, in fact, was virtually the first report confirming the antifertility effect of gossypol. In the late 1960s many rural areas in China that produced cotton happened to be 'infertility villages'. This phenomenon had led Chinese scientists to investigate the possibility of making use of the toxic effects of gossypol on the male sex in particular, since it had always been Chairman Mao's idea that men should share the burden of birth control with their wives.

Animal experiments by Chinese scientists in the late 1960s and early 1970s were not just repetitions of past experiments carried out in the West; in addition, the Chinese scientists paid more attention to the reproductive aspects of the male animals. Gossypol's action was found to be directly on the testis and aimed at the spermatids during their development into living sperms. We also found that the toxicity of gossypol is dose-related—that is, if the dosage is limited to the minimum, gossypol can exert an antifertility effect without producing pronounced toxicity. Studies using male rats, mice, rabbits, hamsters, dogs and monkeys yielded almost identical infertility results[6, 7]. The absorption, distribution and excretion of gossypol were also found to be similar in these animals[6, 7]. The biological half-life of gossypol in the gastrointestinal tract of the rat is 9.6 h. Elimination of gossypol takes place mainly through the bile–faecal pathway, while excretion through the kidney is minimal[8].

Elimination of gossypol from the body is slow. It takes a rat 19 days to eliminate 97% of the dose from its body[8]. Continued administration, therefore, could lead to accumulation.

The order of gossypol distribution throughout the body in all animals is liver, gastrointestinal tract, spleen, lymph nodes, kidneys, heart, lungs, pancreas, salivary glands, muscle, adipose tissue, testes, blood, urinary bladder, brain and spinal cord[8]. Although the testes do not retain much gossypol, sperm cells are vulnerable to the substance. Because gossypol concentration is high in the liver and kidney, there should be special concern about toxic effects on these organs. Fortunately, because of their regenerative and compensatory properties, relatively little harm is done to the liver and kidneys.

Theoretically, gossypol should not affect the endocrine status, since its action on spermatogenesis is directly on the germ cells of the testis. Animal experiments in China, Austria and India showed no difference in serum concentration of testosterone, LH or FSH before and after administration of antifertility doses of gossypol to male rats. In Austria[9] gossypol acetic acid at dosages of 2.5-30 mg/kg for 10-20 weeks did not affect serum concentrations of testosterone and gonadotrophins, weights of the animals and accessory reproductive organs, histology of the accessory sex organs or prostate biochemistry in adult rats. Thus, gossypol evidently does not disturb hypothalamic-pituitary-gonadal communication. Our findings are in agreement with other rat studies also reporting normal hormone concentrations and reproductive organ weights after gossypol treatment. However, Hadley et al.[10] noted that daily administration of 30 mg/kg gossypol for 5 weeks significantly lowered testosterone and LH values and produced a marked reduction of Leydig cell area and epididymal weight.

CLINICAL STUDIES TESTING GOSSYPOL AS A MALE CONTRACEPTIVE

In 1972 scientists in Nanjing[11] felt that it would be safe to start a first-phase clinical study, using the smallest possible gossypol dosage. Volunteers were carefully monitored with periodic interviews and physical and laboratory check-ups, including blood electrolyte estimations, liver and kidney function tests, and ECG. Ordinary gossypol was used at a dosage of 60 mg per day. At the end of 40 days volunteers showed either azoospermia or severe oligospermia. No side-effects were apparent.

In 1973 hospitals and research institutions from all over China joined the clinical study[2]. More than 10 000 volunteers took gossypol in the form of ordinary gossypol or gossypol acetate. Both forms produced similar antifertility effects[2]. For safety reasons the already low dosage was first reduced to 30 mg per day and then to 20 mg per day. In 1975 this dose was considered by most researchers the optimal dose concentration. At the end of 60-75 days most patients showed azoospermia or severe oligospermia[2]. They were then told to reduce their intake to 7 mg per day or 50 mg per week. This was termed the maintenance dosage. The regimen now consisted of a 60-75 day loading phase of 20 mg gossypol per day followed by a 50 mg per week maintenance phase to control the level of infertility[2, 12, 13].

Gossypol has many advantages, making it a prime candidate for fertility control. It has a remarkable effectiveness rate of over 99%[2, 12, 13]. As long as the maintenance dosage is taken, sperm will not appear in the semen. Side-effects are not prominent; there are no alarming symptoms in the loading phase. The cost of gossypol is quite low. Cotton is an abundant natural resource, and the seeds have been discarded in the past.

During a period of about 5 years more than 4000 participants from 14 provinces took part in the clinical trial[2]. Some side-effects were present. It was found that 12% of the subjects complained of fatigue, 5% of decreased libido and 5% of a decrease in appetite[12, 13]. The symptoms usually occurred 2–3 weeks after the beginning of the loading phase. They tended to become less apparent, however, towards the end of the loading phase. The symptoms were attributed to bodily adjustment to the new substances. These mild symptoms usually disappeared after the loading phase. All liver and kidney functions, ECG results, and blood and urine analyses were normal. In most men the side-effects did not recur during the maintenance phase. However, there were occasional cases of hypokalaemia.

Gossypol-induced clinical hypokalemia occurs in about 1% of all cases. Its main manifestation is a weakening of the voluntary muscles. Afflicted patients are sometimes unable even to stand up, to dress themselves or to mount a bicycle. In these instances serum potassium can be as low as 2 mmol/l. There are sometimes bradycardia and typical ECG changes associated with hypokalaemia. Like hypokalaemia produced by other causes, gossypol-induced hypokalaemia usually can be relieved by supplementing potassium salts orally and intravenously.

Gossypol-induced hypokalaemia occurred most often in the southern part of China, in areas such as the Yangtze Valley. This is considered to be due to dietary factors[14]. People in the south of China consume large quantities of rice, while wheat, higher in potassium, is the main grain in the diets of northerners.

The mechanism of gossypol-induced hypokalaemia is not clear. One thing is certain: potassium is lost through the kidneys. It is probably the result of gossypol enhancing prostaglandin biosynthesis, which leads to renal potassium loss[14]. Another possibility is an inhibitory effect of gossypol on sodium/potassium ATPase[14].

Hypokalaemia occurs almost exclusively in the maintenance phase. This may be due to the fact that in the loading phase gossypol has not reached the crucial level of toxicity.

Another problem with gossypol arose when a small percentage of men failed to regain fertility after gossypol treatment ended. In a study of 2067 cases where the standard dose was administered for $\frac{1}{2}$–$4\frac{1}{2}$ years, semen analyses showed a recovery rate of 90.08%, with 9.92% remaining azoospermic years after gossypol withdrawal[15].

Biopsies of gossypol-treated animal and human testes revealed similar damage to the seminiferous epithelia[8]. This phenomenon helps to explain the basis of gossypol's antifertility action. It also explains the reason for irreversibility. Extensive gossypol exposure and subsequent severe damage to the spermatogenic epithelium appears to reduce the chance of recovery of fertility following cessation of treatment. Clinical observations disclosed that more irreversible cases occur in men approximately of 35 years and older[15, 16]. Although men over 35 are still fertile, the ability to recover fertility is less than it is in younger men. An older man's germinal epithelium cannot withstand the same amount of gossypol as a younger man. In order to avoid irreversibility, researchers advise that duration of exposure to gossypol should not exceed 2 years. It is advisable that a patient should not consume more than a total of 6 g gossypol[15, 16].

The effects, if any, of gossypol on offspring is a subject that warrants consideration and further investigation. Following termination of gossypol treatment, experimental animals could have normal pregnancies and normal offspring[17]. Fifty-three women gave birth to normal babies after their husbands ceased to take gossypol. In the areas of epidemic sterility due to cottonseed oil, children born after recovery from azoospermia all appeared quite normal[15].

CONCLUSIONS AND PROGNOSIS

Why do so many researchers consider gossypol the most promising male antifertility agent? One advantage, already mentioned, is its availability and low cost. Of even more interest is its mechanism of action. Gossypol acts locally, at the level of the reproductive organs themselves[17]. It does not act indirectly, interfering with hormone production, as LHRH and steroid hormones do. During the first few weeks of treatment, gossypol attaches to maturing sperms stored in the epididymis and renders them immotile. Later, when gossypol has been taken for longer, the drug also acts in the testes to check sperm production. These characteristics, the direct actions on the motility of mature spermatozoa and on the growth of immature sperm cells, is what sets gossypol apart from other potential chemical fertility-regulating agents. Gossypol acts without interfering with the Leydig cells or with the pituitary–gonadal system. It therefore should not affect a man's sex drive and should not cause profound disturbances of the general hormonal regulatory system.

Gossypol is not without its disadvantages. The slow onset of the antifertility effect is merely inconvenient, but the risks of sterility and hypokalaemia are much graver problems. Toxicity is still the main concern. Gossypol has been considered poisonous since its discovery almost 100 years ago, and toxic effects in certain animal species have further alarmed those who already view gossypol's toxicity as an insurmountable barrier. Gossypol's toxic properties or side-effects should be viewed from a scientific viewpoint. One should remain aware of, though not be alarmed by, the results of animal experiments using dogs and other sensitive species. Other animal species, especially primates, exhibit a much less marked toxic reaction and require a lower antifertility dose. This is not to say that one ought to take the completely optimistic view at the other extreme. One cannot deem gossypol the ideal male antifertility agent, ignoring the occurrence of hypokalaemia, possible toxic manifestations in the heart and muscle, and permanent sterility.

We now should study more in order to discover more. Perhaps supplementing the gossypol dosage with potassium will alleviate the hypokalaemia problem. Gossypol analogues and derivatives, or perhaps other phenolic compounds, may be of use in the future. It is important to recognize that studies on gossypol have created a major new lead in the search for male fertility-regulating agents. We should admit that gossypol has drawbacks, and then we should attempt to overcome them.

Developing a contraceptive requires decades of painstaking research. We are dealing with a drug to be taken by hundreds of thousands of healthy young and middle-aged people. The world population is increasing steadily, however, and always at a faster pace, especially in recent years. The projected world population for the year 2000 is 6 billion. We cannot rely for population control only on the contraceptives already in use. They are not sufficient, and some methods have proved unsatisfactory. At a time when there are not enough male fertility-regulating methods available, gossypol appears to be an agent of promise.

REFERENCES

1. Liu Bao-shan (1957) Control of fertility with cooking oil from cotton seeds. *J. Trad. Med. Shanghai*, **283**, 43
2. National Coordinating Group on Male Antifertility Agents (1978) Gossypol—a new antifertility agent for males. *Chinese Med. J.*, **4**, 417
3. Longmore, J.J. (1886) Cottonseed oil: Its colouring matter mucilage, and description of a new method of recovering the loss occurring in the refining process. *J. Soc. Chem. Ind.*, **5**, 200
4. Marchlewski, L. (1899) Gossypol, ein Bestandteil der Baumwollsamen. *J. Prakt. Chem.*, **60**, 84
5. Adams, R. *et al.* (1960) Gossypol, a pigment of cottonseed. *Chem. Revs.*, **60**, 555
6. Lei Hai Peng (1982) Retrospective and prospective outlook of gossypol as a male contraceptive. *Yi Yao Xue Bao*, **17**, 1
7. Lei Hai Peng (1983) Future prospects of gossypol as a male contraceptive. *Yi Yao Xue Bao*, **18**, 321
8. Xue She Pu (1980) Studies on the antifertility effect of gossypol. A new contraceptive for males. In *Recent Advances in Fertility Regulation*, Proceedings of Symposium, Beijing, September 1980
9. Weinbauer, G.F. *et al.* (1982) The endocrine status of gossypol-treated male rats. *Andrologia*, **15** (special number), 565
10. Hadley, M.A. *et al.* (1981) Effects of gossypol on the reproductive system of male rats. *J. Androl.*, **2**, 190
11. Qian, S.Z. *et al.* (1972) The first clinical trial of gossypol on male antifertility. Presented at *First National Conference on Male Antifertility Agents*, Wuhan
12. Liu, G.Z. (1981) Clinical study of gossypol as a male contraceptive. *Reproduccion*, **5**, 189
13. Liu, Z.Q. *et al.* (1980) Clinical trial of gossypol as a male antifertility agent. In *Recent Advances in Fertility Regulation*, Proceedings of Symposium, Beijing, September 1980
14. Qian, S.Z. *et al.* (1980) Gossypol related hypokalaemia, clinicopharmacological studies. *Chinese Med. J.*, **93**, 477
15. National Coordinating Group on Male Antifertility Agents (1980) Clinical Trial of Gossypol. (Unpublished data)
16. Cao Jian *et al.* (1983) Studies on gossypol reversibility of azoospermia following gossypol withdrawal. *Acta Acad. Med. Sin.*, **5**, 227
17. Wang, N.G. *et al.* (1979) Antifertility effect of gossypol acetic acid on male rats. *Chin. Med. J.*, **59**, 402

12
Antifertility activity of (−)-gossypol

S.A. MATLIN and R.H. ZHOU

Gossypol (**1**) is a yellow, phenolic pigment found in the cotton plant[1]. The compound, both in the free form and as 1:1 complexes with acetic acid and with formic acid, was discovered by the Chinese to be orally active as an antifertility agent in the male[2]. Interference with spermatogenesis has been demonstrated both in clinical trials in China and in laboratory studies in rats and hamsters in several countries[3-9]. The principal side-effects revealed in the Chinese studies were low incidences of hypokalaemia and of failure to regain fertility on ceasing treatment. Gossypol has also been demonstrated to be an active spermicidal agent and there have been trials of its efficacy as a vaginal spermicide[10-17].

$$\underline{1}$$

Gossypol is reported to have a relatively poor stability and is generally handled as a 1:1 complex with acetic acid. Initial concerns about the purity of the material being studied *in vivo* led us to establish suitable HPLC methods for the analysis of gossypol and a number of its chemical derivatives, including gossypolone, anhydrogossypol, gossypol hexa-acetate and Schiff's bases. In addition, mass spectral (including FD and CI) and linked LC/MS methods for the analysis of these compounds have been described[18]. These studies have revealed the complexity of the chemistry of gossypol and its tendency to generate isomeric products as a result of tautomerism.

We also undertook a stability study of gossypol solutions and formulations under a wide variety of conditions, as part of a four-centre collaborative study sponsored by the World Health Organization. This revealed[19] that gossypol has poor stability under many conditions (especially in solutions in alcohols and in bases) but stores well as the pure solid (cold and

237

dark preferred) and in solutions in apolar, aprotic solvents (e.g. benzene, chloroform, dichloromethane: concentrated, cold and dark conditions preferred).

Gossypol is a chiral molecule, as a result of restricted rotation about the bond linking the two naphthyl residues. Cotton plants (*Gossypium* species of the family Malvaceae) produce gossypol which is an equal mixture of the (+) and (−) enantiomers. However, another plant in this family (*Thespesia populnea*) produces (+)-gossypol. It is interesting to note that racemic gossypol can be crystallized as the acetic acid complex, whereas the (+) enantiomer apparently cannot[20-22]. (+)-Gossypol has been shown to be inactive as an antifertility agent when tested in animals under the same conditions as racemic gossypol–acetic acid. It has therefore been proposed that (−)-gossypol should be the sole form which possesses antifertility activity in the male[23-25]. A widespread search for a plant producing (−)-gossypol has so far proved negative.

An attempt was made to resolve gossypol by the classical procedure of fractional recrystallization of diastereomeric derivatives. Gossypol was converted into Schiff's bases by condensation with chiral amines such as 1-phenylethylamine and phenylglycine ethyl ester[18], but no resolution was observed on recrystallization. Attention was therefore directed to the use of chiral HPLC columns for resolution[26]. A series of chiral columns was prepared by reaction of aminopropyl silica with optically pure amino acid derivatives. Initial attempts to resolve gossypol directly on these columns were unsuccessful. However, the Schiff's base (2) formed by reaction of gossypol with (+)-1-phenylethylamine gave good resolution of the diastereoisomers on a variety of chiral columns, and the column containing the salt of D-(−)-phenylglycine 3,5-dinitrobenzamide (3) on aminopropyl silica

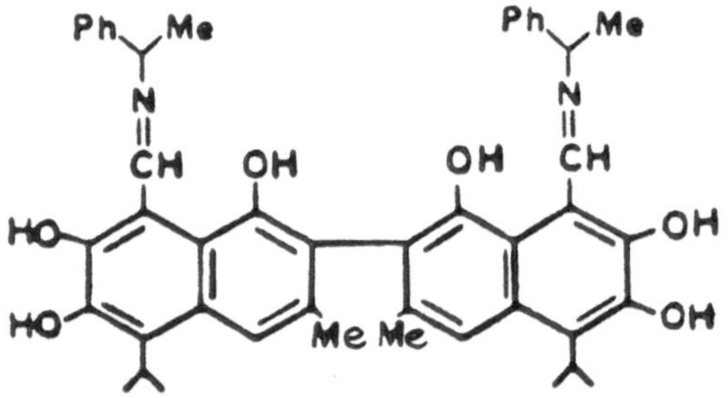

2

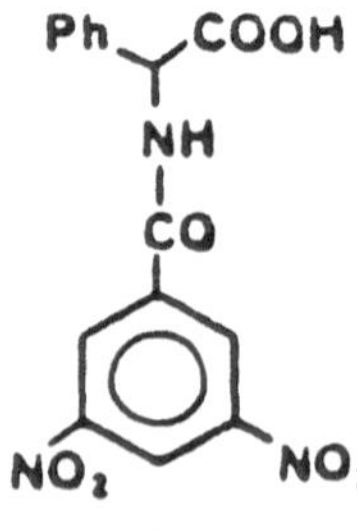

3

was selected as the most convenient for further study. It was subsequently found that Schiff's bases of gossypol with a variety of achiral amines (e.g. propylamine, aniline) also resolved well on this column[27]. Preparative HPLC isolation of the resolved Schiff's bases on a multigram scale, followed by hydrolysis, afforded gram quantities of (−)-gossypol (and also the (+) enantiomer)[28].

Antifertility studies in male hamsters[28] show that (−)-gossypol is active at half the dose of the racemate (Table 1) and is clearly the sole enantiomer possessing activity. A slightly slower rate of response, for both the (−) isomer and the free racemate, compared with the 1:1 complex with acetic acid, suggests an effect of the physical form of the oral dosage on bioavailability.

Table 1   Effects of gossypol isomers on fertility of male hamsters after dosing for 40 days

Day of mating	Treatment/day	No. of males that mated	No. of males fertile	Mean no. of implants Normal	Abnormal
49	control	5/5	5/5	10.1	0
	(±)-gossypol-AcOH, 16 mg/kg	5/5	1/5	0	0.2
	(−)-gossypol, 8 mg/kg	3/5	1/3	0	0.4
	(±)-gossypol, 16 mg/kg	5/5	3/5	1.1	1.2

The direct effect of the gossypol enantiomers on sperm function has also been examined. At concentrations at which (+)-gossypol is less active, (−)-gossypol causes loss of motility, velocity, linearity of progression and zona-free ovum penetrating capacity[29].

(−)-Gossypol has emerged as the enantiomer possessing all the important antifertility effects previously associated with the racemate, and will be an important focus of future work in the search for a safe oral antifertility agent for men.

A multinational programme for the synthesis of analogues of gossypol has recently been initiated by WHO[30]. Although there are literature reports of hemigossypol derivatives with *in vitro* spermicidal activity[31], no analogues or derivatives of gossypol have so far been shown to have substantial *in vivo* activity in the male[32]. A large number of compounds are currently being synthesized for screening in the WHO programme, and it is hoped that this will lead to the identification of more active and/or less toxic compounds.

ACKNOWLEDGEMENTS

We thank the World Health Organization for financial support (SAM) and for a Research Training Grant (RZ); Dr R.J. Aitken and Dr G. Bialy for the biological assays; and The City University for an equipment grant for HPLC.

REFERENCES

1. Adams, R., Geissman, T.A. and Edwards, J.D. (1960). Gossypol, a pigment of cottonseed. *Chem. Rev.*, **60**, 555
2. National Coordinating Group on Male Antifertility Agents (1978). Gossypol, a new antifertility agent for males. *Chinese Med. J.*, **6**, 417
3. Liu, Z., Liu, G., Hei, L., Zhang, R. and Yu, C. (1981). Clinical trial of gossypol as a male antifertility agent. In *Recent Advances in Fertility Regulation, Beijing, 1980*, pp. 160–163. (Geneva: World Health Organization)
4. Prassad, M.R.N. and Diczfalusy, E. (1982). Gossypol. *Int. J. Androl. Suppl.*, **5**, 53
5. Jackson, H. (1982). Gossypol. In Jeffcoate, S.L. and Sandler, M. (eds.) *Progress Towards a Male Contraceptive*, pp. 145–157. (Chichester: Wiley)
6. Qian, S.-Z. and Wang, Z.-G. (1984). Gossypol: A potential antifertility agent for males. *Ann. Rev. Pharmacol. Toxicol.*, **24**, 329
7. Waller, D.P., Fong, H.H.S., Cordell, G.A. and Soejarto, D.D. (1981). Antifertility effects of gossypol and its impurities on male hamsters. *Contraception*, **23**, 653
8. Chang, M.C., Gu, Z. and Saksena, S.K. (1980). Effects of gossypol on the fertility of male rats, hamsters and rabbits. *Contraception*, **21**, 461
9. Hahn, D.W., Rusticus, C., Probst, A., Homm, R. and Johnson, A.N. (1981). Antifertility and endocrine activities of gossypol in rodents. *Contraception*, **24**, 97
10. Waller, D.P., Zaneveld, L.J.D. and Fong, H.H.S. (1980). In vitro spermicidal activity of gossypol. *Contraception*, **22**, 183
11. Williams, W.L. (1980). New antifertility agents active in rabbit vaginal contraception method. *Contraception*, **22**, 659
12. Ridley, A.J. and Blasco, L. (1981). Testosterone and gossypol effects on human sperm motility. *Fertil. Steril. Suppl.*, **35**, 244
13. Tso, W.W. and Lee, C.S. (1981). Effect of gossypol on boar spermatozoa in vitro. *Arch. Androl.*, **7**, 85
14. Tso, W.W. and Lee, C.S. (1982). Cottonseed oil as a vaginal contraceptive. *Arch. Androl.*, **8**, 11
15. Cameron, S.M., Waller, D.P. and Zaneveld, L.J.D. (1982). Vaginal spermicidal activity of gossypol in *Macaca arctoides. Fertil. Steril.*, **37**, 273
16. Aitken, R.J., Liu, J., Best, F.S.M. and Richardson, D.W. (1983). An analysis of the direct effects of gossypol on human spermatozoa. *Int. J. Androl.*, **6**, 157
17. Ratsula, K., Haukkamaa, M., Wichmann, K. and Luukkainen, T. (1983). Vaginal contraception with gossypol: a clinical study. *Contraception*, **27**, 571
18. Matlin, S.A., Zhou, R., Games, D.E., Jones, A. and Ramsey, E.D. (1984). HPLC, MS and LC/MS of gossypol and its derivatives. *J. High Res. Chromatogr. Chromatogr. Commun.*, **7**, 196
19. Details of the stability study will be published in the near future
20. King, T.J. and de Silva, L.B. (1968). Optically active gossypol from *Thespesia populnea. Tetrahedron Lett.*, 261
21. Dechary, J.M. and Pradel, P. (1971). The occurrence of (+)-gossypol in *Gossypium* species. *J. Am. Oil Chem. Soc.*, **48**, 563
22. Datta, S.C., Murti, V.V.S. and Sheshadri, T.R. (1972). Isolation and study of (+)-gossypol from *Thespesia populnea. Indian J. Chem.*, **10**, 263
23. Wang, Y.E., Luo, Y.D. and Tang, X.C. (1979). Studies on the antifertility action of cottonseed meal and gossypol. *Acta Pharmacol. Sinica*, **14**, 662
24. Yao, X.Y. (1981). Studies on the isolation and the antifertility effect of (+)-gossypol. *Reprod. Contracep. China*, **2**, 51
25. Waller, D.P., Bunyapraphatsara, N., Martin, A., Vournazos, C.J., Ahmed, M.S., Soejarto, D.D., Cordell, G.A. and Fong, H.H.S. (1983). Effect of (+)-gossypol on fertility in male hamsters. *J. Androl.*, **4**, 276
26. Pirkle, W.H. and Finn, J.M. (1982). Preparative resolution of racemates on a chiral liquid chromatography column. *J. Org. Chem.*, **47**, 4037
27. Matlin, S.A. and Zhou, R. (1984). Resolution of gossypol by HPLC. *J. High Res. Chromatogr. Chromatogr. Commun.* (Submitted)
28. Matlin, S.A., Zhou, R. and Bialy, G. (1984). (−)-Gossypol: an active male oral antifertility agent. *Contraception.* (Submitted)
29. Aitken, R.J., Matlin, S.A. *et al.* (1984). Manuscript in preparation

30. WHO (1983). Special Programme of Research, Development and Research Training in Human Reproduction. In *12th Annual Report*. (Geneva: World Health Organization)
31. Manmade, A., Herlihy, P., Quick, J., Burgos, M. and Hoffer, A.P. (1984). Gossypol. Synthesis and in vitro spermicidal activity of isomeric hemigossypol derivatives. *Experientia*, **39**, 1276
32. Wu, G., Wang, W., Ying, H. and Yan, Z. (1981). A preliminary report on the synthesis and screening of gossypol derivatives and analogues—an attempt to simplify the gossypol molecule. *Recent Advances in Synthetic Chemistry for Fertility Regulating Agents. J. Reprod. Contracep.*, 71

13
Monoclonal antibodies directed against human sperm antigens

N.J. ALEXANDER

INTRODUCTION

During spermatogenesis, after germinal cells leave the basal compartment, testicular germ cells begin to express gene products not found elsewhere in the body. Novel surface constituents called differentiation antigens are inserted during both meiosis and the spermatid stages as the cells undergo remodelling. Germ cell antigens are inserted in a precise temporal sequence. Specific germ cell antigens have been identified as early as the pachytene stage of meiosis in mice[1, 2], and a glycolipid, sulphatoxygalactosylacylalkylglycerol, first appears on the surface of early spermatocytes in rats[3, 4].

Many of these determinants are integral parts of the sperm structure, and they persist on epididymal sperm. During epididymal transit, a period when these gametes gain the ability to fertilize, the sperm surface undergoes chemical and functional modifications. Among the maturational changes that occur are: changes in electrophoretic characteristics and increases in negative charge[5]; changes in lectin binding patterns[6]; and alterations in the amount and type of surface glycoproteins[7]. During this period some testicular proteins become lost or masked. Brooks and Tiver[8] have described three proteins of 130 ku, susceptible to labelling with tritiated borohydride in the presence of galactose oxidase, which fall into this category. Secretions from the epididymal epithelium may become attached. Therefore, the surface polypeptide composition of caudal spermatozoa markedly differs from that of testicular spermatozoa[9, 10].

The sperm surface undergoes further alterations when coated by seminal plasma. Such coating antigens from seminal plasma may affect sperm function. Shigeta et al.[11] have developed a complement-dependent sperm-immobilizing monoclonal; the antigen to which it is directed may be similar to seminal plasma lactoferrin.

Sperm surface change continues during capacitation, when some antigens become exposed and altered. Finally, sperm binding to the egg entails interaction with several oocyte investments and the ooplasm itself.

An understanding of the composition of the sperm plasma membrane is essential for deducing the role of specific sperm antigens in germ cell differentiation, sperm maturation, sperm capacitation and gamete interactions.

Monoclonal antibodies, which are highly specific immunoglobulins, recognize components of the cell surface and have been used to examine sperm surfaces in several species[12-15].

My colleagues and I, as well as others, have generated hybridoma cell lines secreting antibodies against spermatozoal antigens. Definition and characterization of these antibodies will aid in the understanding of sperm function and fertilization.

METHODS

My co-workers and I used a standard technique[16] to prepare antibody-synthesizing hybridoma cultures. The mice were immunized with 10^6 washed ejaculated sperm in Complete Freund Adjuvant. Each mouse received a booster injection on days 21 and 42, and was bled on day 50. A final intravenous injection of antigen in saline was given 4 days before the fusion. From 10 to 14 days after hybridization, the supernatants of all the wells were sampled and screened for antisperm activity by means of an enzyme-linked immunosorption assay (ELISA)[17]. The contents that were of interest were cloned, the supernatants were collected, and the cells were injected into mice so that ascites fluid could be produced. The site of antigen binding to spermatozoa was tested by means of indirect immunofluorescence. Absorption tests for species and tissue specificities, agglutination tests and immobilization tests were performed. Proteins were detected immunologically on nitrocellulose paper. A more complete description of our methods has been published elsewhere[18].

RESULTS AND DISCUSSION

We currently have about 30 cell lines that produce antibodies against whole human sperm (verified in an initial ELISA) and a lithium 3,5-di-iodosalicylate sperm membrane extract[17]. A lymphoblastoid cell line is used for a negative control. Immunofluorescence assays on methanol-fixed sperm have revealed that about 70% of the monoclonal antibodies are directed against the acrosomal region. It is not uncommon for binding to occur also in the neck region. Examples of monoclonal antibody binding patterns are depicted in Figure 1. Most antibodies bind to the same region of both fixed and unfixed samples, but the fluorescence is patchier when living spermatozoa are used. Western blot techniques have revealed that, even though an antibody reacts to what appears to be the entire acrosome (immunofluorescence data), antigens of differing molecular weights may be involved. Primakoff and Myles[19] have found guinea-pig sperm head antigens ranging from 18 to 70 ku, and we have observed human sperm acrosomal antigens varying from 34 to 240 ku. In elegant studies Reynolds and Oliphant[20] have used monoclonal antibodies to characterize an acrosome-stabilizing factor, a 360 ku dimer synthesized in the corpus epididymidis and found in seminal plasma and caudal epididymal fluid. This substance maintains the acrosome during epididymal storage by preventing the acrosome reaction.

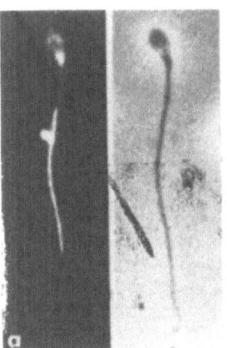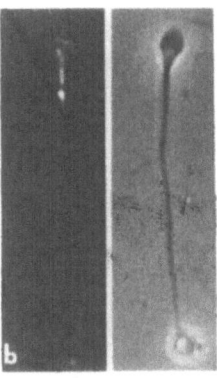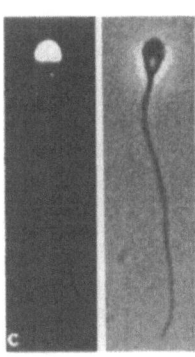

Figure 1 Examples of monoclonal antibody binding patterns on human spermatozoa. The left frame is by fluorescence microscopy; the right by phase microscopy. Washed spermatozoa were methanol-fixed and air-dried. A 1:500 dilution of ascites fluid antibody is incubated with the spermatozoa. After washing in phosphate-buffered saline, the slides are incubated with a fluorescein-conjugated second antibody. (a) Reveals binding to the principal piece of the tail and postacrosome, (b) binding to the equatorial region and to the midpiece, (c) binding to the acrosome

Antibodies to human spermatozoa have been implicated in immunologically mediated infertility in both men and women. Because the presence of antisperm antibodies in patients frequently results in sperm agglutination or cytotoxicity, we use these tests routinely both clinically and to test for antisperm monoclonal antibodies. Monoclonal antibodies exhibit actions and specificities similar to those of naturally occurring antisperm antibodies in human beings. MA-5, for instance, has been found to cause complement-dependent immobilization but not agglutination of human sperm[18]. Our studies suggest that at least three different acrosomal antigens on human sperm are involved in head-to-head agglutination.

Extensive testing for tissue specificity is an important consideration during the development of monoclonal antibodies, since spermatozoa have many constituents common to all mammalian cells, in addition to unique antigens. For example, for a monoclonal to be of interest to us, it must not react with human lymphocytes, erythrocytes, lymphoblastoid cells or K5262 leukaemia cells, but Mettler et al.[21] have found only 4 of 149 hybridoma cell lines secreting antisperm antibodies that do not also react with spleen and tonsil. Most (91%) of the clones studied by Mettler et al.[21] produced antibodies that reacted with seminal plasma. Such findings emphasize the importance of tissue specificity studies.

The state of the spermatozoon can affect the binding pattern. For example, indirect immunofluorescence has indicated that MA-5 reacts with the equatorial region and is weakly bound to the tails of ejaculated sperm (Figure 2), but when sperm are incubated in a capacitation medium, they lose this equatorial binding. We have found a significant correlation between lack of equatorial fluorescence and the frequency with which sperm penetrate denuded hamster eggs. Increasing the osmolarity of NaCl in the capacitation medium increases the egg penetration rate and decreases binding of antibody to the equatorial region (Naz and Alexander, in preparation). The mobility of antigens on lymphocytes has long been known. Surface

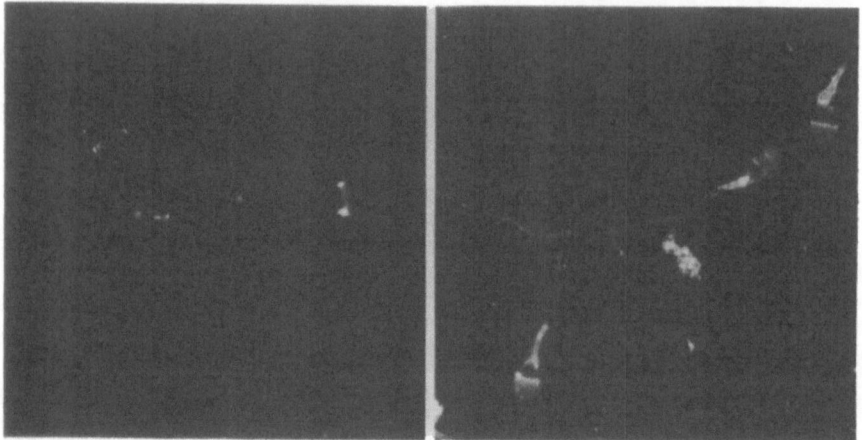

Figure 2 An example of a monoclonal antibody that reacts with the equatorial region of freshly ejaculated sperm (left) but to the equatorial plus postacrosome and midpiece of spermatozoa that have been incubated to effect capacitation (right). Samples have been prepared for immunofluorescence as in Figure 1

receptors on spermatozoa may also exhibit mobility and are susceptible to antibody-induced patching[22]. Gaunt et al.[22] found mobile antigens distributed over the entire sperm flagellum, whereas the mobile antigens that we have observed are associated with changes in head membranes most probably involved in capacitation. Blocking with azide, a procedure routinely used by scientists checking for lymphocyte capping, will be an important step in determining whether the antigen recognized by MA-5 is shed, modified or masked.

MA-5 appears to recognize a labile antigen possibly associated with capacitation, but MA-5 does not impede fertilization when added to sperm prior to exposure to hamster eggs. Other monoclonal antibodies studied in our laboratory do prevent gamete interaction. MA-24, which is of the 2a subclass of immunoglobulin G, falls into this category. It causes neither sperm agglutination nor sperm immobilization. It is specific for germ cells and binds to the postacrosomes, midpieces and tails of both viable and methanol-fixed human spermatozoa (Figure 3). The binding patterns are similar on non-capacitated, capacitated and reduced (swollen-head) sperm treated with dithiothreitol plus Triton X-100. The antibody reacts not only with human sperm, but also with ejaculated rhesus sperm and murine epididymal sperm. With the Western blot enzyme immunobinding assay, we can begin to determine the molecular identity. MA-24 reacts with a single 23 ku protein band when a detergent-solubilized membrane preparation of human testis is used[23]. MA-24 completely blocks binding and penetration of zona-free hamster ova and significantly inhibits in vitro fertilization of mouse eggs by murine sperm[23].

Many antigens may be involved in fertilization. For example, O'Rand and co-workers[24, 25] have described a family of rabbit sperm antigens of low molecular weight which exhibit similar physicochemical and immunological properties. These plasma membrane glycoproteins play an important role in zona penetration. Immunoadsorption chromatography and sodium

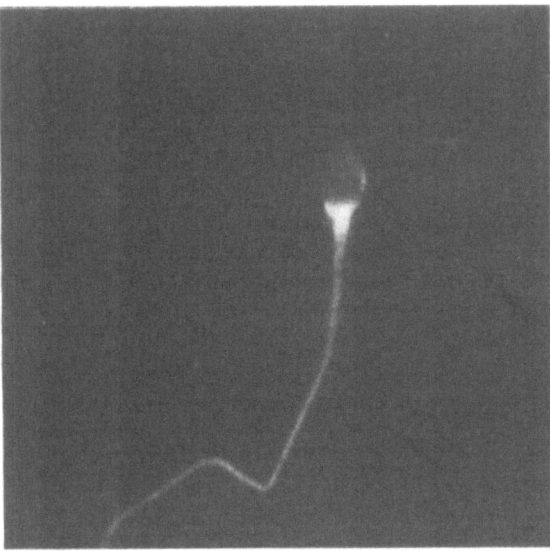

Figure 3 The binding pattern as revealed by immunofluorescence of MA-24, a monoclonal antibody that impedes fertilization. Sample was prepared for immunofluorescence as in Figure 1

dodecyl sulphate–polyacrylamide gel electrophoresis studies have identified three antigens of 87, 15 and 13 ku on the tail, midpiece and, to a lesser extent, head region. Our studies and those of O'Rand's group[24, 25], Schmell et al.[26] and Moore and Hartman[27] indicate that monoclonal antibodies directed against the sperm head or the sperm head and tail can inhibit *in vitro* fertilization.

The antigen that forms a complex with MA-24 is associated with human involuntary immuno-infertility[23]. Serum from some infertile patients with evidence of circulating antisperm antibodies shows strong binding to purified antigen in an ELISA. Although the relationship between human infertility and the presence of antibodies to sperm is well documented, it has been difficult to characterize sperm antibodies in order to understand immunologically mediated infertility. When human spermatozoa were tested for the ability to penetrate hamster eggs after being exposed to antisperm antibodies from patients presumed to have immunologically mediated infertility, the penetration rate was reduced by 44%. Six serum samples totally blocked egg penetration, ten significantly reduced it, and only two samples yielded results comparable with those for normal serum[28]. In that study no particular antibody type was observed to always prevent either cervical mucus or egg penetration—an indication of the usefulness of monoclonal antibodies for attempts to determine which antigens are involved in fertilization and to develop tests to diagnose immune infertility.

MA-24 reacts with sperm from several species—an advantage for studying human antigens that may be important in fertilization. Since sperm exhibit many ultrastructural similarities in the acrosome, the equatorial segment and the postnuclear cap[29–31], it is not surprising that they have antigenically similar determinants. Antigenic similarities were observed as early as 1900, when von Moxter[32] noted that serum from rabbits immunized with sheep semen had antibodies that immobilized rat sperm. Guyer[33] observed that chickens immunized with rabbit sperm had immobilizing antibodies against not only rabbit sperm, but also guinea-pig sperm. Some of our monoclonal antibodies react with the surfaces of human, monkey, dog, rabbit, rat and mouse sperm[18]. If certain antigenic determinants are part of a surface component having a particular role in sperm function, and similar sperm-specific antigenic determinants can be segregated into identical domains, the two determinants probably have a common sperm function. One such sperm antigen is lactate dehydrogenase C-4, which is antigenically and functionally similar in several mammalian species[34].

The cross-reactivity that we have observed is not an artifact. Quantitative tissue absorption data indicate that the antibody reactivity is not due to cross-reacting antigens of mammalian sperm, kidney and central nervous system[35, 36], but is specific for male germ cells. Isahakia and I[18] found that cross-reactivity data obtained with immunofluorescence and quantitative absorption techniques are identical. The activity is not due to non-specific binding of the Fc region of antibodies[37], since some of the monoclonal antibodies react only with human sperm. The fact that some monoclonal antibodies have similar agglutinating and immobilizing effects on human and monkey sperm further indicates the specificity of the observed cross-reactivity. By the technique of Western blotting, Isahakia and I[18] have shown that one of our monoclonal antibodies recognizes antigens of similar molecular weights on human (84 ku), bull (82 ku) and mouse (82 ku) sperm.

The structural and functional characteristics of the human sperm surface are at present little understood, and monoclonal antibodies are useful as probes for studies designed to delineate them. It has become apparent that the spermatozoon maintains contiguous domains of differing compositions, each of which may contain several localized antigens[19]. The identification of sperm-specific antigens and their respective roles in fertility will greatly facilitate development of contraceptive vaccines.

ACKNOWLEDGEMENTS

The work described in this chapter, Publication no. 1357 of the Oregon Regional Primate Research Center, was supported by National Institutes of Health grants RR-00163, HD-14572 and RR-05694.

REFERENCES

1. Millette, C.F. and Bellvé, A.R. (1977). Temporal expression of membrane antigens during mouse spermatogenesis. *J. Cell Biol.*, **74**, 86
2. O'Brien, D.A. and Millette, C.F. (1984). Identification and immunochemical characterization of spermatogenic cell surface antigens that appear during early meiotic prophase. *Dev. Biol.*, **101**, 307
3. Kornblatt, M.J. (1979). Synthesis and turnover of sulfogalactoglycerolipid, a membrane lipid, during spermatogenesis. *Can. J. Biochem.*, **57**, 255
4. Lingwood, C. and Schachter, H. (1981). Localization of sulfatoxygalactosylacylalkylglycerol at the surface of rat testicular germinal cells by immunocytochemical tech-

niques: pH dependence of a nonimmunological reaction between immunoglobulin and germinal cells. *J. Cell Biol.*, **89**, 621

5. Bedford, J.M. (1963). Changes in the electrophoretic properties of rabbit spermatozoa during passage through the epididymis. *Nature (London)*, **200**, 1178

6. Koehler, J.K. (1981). Lectins as probes of the spermatozoon surface. *Arch. Androl.*, **6**, 197

7. Fournier-Delpech, S., Banzo, B.J. and Orgebin-Crist, M.-C. (1977). Extraction of concanavalin A affinity material from rat testicular and epididymal spermatozoa. *Ann. Biol. Anim. Biochim. Biophys.*, **17**, 207

8. Brooks, D.E. and Tiver, K. (1984). Analysis of surface proteins of rat spermatozoa during epididymal transit and identification of antigens common to spermatozoa, rete testis fluid and cauda epididymal plasma. *J. Reprod. Fertil.*, **71**, 249

9. Brooks, D.E. and Tiver, K. (1983). Localization of epididymal secretory proteins on rat spermatozoa. *J. Reprod. Fertil.*, **69**, 651

10. Echeverria, F.G., Cuasnicú, P.S., Piazza, A., Piñeiro, L. and Blaquier, J.A. (1984). Addition of an androgen-free epididymal protein extract increases the ability of immature hamster spermatozoa to fertilize *in vivo* and *in vitro*. *J. Reprod. Fertil.*, **71**, 433

11. Shigeta, M., Watanabe, T., Maruyama, S., Koyama, K. and Isojima, S. (1980). Sperm-immobilizing monoclonal antibody to human seminal plasma antigens. *Clin. Exp. Immunol.*, **42**, 458

12. Feuchter, F.A., Vernon, R.B. and Eddy, E.M. (1981). Analysis of the sperm surface with monoclonal antibodies: Topographically restricted antigens appearing in the epididymis. *Biol. Reprod.*, **24**, 1099

13. Myles, D.G., Primakoff, P., and Bellvé, A.R. (1981). Surface domains of the guinea pig sperm defined with monoclonal antibodies. *Cell*, **23**, 433

14. Lee, C.-Y.G., Huang, Y.-S., Huang, C.-H., Hu, P.-C. and Menge, A.C. (1982). Monoclonal antibodies to human sperm antigens. *J. Reprod. Immunol.*, **4**, 173

15. Lee, C.-Y.G., Wong, E. and Menge, A.C. (1984). Monoclonal antibodies to rabbit sperm autoantigens. *Fertil. Steril.*, **41**, 131

16. Kohler, G. and Milstein, C. (1975). Continuous cultures of fused cells secreting antibody of predefined specificity. *Nature (London)*, **256**, 495

17. Alexander, N.J. and Bearwood, D. (1984). An immunosorption assay for antibodies to spermatozoa: Comparison with agglutination and immobilization tests. *Fertil. Steril.*, **41**, 270

18. Isahakia, M. and Alexander, N.J. (1984). Interspecies cross-reactivity of monoclonal antibodies directed against human sperm antigens. *Biol. Reprod.*, **30**, 1015

19. Primakoff, P. and Myles, D.G. (1983). A map of the guinea pig sperm surface constructed with monoclonal antibodies. *Dev. Biol.*, **98**, 417

20. Reynolds, A.B. and Oliphant, G. (1984). Production and characterization of monoclonal antibodies to the sperm acrosome stabilizing factor (ASF): Utilization for purification and molecular analysis of ASF. *Biol. Reprod.*, **30**, 775

21. Mettler, L., Paul, S., Baukloh, V. and Feller, A.C. (1984). Monoclonal sperm antibodies: Their potential for investigation of sperms as target of immunological contraception. *Am. J. Reprod. Immunol.*, **5**, 125

22. Gaunt, S.J., Brown, C.R. and Jones, R. (1983). Identification of mobile and fixed antigens on the plasma membrane of rat spermatozoa using monoclonal antibodies. *Exp. Cell Res.*, **144**, 275

23. Naz, R.K., Alexander, N.J., Isahakia, M. and Hamilton, M.S. (1984). Monoclonal antibody to a human germ cell membrane glycoprotein that inhibits fertilization. *Science, N.Y.*, **225**, 342

24. O'Rand, M.G. and Irons, G.P. (1984). Monoclonal antibodies to rabbit sperm autoantigens. II. Inhibition of human sperm penetration of zona-free hamster eggs. *Biol. Reprod.*, **30**, 731

25. O'Rand, M.G., Irons, G.P. and Porter, J.P. (1984). Monoclonal antibodies to rabbit sperm autoantigens. I. Inhibition of in vitro fertilization and localization on the egg. *Biol. Reprod.*, **30**, 721

26. Schmell, E.D., Yuan, L.C., Gulyas, B.J. and August, J.T. (1982). Identification of mammalian sperm surface antigens. I. Production of monoclonal anti-mouse sperm antibodies. *Fertil. Steril.*, **37**, 249

27. Moore, H.D.M. and Hartman, T.D. (1984). Localization by monoclonal antibodies of various surface antigens of hamster spermatozoa and the effect of antibody on fertilization *in vitro*. *J. Reprod. Fertil.*, **70**, 175

28. Alexander, N.J. (1984). Antibodies to human spermatozoa impede sperm penetration of cervical mucus or hamster eggs. *Fertil. Steril.*, **41**, 433
29. Fawcett, D.W. (1958). The structure of the mammalian spermatozoon. *Int. Rev. Cytol.*, **7**, 195
30. Bedford, J.M. (1964). Fine structure of the sperm head in ejaculate and uterine spermatozoa of the rabbit. *J. Reprod. Fertil.*, **7**, 221
31. Pedersen, H. (1969). Ultrastructure of the ejaculated human sperm. *Z. Zellforsch. Mikrosk. Anat.*, **94**, 542
32. von Moxter, D. (1900). Uber ein spezifisches Immunserum gegen Spermatozoen. *Dtsch. Med. Wochenschr.*, **26**, 21
33. Guyer, M.P. (1922). Studies on cytolysins. III. Experiments with spermatoxins. *J. Exp. Zool.*, **35**, 207
34. Erickson, R.P., Friend, D.S. and Tennenbaum, D. (1975). Localization of lactate dehydrogenase-X on the surfaces of mouse spermatozoa. *Exp. Cell Res.*, **91**, 1
35. Schachner, M., Wortham, K.A., Carter, L.D. and Chaffee, J.K. (1975). NS-4 (nervous system antigen-4), a cell surface antigen of developing and adult mouse brain and sperm. *Dev. Biol.*, **44**, 313
36. Chaffee, J.K. and Schachner, M. (1978). NS-6 (nervous system antigen-6): A new cell surface antigen of brain, kidney, and spermatozoa. *Dev. Biol.*, **62**, 173
37. Allen, G.J. and Bourne, F.J. (1978). Interaction of immunoglobulin fragments with the mammalian sperm. *J. Exp. Zool.*, **203**, 271

14
Influence of psychotropic drugs, gossypol and acetylcholine receptor blockers on the motility of human spermatozoa *in vitro*

F. KRASSNIGG, R. PLACZEK, R. ENGL, J. FRICK and W.-B. SCHILL

INTRODUCTION

Inhibition of spermatogenesis, sperm transport and also interference with sperm maturation and viability are the steps in reproduction where inhibition of male fertility seems to be possible. However, apart from gossypol, a sesquiterpene derivative detectable in several plants, no drug has so far reached the stage of clinical trial. In this study the motility-inhibiting effect on spermatozoa of gossypol acetic acid (racemic mixture) and (+)-gossypol, and also of psychotropic drugs, e.g. trifluoperazine, regarded as inhibitor of the calcium-binding protein calmodulin, was investigated. In addition, the sperm-immobilizing effect of acetylcholine receptor-blocking substances such as the neurotoxin alpha-bungarotoxin was measured.

The inhibitory effect of gossypol on lactate dehydrogenase X (E.C.1.1.1.27), detectable only in mammalian spermatozoa and spermatogenic cells, was reported (Stephens *et al.*, 1983). In the light of these findings, we have examined the influence of gossypol on components of the kallikrein–kinin system. Their involvement in sperm motility regulation was demonstrated previously (Schill and Haberland, 1974). Our investigations were mainly focussed on the angiotensin converting enzyme (E.C.3.4.15.1), which is regarded as the regulatory link between the kallikrein–kinin and the renin–angiotensin systems and is detectable in seminal plasma in significantly higher amounts than in all other human body fluids and tissues.

MATERIALS AND METHODS

Semen samples were collected from patients of our Andrological Unit, after liquefaction freed from seminal plasma by several washings with a modified Tyrode's solution. Motility measurements were carried out by multiple exposure photography (Makler, 1980). After pretreatment the semen samples were placed in a Makler chamber (SEF1 Medical Instruments, Haifa, Israel). Using a phase contrast microscope, the sample was photographed by opening the shutter for a second, during which it is illuminated by six light pulses. Motile sperms appear on the frame as six-ringed chains. After development of the exposed film, the photographs are projected for analysis onto a screen. Each measurement of sperm motility was carried out in triplicate with different spermatozoa. The results presented in Figures 1-5 represent the mean values of the three measurements.

Gossypol acetic acid (racemic mixture) and alpha-bungarotoxin were purchased from Sigma, Munich, West Germany. (+)-Gossypol was a generous gift from Dr N. Kalla, Department of Biophysics, Punjab University, Chandigarh, India. Captopril was a gift of the Von Heyden Co., Munich, West Germany. Trifluoperazine was received from Boehringer Biochemicals, Mannheim, West Germany.

Angiotensin converting enzyme activity was estimated with hippuryl-L-His, L-Leu as substrate (Cushman and Cheung, 1971). All other chemicals used were of analytical grade.

RESULTS

The inhibition of sperm motility by trifluoperazine is shown in Figure 1. At a concentration of $10^{-4} M \times 1^{-1}$ the complete inhibition of the total motility was achieved. In Figure 2 the influence of the neurotoxin alpha-bungarotoxin on sperm motility is demonstrated. At a concentration of $10^{-4.3} M \times 1^{-1}$ nearly complete immobilization of the treated spermatozoa was reached. Figure 3 shows the inhibitory action of gossypol acetic acid on the sperm motility. At $10^{-4.3} M \times 1^{-1}$ more than 90% inhibition was detectable. Figure 4 demonstrates more than 90% inhibition of the sperm

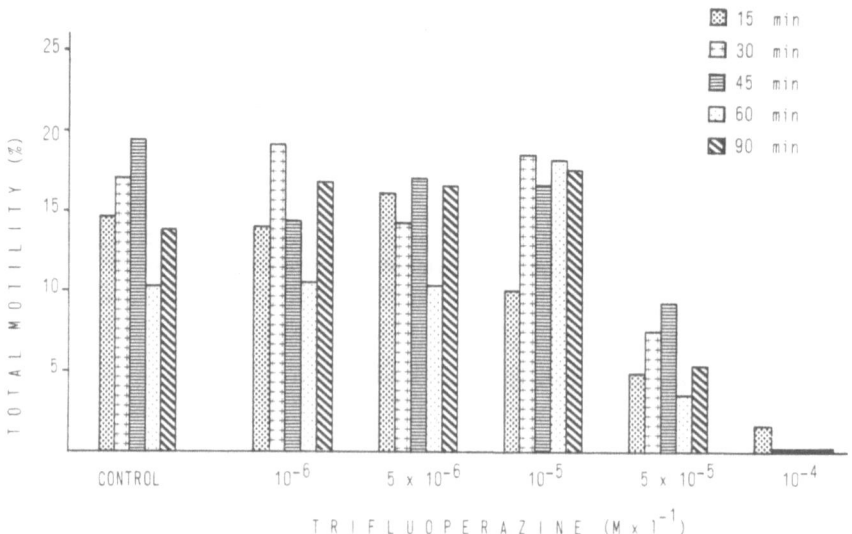

Figure 1   Inhibition of the total motility of washed human spermatozoa: concentration $1.0 \times 10^7 \times ml^{-1}$; incubation temperature 37°C

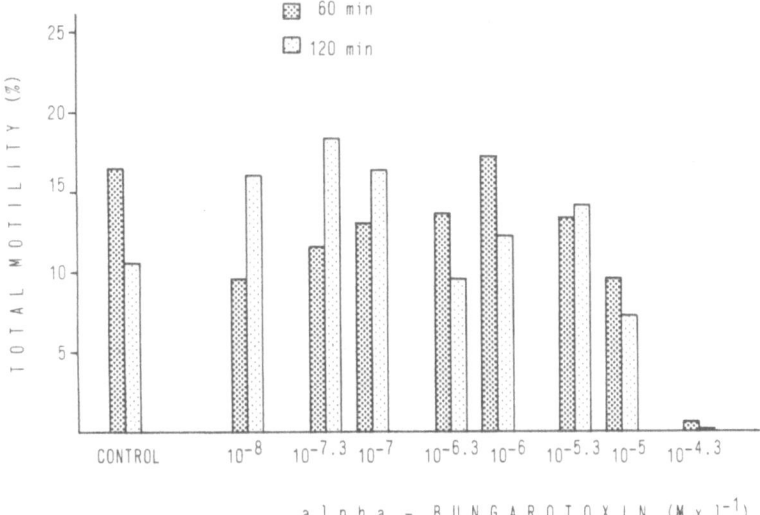

Figure 2 Total inhibition of motility by alpha-bungarotoxin at 37°C: sperm concentration $1.0 \times 10^7 \times ml^{-1}$

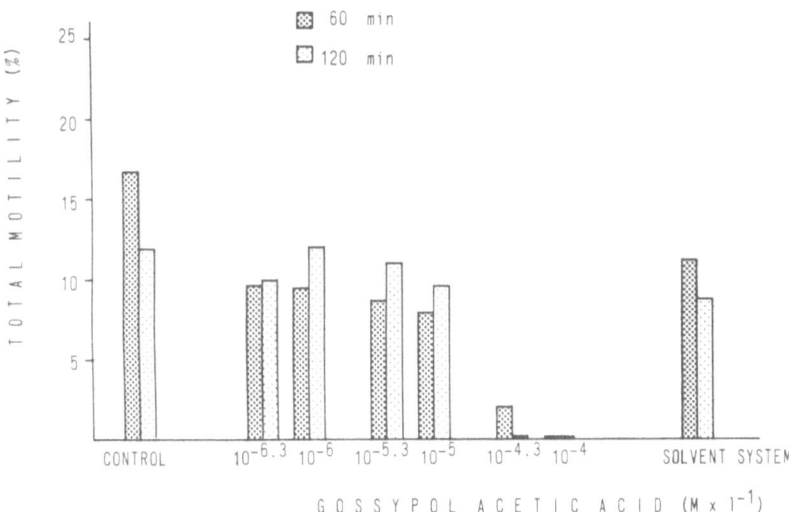

Figure 3 Inhibition of total motility by gossypol acetic acid (racemic mixture). Sperm concentration $1.0 \times 10^7 \times ml^{-1}$. Solvent system for gossypol acetic acid: N,N'-dimethylformamide 5% (v/v) in modified Tyrode's solution. Incubation at 37°C

motility by (+)-gossypol at a concentration of $10^{-4.3} M \times l^{-1}$. Figure 5 demonstrates the lack of inhibitory effect of the specific angiotensin converting enzyme inhibitor captopril on the sperm motility. On the contrary, at concentrations of more than $10^{-4} M \times l^{-1}$ a motility-stimulating effect could be demonstrated. In all our preparations of spermatozoa angiotensin converting enzyme activity was still detectable after several washings.

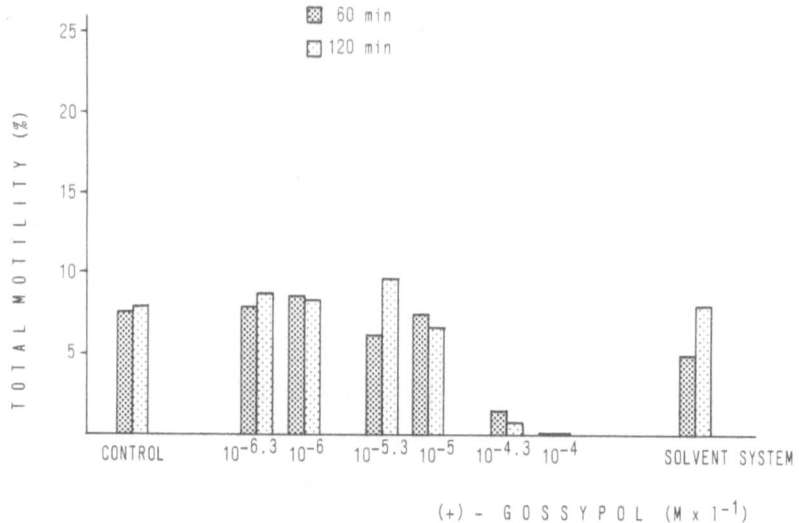

Figure 4 Total motility inhibition by (+)-gossypol. Sperm concentration $1.0 \times 10^7 \times ml^{-1}$. Solvent system: see Figure 3. Incubation temperature 37°C

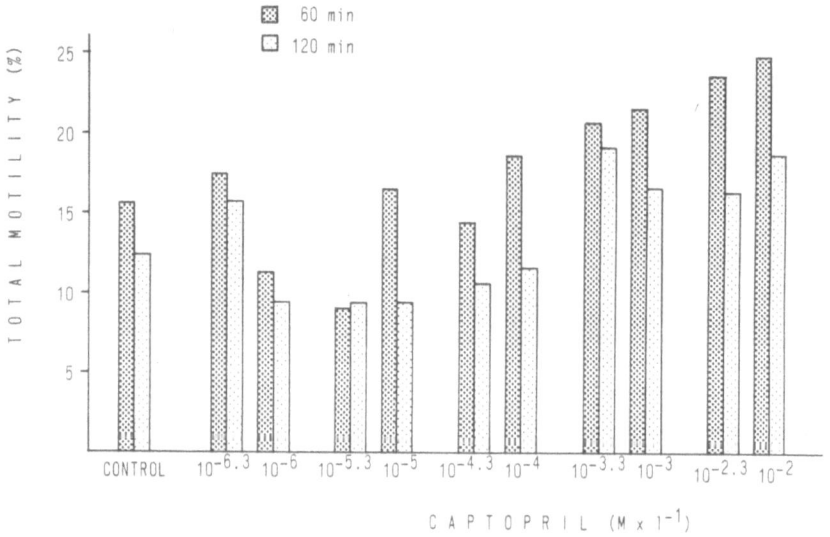

Figure 5 Influence of captopril on total motility: sperm concentration $1.0 \times 10^7 \times ml^{-1}$; incubation temperature 37°C

DISCUSSION

A variety of animal studies with gossypol and gossypol acetic acid have shown that gossypol reduced fertility in many but not in all mammalian species. Gossypol inhibits the motility of spermatozoa both *in vitro* (Kalla and Vasudev, 1980) and *in vivo* (Cameron *et al.*, 1982). We were able to demonstrate that gossypol is also a potent inhibitor of the angiotensin converting enzyme (ACE).

To answer the question whether ACE is involved in the regulation of sperm motility, the influence of the specific ACE inhibitor captopril on sperm motility was estimated. As the results indicate, any direct involvement of ACE in sperm motility mechanisms seems improbable. However, ACE is possibly of indirect importance for its kinin-degrading potency.

The immobilization of spermatozoa by calmodulin-inhibiting drugs acts via the inhibition of membrane-located ion transport mechanisms. Our results produced strong evidence that the inhibition of membrane-based ion transport could be, in general, a useful method for the inhibition of sperm motility.

To evaluate this conclusion, spermatozoa were incubated with alpha-bungarotoxin, a peptide isolated from snake venom (*Bungarus multicinctus*) and well characterized as a specific blocker of the membrane-located acetyl-choline receptor. The application of alpha-bungarotoxin resulted in a complete inhibition of the sperm motility. This points to the fact that acetyl-choline receptor blocking drugs might also be interesting substances for the study of molecular mechanisms involved in the regulation of sperm motility, as well as for practical purposes of antifertility treatment.

In addition, the inhibition of sperm motility by gossypol, trifluoperazine and acetylcholine receptor-blocking drugs makes these substances possibly interesting agents for local application as contraceptives in females.

ACKNOWLEDGEMENT

This work was supported by the Deutsche Forschungsgemeinschaft (SFB 0207, LP-20).

REFERENCES

Cameron, S.M., Waller, D.P. and Zaneveld, L.J. (1982). *Fertil. Steril.*, **37,** 273
Cushman, D.W. and Cheung, H.S. (1971). *Biochem. Pharmacol.*, **20,** 1637
Kalla, N.R. and Vasudev, M. (1980). *IRCS Med. Sci. Biochem.*, **8,** 375
Makler, A. (1980). *Fertil. Steril.*, **33,** 160
Schill, W.-B. and Haberland, G.L. (1974). *Hoppe-Seyler's Z. Physiol. Chem.*, **355,** 229
Stephens, D.T., Critchlow, L.M. and Hoskins, D.D. (1983). *J. Reprod. Fertil.*, **69,** 447

15
Investigations on the spermicidal action of cellulose trisulphuric acid ester

W.-B. SCHILL and H.H. WOLFF

Most vaginal contraceptives contain potent spermicides which cause irreversible membrane alterations of the spermatozoa leading to an immediate devitalization of the ejaculated sperm cells. One of the most effective spermicides is the non-ionic surface-active compound nonoxinol-9[1], which leads to an immediate immobilization of the spermatozoa even in concentrations between 0.05% and 0.2%[2]. Simultaneously, the penetration enzyme acrosin is detached from the acrosome as a result of a removal of the acrosomal membranes by detergent treatment[3, 4].

The aim of the following study was to investigate the spermicidal effects of another active compound of a vaginal contraceptive which is frequently used in spermicidal preparations. This substance is the polysaccharide polysulphuric acid ester CTSA (trisodium salt of cellulose trisulphuric acid ester) in which three sodium sulphate residues are esterified to one molecule of glucose, which is linked to other glucose molecules in the form of a β-glycoside (Figure 1).

MATERIAL AND METHODS

CTSA was obtained in pharmaceutical quality from EGA Chemie, West Germany. In addition, the polysaccharide polysulphuric acid ester was isolated from frequently used vaginal contraceptives, i.e. CTSA-containing suppositories (A-gen 53, Deutsche Chefaro Pharma), where it should be effective in intravaginal concentrations between 1% and 2%. The identity of both substances was confirmed by NMR and infrared studies performed by Professor Dr H. Kessler, Institute for Organic Chemistry, Frankfurt University. In what follows, therefore, both substances are treated as one compound if there is no specific indication to the contrary.

To study the effects of CTSA on spermatozoa, the following parameters were investigated: the motility and ultrastructure of human spermatozoa, and the activity of the acrosomal penetration enzyme acrosin.

Total and progressive sperm motility was determined under a phase contrast microscope at an incubation temperature of 37°C during different time

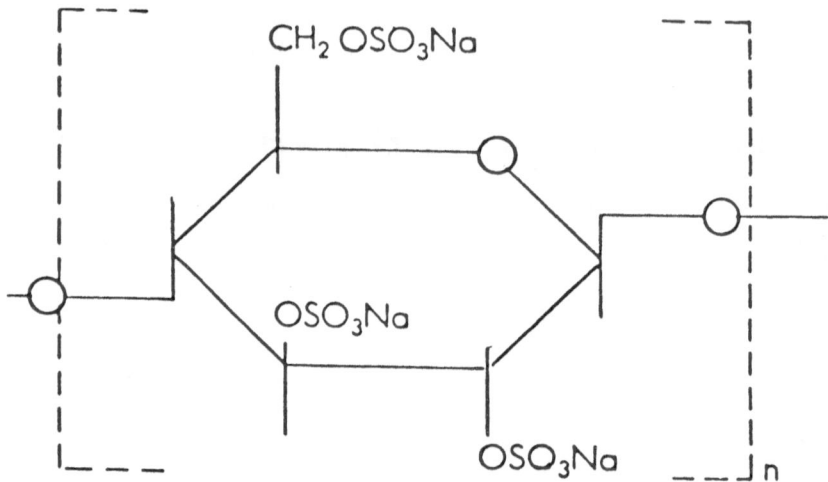

Figure 1   Structure of CTSA

periods[7]. In addition, the IPPF-approved Sander–Cramer test was used, which is performed at room temperature conditions[8]. Acrosin activity was determined after acid extraction from the spermatozoa by a spectrophotometric assay using BAEE as substrate as well as by the method of gelatinolysis[5, 6]. Transmission electron microscopy was performed according to a previously published procedure[2]. In these studies a 1.7% CTSA concentration was employed which corresponds to the mean vaginal concentration present under *in vivo* conditions, taking into account the vaginal suppository, a 3 ml ejaculate volume and a 0.7 ml volume of vaginal secretion. Both commercial and isolated CTSA were incubated for 10 min at 37°C with the semen of a fertile man. After fixation according to the method of Stefanini, thin sections were stained with uranyl acetate and lead citrate, and viewed and photographed under a Zeiss electron microscope.

RESULTS

With donor semen of good quality, commercial CTSA effected an immediate complete immobilization of the spermatozoa at a concentration of 10% (Figure 2). However, the eosin supravital staining technique revealed that 20% of the non-motile spermatozoa were still alive. Five per cent CTSA yielded a complete immobilization only after 1 h of incubation. In the presence of 1% CTSA, which corresponds to the vaginal concentration present under *in vivo* conditions, motile spermatozoa were still observed after an incubation period of 4 h. In the presence of 0.5% CTSA, spermatozoa with excellent progressive motility were observed even at the end of the 4 h incubation period.

Table 1 summarizes the results of various experiments. It shows that the marketed product CTSA induces an immediate sperm immobilization only at extremely high concentrations, while sperm motility is only slightly impaired in concentrations used for vaginal contraception. The surface-active

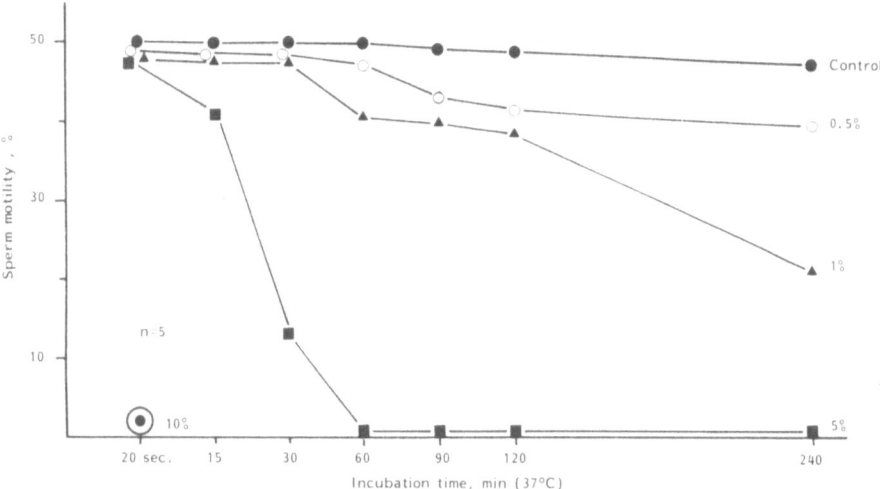

Figure 2   Sperm motility in presence of CTSA (commercial product)

Table 1   Cellulose trisulphuric acid ester and sperm motility

Concentration	Complete immobilization
CTSA (EGA 18099-8)	
10%	immediate (20 s)
5%	after 1 h
≤1%	>4 h
Nonoxinol-9	
0.05–10%	immediate (10 s)

Table 2   Sander–Cramer test

Agent	Source	*Time of complete immobilization* (s)					
		Concentration					
		1/5 (2%)	1/10 (1%)	1/25 (0.4%)	1/50 (0.2%)	1/150 (0.07%)	1/250 (0.04%)
(no. of experiments)	*isolated from*	Conc. range in vivo					
CTSA (6) 100 mg	vaginal suppositories A-gen 53 batch no. 75242 1, 22101 K	>600	>600	>600	>600	>600	>600
Nonoxinol-9 (3) 75 mg	batch no. HV 8448	(1.5%) <30	(0.75%) <30	(0.3%) <30	(0.15%) <30	(0.05%) <30	(0.03%) <30

spermicide nonoxinol-9, on the other hand, leads to an immediate immobilization of spermatozoa under the same experimental conditions within a concentration range 0.05–10%.

With isolated CTSA from vaginal suppositories in concentrations up to 2%, the Sander–Cramer test showed no sperm immobilization within an observation period of 10 min (Table 2). Motile spermatozoa were still observed after a 48 h incubation period in the presence of *in vivo* concentrations of CTSA. The surface-active spermicide nonoxinol-9, on the other hand, yielded an immediate sperm immobilization in concentrations of 1.5–0.03%. Observation of sperm motility in the presence of vaginally relevant concentrations of isolated CTSA showed no significant motility inhibition as compared with the untreated controls during an observation period of up to 6 h (Figure 3).

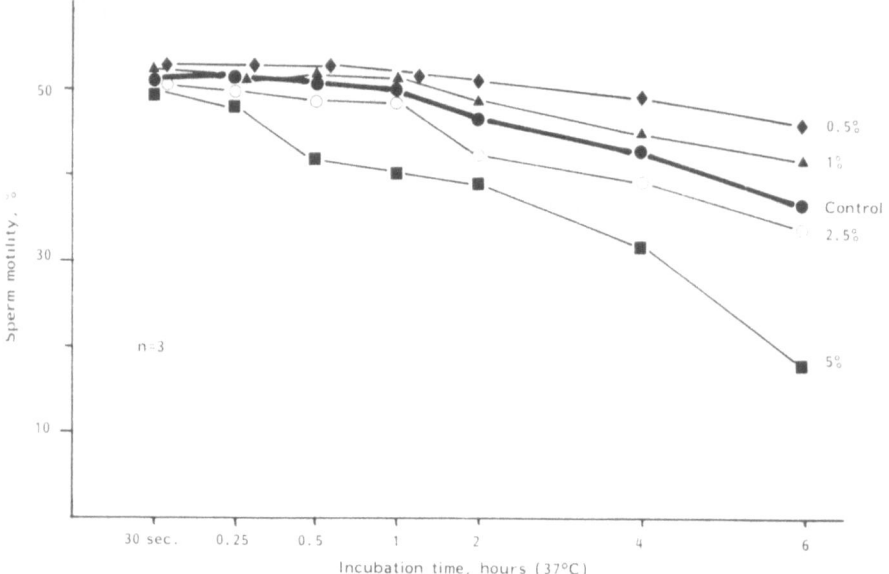

Figure 3   Sperm motility in presence of CTSA (isolated product)

Only 5% CTSA led to a slight impairment of total and progressive sperm motility, whereas concentrations below 2.5% even showed a tendency towards greater motility as compared with the untreated controls. This indicates that the isolated CTSA is still less effective than the commercially available product with respect to its interference with sperm motility.

The behaviour of the acrosomal penetration enzyme acrosin in the presence of the polysaccharide polysulphuric acid ester will now be considered.

The influence of CTSA on the BAEE-splitting activity of human spermatozoa is illustrated in Table 3. After incubation of washed spermatozoa with different CTSA concentrations, no difference in acrosin activity is found in spermatozoa treated with CTSA as compared with the control. In addition, no acrosin will be released from the sperm acrosome into the supernatant fluid.

The surface-active nonoxinol-9, on the other hand, leads to a complete

Table 3 BAEE-splitting activity of washed human spermatozoa

Concentration (%)	Acrosin activity (mU/10^6 spermatozoa)		
	Sperm pellet	Supernatant	Total activity
CTSA: 1	1.84	0.17	2.01
0.7	1.77	0.20	1.97
0.5	1.79	0.25	2.04
0.3	1.81	0.25	2.06
0.1	1.91	0.13	2.04
0.01	1.82	0.07	1.89
Nonoxinol-9:			
0.1	0.25	2.53	2.78
Control:	1.78	0.21	1.99

liberation of acrosin into the supernatant fluid. Only traces of the enzyme can be determined within the sperm pellet. Detachment of acrosin under these conditions is due to a removal of the acrosomal cap by detergent action which has already been investigated by us in more detail[2-4].

Determination of acrosin activity of individual spermatozoa by the gelatine film technique showed that pretreatment of washed spermatozoa with different concentrations of CTSA was without effect on the acrosin-induced halo formation (Figure 4). This indicates that no severe alterations of the

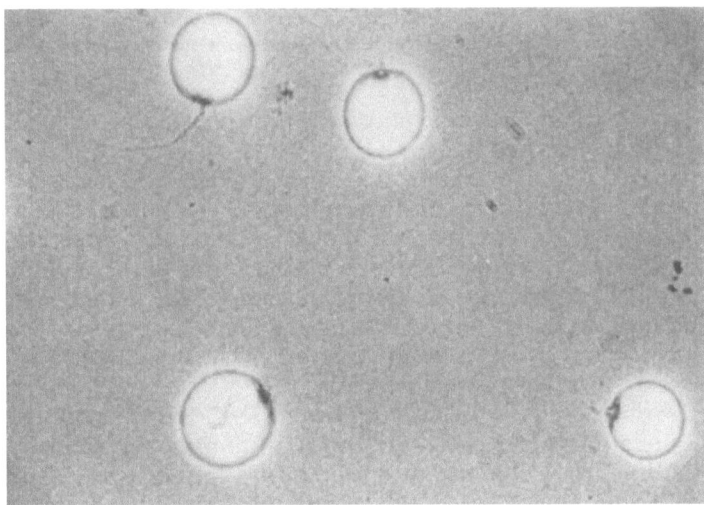

Figure 4 Gelatinolytic (acrosin) activity of washed human spermatozoa incubated for 30 min at 37°C in the presence of 1% CTSA. Magnification × 400. Compared with the controls, halo formation was not inhibited

Table 4 Gelatinolytic activity of washed human spermatozoa

Concentration	Gelatinolysis
CTSA: 0.01–1%	no inhibition
Nonoxinol-9: 0.01–1%	complete inhibition

acrosomal membranes will occur, as was found in the case of nonoxinol-9 treatment (Table 4), where a complete inhibition of halo formation was observed which is due to a complete detachment of acrosin from the acrosome by the spermicide.

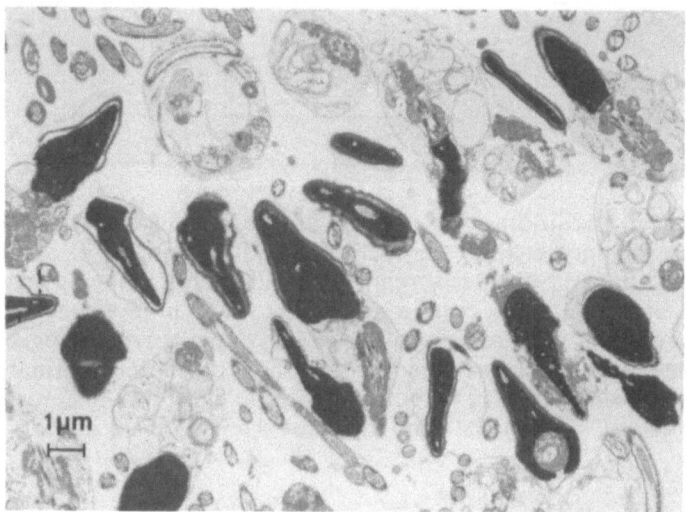

Figure 5 Electron microscopy of human spermatozoa before treatment with CTSA

The biochemical studies were accomplished by investigations using transmission electron microscopy.

As compared with the control experiments (Figure 5), no significant differences could be observed in the presence of 1.7% of commercial or isolated CTSA (Figures 6, 7). Spermatozoa showed normal ultrastructure, with an intact plasma membrane which sometimes had irregular discontinuities due to the washing procedure. The acrosomal membrane complex was intact. The same holds true for the equatorial segment, the nucleus, the nuclear membrane and the postacrosomal structures. The middle piece, the principal piece and the end piece were normal.

The described findings are in contrast to the severe membrane and acrosomal alterations induced by low concentrations of surface-active spermicides leading to an immediate killing of spermatozoa. Addition of nonoxinol-9 in a final concentration of 1.25% led to significant changes in the ultrastructure of the spermatozoa. These changes were uniform throughout the preparations (Figure 8). The plasma membrane was completely removed, and the acrosomal complex disappeared, with the excep-

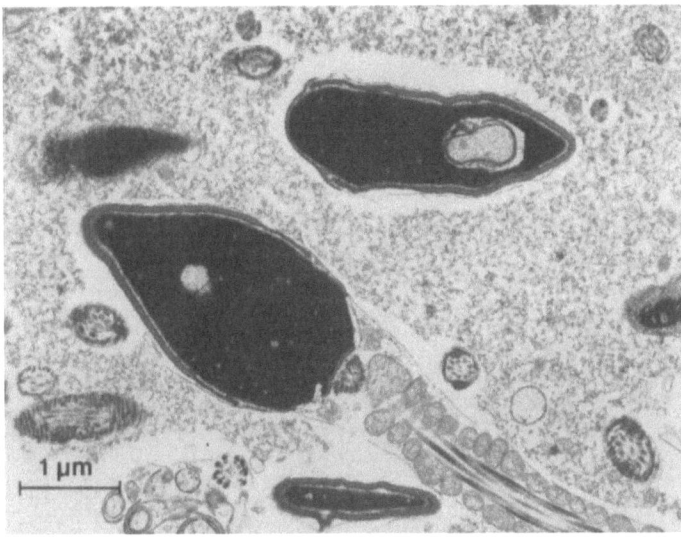

Figure 6 Ultrastructure of human spermatozoa after treatment with 1.7% CTSA commercially obtained in pharmaceutical quality

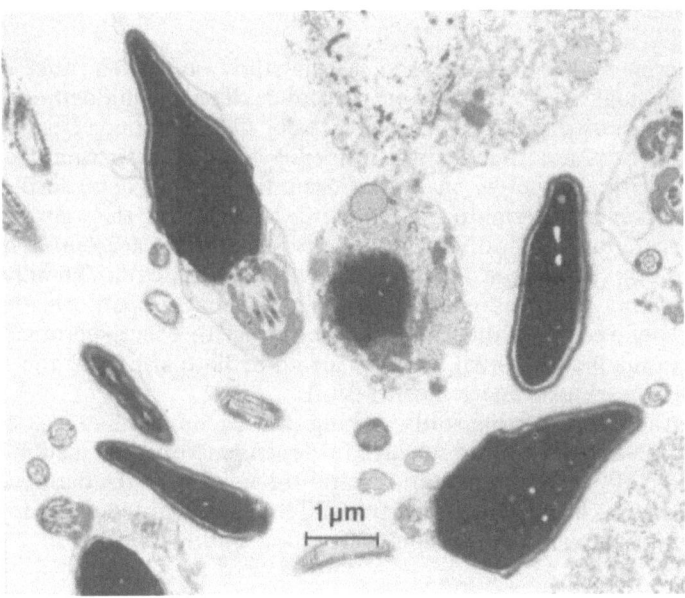

Figure 7 Ultrastructure of human spermatozoa after treatment with 1.7% CTSA isolated from vaginal suppositories

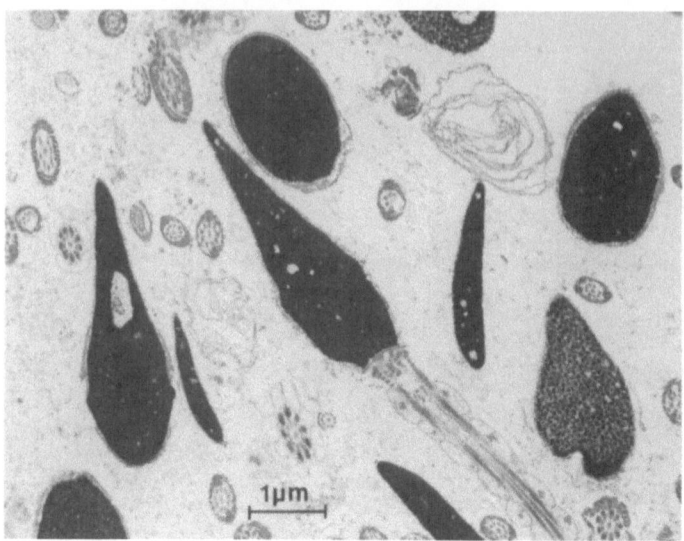

Figure 8　Ultrastructure of human spermatozoa after treatment with 1.25% nonoxinol-9

tion of some irregularly scattered membrane remnants. The nucleus sometimes showed all steps of nuclear decondensation. Within the middle piece
the mitochondriae were empty, without cristae, and contained fine granular
electron-dense material.

DISCUSSION

The experimental conditions used in this study are of relevance in judging
the spermicidal action of a given substance. The results demonstrate that
the polysaccharide polysulphuric acid ester CTSA cannot be a spermicide
and that it does not significantly influence ejaculated spermatozoa in concentrations used under *in vivo* conditions for vaginal contraception, i.e. it
does not prevent spermatozoa from migrating from the vaginal into the
cervical secretions. In addition, it will alter neither the acrosomal membrane
structure nor the plasma membrane of the spermatozoa. Therefore, interaction—if any—with acrosomal penetration enzymes or other sperm enzymes is not very probable. This is in contrast to other spermicidal agents
such as nonoxinol-9, which leads to an immediate killing of the spermatozoa under the same *in vivo* concentrations.

　From the results of this study, taking into account the *in vivo* concentrations of spermicidal agents which are dependent on the ejaculate volume,
the volume of the vaginal secretions and the volume of the dissolved vaginal
suppository, it can be concluded that CTSA is not suited for incorporation
into vaginal suppositories to be used for local contraception.

ACKNOWLEDGEMENTS

We acknowledge the excellent technical assistance of Mrs M. Feifel and Mrs E. Januschke. This study was supported by a grant of the Deutsche Forschungsgemeinschaft Schi 86/7-4.

REFERENCES

1. United States. Department of Health and Human Services. Food and Drug Administration (1980). Vaginal contraceptive drug products for over-the-counter human use; establishment of a monograph; proposed rulemaking. *Federal Register*, **45** (241), 82014
2. Schill, W.-B., Mueller-Esterl, W. and Wolff, H. H. (1983). The effect of nonoxinol-9 on sperm ultrastructure, acrosin and sperm motility. In Adimoelja, F.X.A. and Karundeng, E. (eds.) *Andrology in Perspective*, pp. 148–154. (Denpasar, Bali: P.T. Kenrose)
3. Schill, W.-B. and Wolff, H.H. (1981). Ultrastructure of human spermatozoa in the presence of nonoxinol-9 and a vaginal contraceptive containing nonoxinol-9. *Andrologia*, **13**, 42
4. Mueller-Esterl, W. and Schill, W.-B. (1982). Sperm acrosin: Liberation from the acrosome and activity of the free proteinase in the presence of nonoxinol-9. *Andrologia*, **14**, 309
5. Schill, W.-B. (1973). Acrosin activity in human spermatozoa: methodological investigations. *Arch. Dermatol. Res.*, **248**, 257
6. Schill, W.-B., Feifel, M., Fritz, H. and Hammerstein, J. (1981). Inhibitors of acrosomal proteinase as antifertility agents. A problem of acrosomal membrane permeability. *Int. J. Androl.*, **4**, 25
7. Makler, A., Deutsch, M., Vilensky, A. and Palti, Y. (1981). Factors affecting sperm motility. VIII. Velocity and survival of human spermatozoa as related to temperatures above zero. *Int. J. Androl.*, **4**, 559
8. Sander, F.V. and Cramer, S.D. (1941). A practical method for testing the spermicidal action of chemical contraceptives. *Hum. Fertil.*, **6**, 134

Index of contraceptive agents*

* Chemical names are listed only where they are significant and no pharmaceutical and/or proprietary name is mentioned.